T0075161

OXFORD HANDBOOK FOR

The Dental Foundation and Core Training Programmes

Published and forthcoming Oxford Handbooks

Oxford Handbook for the Foundation Programme 5e

Oxford Handbook of Acute Medicine 4e

Oxford Handbook of Anaesthesia 5e

Oxford Handbook of Cardiology 2e

Oxford Handbook of Clinical and Healthcare Research

Oxford Handbook of Clinical and Laboratory Investigation 4e

Oxford Handbook of Clinical Dentistry 7e

Oxford Handbook of Clinical Diagnosis 3e

Oxford Handbook of Clinical Examination and Practical Skills 2e

Oxford Handbook of Clinical Haematology 4e

Oxford Handbook of Clinical Immunology and Allergy 4e

Oxford Handbook of Clinical Medicine – Mini Edition 10e

Oxford Handbook of Clinical Medicine 10e

Oxford Handbook of Clinical Pathology

Oxford Handbook of Clinical Pharmacy 3e

Oxford Handbook of Clinical Specialties 11e

Oxford Handbook of Clinical Surgery 5e

Oxford Handbook of Complementary Medicine

Oxford Handbook of Critical Care 3e

Oxford Handbook of Dental Patient Care

Oxford Handbook of Dialysis 4e

Oxford Handbook of Emergency Medicine 5e

Oxford Handbook of Endocrinology and Diabetes 4e

Oxford Handbook of ENT and Head and Neck Surgery 3e

Oxford Handbook of Epidemiology for Clinicians

Oxford Handbook of Expedition and Wilderness Medicine 3e

Oxford Handbook of Forensic Medicine

Oxford Handbook of Gastroenterology & Hepatology 3e

Oxford Handbook of General Practice 5e

Oxford Handbook of Genetics

Oxford Handbook of Genitourinary Medicine, HIV, and Sexual Health 3e

Oxford Handbook of Geriatric Medicine 3e

Oxford Handbook of Infectious Diseases and Microbiology 2e

Oxford Handbook of Integrated Dental Biosciences 2e

Oxford Handbook of Head and Neck Anatomy

Oxford Handbook of Humanitarian Medic

Oxford Handbook of Key Clinical Evidence

Oxford Handbook of Medical Dermatolog

Oxford Handbook of Medical Ethics and L

Oxford Handbook of Medical Imaging

Oxford Handbook of Medical Sciences 3e

Oxford Handbook for Medical School

Oxford Handbook of Medical Statistics 2e

Oxford Handbook of Neonatology 2e

Oxford Handbook of Nephrology and Hypertension 2e

Oxford Handbook of Neurology 2e

Oxford Handbook of Nutrition and Dietetics 3e

Oxford Handbook of Obstetrics and Gynaecology 3e

Oxford Handbook of Occupational Health

Oxford Handbook of Oncology 3e

Oxford Handbook of Operative Surgery 3

Oxford Handbook of Ophthalmology 4e

Oxford Handbook of Oral and Maxillofacia Surgery 2e

Oxford Handbook of Orthopaedics and Trauma

Oxford Handbook of Paediatrics 3e

Oxford Handbook of Pain Management

Oxford Handbook of Palliative Care 3e

Oxford Handbook of Practical Drug Therapy 2e

Oxford Handbook of Pre-Hospital Care 2e

Oxford Handbook of Psychiatry 4e

Oxford Handbook of Public Health Practic

Oxford Handbook of Rehabilitation Medicine 3e

Oxford Handbook of Reproductive Medic & Family Planning 2e

Oxford Handbook of Respiratory Medicine

Oxford Handbook of Rheumatology 4e

Oxford Handbook of Sleep Medicine

Oxford Handbook of Sport and Exercise Medicine 2e

Handbook of Surgical Consent

Oxford Handbook of Tropical Medicine 5e

Oxford Handbook of Urology 4e

Oxford Handbook for the Dental Foundat and Core Training Programmes

OXFORD HANDBOOK FOR

The Dental Foundation and Core Training Programmes

EDITED BY

Chris Barker

Consultant in Orthodontics, Pinderfields General Hospital;
Former Training Programme Director for Dental Core Training,
Pinderfields General Hospital, Wakefield; Honorary Senior
Lecturer in Orthodontics, School of Dentistry, Faculty of
Medicine and Health, University of Leeds, Leeds, UK;
Specialist Orthodontic Practitioner, Yorkshire, UK

Hemash Shah

General Dental Practitioner, London; Educational Supervisor for
Dental Foundation Training, London, UK

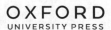

OXFORD
UNIVERSITY PRESS

OXFORD
UNIVERSITY PRESS

Great Clarendon Street, Oxford, OX2 6DP,
United Kingdom

Oxford University Press is a department of the University of Oxford.
It furthers the University's objective of excellence in research, scholarship,
and education by publishing worldwide. Oxford is a registered trade mark of
Oxford University Press in the UK and in certain other countries

© Oxford University Press 2023

The moral rights of the authors have been asserted

First Edition published in 2023

All rights reserved. No part of this publication may be reproduced, stored in
a retrieval system, or transmitted, in any form or by any means, without the
prior permission in writing of Oxford University Press, or as expressly permitted
by law, by licence or under terms agreed with the appropriate reprographics
rights organization. Enquiries concerning reproduction outside the scope of the
above should be sent to the Rights Department, Oxford University Press, at the
address above

You must not circulate this work in any other form
and you must impose this same condition on any acquirer

Published in the United States of America by Oxford University Press
198 Madison Avenue, New York, NY 10016, United States of America

British Library Cataloguing in Publication Data
Data available

Library of Congress Control Number: 2022946818

ISBN 978–0–19–876782–4

DOI: 10.1093/med/9780198767824.001.0001

Printed and bound in Turkey by Promat

Oxford University Press makes no representation, express or implied, that the
drug dosages in this book are correct. Readers must therefore always check
the product information and clinical procedures with the most up-to-date
published product information and data sheets provided by the manufacturers
and the most recent codes of conduct and safety regulations. The authors and
the publishers do not accept responsibility or legal liability for any errors in the
text or for the misuse or misapplication of material in this work. Except where
otherwise stated, drug dosages and recommendations are for the non-pregnant
adult who is not breast-feeding

Links to third party websites are provided by Oxford in good faith and
for information only. Oxford disclaims any responsibility for the materials
contained in any third party website referenced in this work.

For JLB

Foreword

The first few steps of any professional career are daunting and challenging in equal measure. This is a vital time for any individual and can potentially shape their future careers in both a positive and a negative way. Any support or guidance during the early stages of a career can have a profound influence on an individual. I was fortunate enough to have mentors throughout my career who helped and guided me but the concurrent challenge of finding accurate contemporaneous information was a significant challenge.

This handbook provides an excellent resource for both those just starting their career as a dentist and those who are involved in their training and mentorship. Everyone's career journey and trajectory is different and so easy access to expert advice is vital.

Covering all aspects of dentistry and training, this guide acts as an extremely comprehensive resource covering not only all clinical disciplines but also wider leadership, management, and governance skills that any young professional and their mentors will need to be aware of.

James Spencer
Postgraduate Dental Dean
HEE Yorkshire and the Humber

Preface

This handbook has been written for trainees and those in the early stages of their career.

Your undergraduate training has given you exposure to all the disciplines within dentistry and provided you with the basic skills to be a competent beginner. Many of you will have developed areas in which you wish to increase your knowledge and competencies, while others may still wish to gain further experience in all areas.

The amount of literature that is available on Dental Foundation and Core Training programmes is currently very limited. This can lead to many misconceptions about what is involved and the experience that can be gained by undertaking additional training.

As a trainee, you will be placed in an approved training unit/practice and provided with the opportunities to develop your skills in that particular area. You can gain as much or as little experience as you desire throughout your training programme and it is up to you as the trainee to take advantage of these opportunities that are presented to you. There are going to be obvious limitations of some placements (e.g. your crown preparations are unlikely to improve after completing a year in oral and maxillofacial surgery) and there may be certain experiences that individual placements may not be able to accommodate. However, the more proactive the trainee is, the more they stand to gain. If an opportunity does not seem obvious or is not presented to you then it is always worthwhile asking more senior colleagues, educational or clinical supervisors, consultants, or training programme directors about additional experiences you would like to gain within your training.

The authors have tried to highlight the different aspects of Dental Foundation and Core Training programmes to enable the trainee to make the most of their training and develop their skills for their future practising careers.

We hope you enjoy your training and your career as a dental professional.

Hemash Shah
Chris Barker

Acknowledgements

We would like to thank all the contributory authors for their time and effort in providing their expertise and knowledge to each of the sections: Daniel Brierley, Amy Hollis, Caroline McCarthy, Amy Robbins, Zahra Shehabi, Robert Williams, and Amanda Willis.

Many thanks to Amardip Singh Kalsi for support with the Restorative Dentistry Dental Core Training sections in Chapter 5 on restorative dentistry.

We would also like to thank our families for their continued support throughout our careers and the writing of this handbook.

Our thanks to Michael Hawkes and Elizabeth Reeves from OUP who have provided a huge amount of support in producing this publication.

Acknowledgements

Contents

Contributors

Daniel J. Brierley

Senior Clinical Teacher and Honorary Consultant in Oral and Maxillofacial Pathology, University of Sheffield, Sheffield, UK

Amy Hollis

Consultant and Honorary Clinical Lecturer in Paediatric Dentistry, Bristol Dental Hospital, Bristol, Co-Specialty Tutor for Dental Core Trainees, UK

Caroline McCarthy

Academic Lecturer in Oral Medicine, School of Clinical Dentistry and Department of Oral Medicine, Liverpool University Dental Hospital, Liverpool, UK.

Amy Robbins

General Dental Practitioner and Advanced Facial Aesthetician, General Dental Practice, Yorkshire, UK

Zahra Shehabi

Consultant in Special Care Dentistry, Barts Health Dental Hospital, London, UK

Robert G. M. Williams

Specialist Oral Surgeon, Wirral University Teaching Hospital NHS Foundation Trust, Birkenhead, UK

Amanda Willis

Clinical Senior Lecturer, Consultant in Oral Medicine, Queens University Belfast and Belfast Health and Social Care Trust, Belfast, UK

Symbols and abbreviations

⊃	cross-reference
℘	website
$	supernumerary teeth
±	with or without
2D	two-dimensional
3D	three-dimensional
ABCDE	Airway, Breathing, Circulation, Disability, Exposure
ABH	angina bullosa haemorrhagica
AC	aesthetic component
AI	amelogenesis imperfecta
AP	anteroposterior
ARCP	Annual Review of Competence Progression
ASA	American Society of Anesthesiologists
AVPU	alert, verbal, pain, and unresponsive
BMI	body mass index
BPE	basic periodontal examination
BW	bitewing
CAL	clinical attachment loss
CBCT	cone-beam computed tomography
CCST	certificate of completion of specialist training
CEJ	cementoenamel junction
CL	cleft lip
CLP	cleft lip and palate
CL/P	cleft lip or palate
CMC	chronic mucocutaneous candidiasis
CN	cranial nerve
CNS	central nervous system
COPDEND	UK Committee of Postgraduate Dental Deans and Directors
CP	cleft palate
CPD	continuing professional development
CPOSHH	Control of Substances Hazardous to Health
CQC	Care Quality Commission
CT	computed tomography
CV	*curriculum vitae*
CVS	cardiovascular system
DBS	Disclosure and Barring Service
DCT	Dental Core Training
DCT1	Dental Core Training Year 1
DCT2	Dental Core Training Year 2
DCT3	Dental Core Training Year 3
DF	Dental Foundation
DFT	Dental Foundation Training
DHC	dental health component
DI	dentinogenesis imperfecta
DMFR	dental and maxillofacial radiology
DOB	date of birth
DOPS	direct observation of procedural skills
DPT	dental panoramic tomography
EBV	Epstein–Barr virus
EM	erythema multiforme
ENT	ear, nose, and throat
ePortfolio	electronic portfolio
ESPR	early-stage peer review
EWS	Early Warning Score
FBC	full blood count
FDS	Faculty of Dental Surgery
FGDP (UK)	Faculty of General Dental Practice (UK)
FPM	first permanent molar
FRCP	Final Review of Competence Progression
GA	general anaesthetic/anaesthesia
GDC	General Dental Council
GI	glass ionomer
GIC	glass ionomer cement
GMP	general medical practitioner
GP	gutta-percha
GVHD	graft-versus-host disease
H&E	haematoxylin and eosin
HA	hyaluronic acid
HEE	Health Education England
HEIW	Health Education and Improvement Wales
HHV	human herpesvirus
HIV	human immunodeficiency virus

HMRC	His Majesty's Revenue and Customs	OMFP	oral and maxillofacial pathology
HSE	Health and Safety Executive	OMFS	oral and maxillofacial surgery
HSV	herpes simplex virus	OPG	orthopantomogram
IELTS	International English Language Testing System	ORIF	open reduction and internal fixation
Ig	immunoglobulin	ORNJ	osteoradionecrosis of the jaw
IMCA	independent mental capacity advocate	OSCE	Objective Structured Clinical Exam
IOTN	Index of Orthodontic Treatment Need	PA	periapical
		PAS	periodic–acid Schiff
IRCP	Interim Review of Competence Progression	PCO	pulp canal obliteration
		PDL	periodontal ligament
IRMER	Ionising Radiation (Medical Exposure) Regulations	PDP	personal development plan
		PEB	post-eruptive breakdown
IV	intravenous	PEG	percutaneous endoscopic gastrostomy
JDFCT	Joint Dental Foundation Core Training	PMC	preformed metal crown
LA	local anaesthetic/anaesthesia	ppmF	parts per million of fluoride
LDC	Local Dental Committee	QI	quality improvement
LGE	linear gingival erythema	RAC	retruded arc of closure
LL	lower left	RCP	Royal College of Pathologists or retruded contact position
LPA	lasting power of attorney		
LR	lower right	RCS England	Royal College of Surgeons of England
MCA	Mental Capacity Act		
MDT	multidisciplinary team	RMGIC	resin-modified glass ionomer cement
MET	medical emergency team		
MEWS	Modified Early Warning Score	RTT	referral to treatment time
MFDS	Membership of the Faculty of Dental Surgery	SALT	speech and language therapist
		SCD	special care dentistry
MH	medical history	SLE	supervised learning event
MIH	molar incisor hypomineralization	SMART	Specific, Measurable, Attainable, Relevant, and Timely
MJDF	Membership of the Joint Dental Faculties		
		SPM	second primary molar
MRONJ	medication-related osteonecrosis of the jaw	SpO_2	oxygen saturation
		ST	specialist trainee
MS	multiple sclerosis	TMJ	temporomandibular joint
MTA	mineral trioxide aggregate	TPD	training programme director
NBM	nil by mouth	TTO	to take out
NES	NHS Education for Scotland	U&E	urea and electrolytes
NICE	National Institute for Health and Care Excellence	UDA	units of dental activity
		UL	upper left
NPBMT	non-pharmacological behaviour management technique	UR	upper right
		VSD	ventriculoseptal defect
		VTE	venous thromboembolism
NSCH	non-setting calcium hydroxide	VZV	varicella zoster virus
NTN	National Training Number	WBA	workplace-based assessment
OI	osteogenesis imperfecta		

Introduction

The start of the safe beginner

This handbook is intended for those who are either at the early stages of their professional career as a dentist or are involved in the training of such individuals.

Dentistry has changed dramatically over the last few decades, with changes in training, funding, advancing techniques, and the need for dental professionals to maintain and increase their knowledge across all the different disciplines of dentistry. Many dentists may not feel comfortable in providing all the different types of treatment and care to the highest level of complexity. Patients expect that any treatment provided to them should be done to a reasonably high standard of quality and the operator to have competency in the treatment they are providing.

It is very difficult to be able to practise and stay up to date in the full range of dental disciplines and to do this to a high standard of quality. For this reason, most dentists chose to either practise a wide breadth of dentistry or restrict their practice, carrying out treatment of greater complexity, or possibly specializing in one of the dental specialisms.

With the introduction of vocational dental training in the early 1990s to the development of the General Dental Council (GDC) learning outcomes, it has been generally recognized that while an individual may be safe to practise independently following completion of undergraduate training, there is a long path ahead with continued learning.[1]

The GDC issued 'Scope of Practice' guidance describing the abilities and skills that each different dental care professional and dentists should have.[2] This was then later revised with the addition of the text 'you can undertake the following if you are trained, competent and indemnified' preceding the list of skills and abilities.[3]

It is therefore expected that the new graduate will be an independent practitioner who is a safe beginner and may not be in a position to deliver all aspects of treatment to a patient, but they should be able to judge their own competence and seek help, supervision, or referral where appropriate. Alternatively the term "Safe Practitioner" is being considered as more appropriate.

The start of Dental Foundation Training marks the first stage in life-long learning, to develop proficiency through training and experience and to become a well-rounded dental professional in one's chosen area of practice.

It is hoped that by reading this handbook as a trainee, you will be in a much stronger position to maximize your training opportunities in whatever role you are in, as well as use it as a reference throughout to aid with decision-making, writing up projects or completing a portfolio of training.

---

1 GDC (May 2011). *Learning Outcomes.*

2 GDC (April 2009). *Scope of Practice.*

3 GDC (September 2013). *Scope of Practice.*

It will not substitute for any hands-on experience that can be gained, but it should serve you well in professional development for these first vital years.

Tips on enjoying your dental career

In no particular order, here are a few tips to help you along your way:

- The first principle of the GDC standards is 'Putting patients' interests first'. When there are pressures to meet financial or activity targets, it can be very easy to forget this principle; however, in doing so, not only could you put patients at risk, which could affect your registration, it will also affect overall morale and job satisfaction. In short, ensure patients' interests are put at the forefront of anything you do.[4]

- Ensure a good work–life balance: in most units you would normally have to give 6 weeks' notice to take leave and have adequate cover in place where appropriate. Try to plan ahead. There may be certain times of the year where several people wish to take leave. In training posts, you are employed and so the set annual leave is paid; however, employers will not pay for any unused annual leave.

- Dentists are competitive. During your undergraduate training there may be a large variation among graduates about the number and complexity of procedures performed. Where you feel there may be a deficiency, use the early years to remedy this. You should find that the degree of exposure that is available during your postgraduate training is far greater than what would have been available as an undergraduate so there is opportunity to remedy any perceived deficiencies. Self-reflection is important along with the ability to identify your areas of need to develop your skills and knowledge.

- Stay organized and decide what you want to achieve for each training programme even before you apply. Other people will tend to be very busy and will not search you out to give opportunities, projects, or cases. Decide what you want to develop, whether that is more experience in certain treatments, publications, audits, or presentations. Establish exactly what this is and seek out people who will be able to guide and enable you early in your training placement.

- Be prepared for setbacks. There are many situations when audit projects, publications, or research ideas may be rejected. The best thing to do is learn from any feedback and use this to progress. Be realistic about your targets. Time constraints within your placements are often some of the major difficulties in developing research projects.

- As a trainee, you are also an employee and are expected to contribute positively to the service of the practice/department. If you have some free time and another colleague is running late or needs assistance, then it is often courteous to make yourself available. Doing this will often not go unnoticed and you will also gain further experience.

- Ask for help. As a trainee you may be handling cases of high complexity and therefore your supervising colleagues will expect you to ask for help at some stage.

4 GDC (September 2013). *Standards for the Dental Team.*

- Plan appropriately for your required competencies of training. Your portfolio is the evidence of your training and progression. Without the evidence of these, you will not progress to the next stage. Work-based assessments and structured learning events need to be planned and regularly completed. They can seem burdensome at times; however, you need to change your mindset about these. They are not to show you are competent in everything. They are useful events to show progression of skills and knowledge, to enable feedback on your abilities, and to develop strategies to improve. Ensure you are on track and spread them out across the year. You will have a certain number to complete. Do not see this number as the 'most' you can do. Do as many as you can. You will not be in this position again, where someone is able to advise you on a one-to-one basis to develop your skills and attitudes as a competent professional. If you find you are falling behind, then make arrangements to remedy this. If you leave them to the end of the year, it can lead to a very stressful time for you and your supervisors.
- Be a personable colleague. There will always be challenging personalities to deal with, and you will need to develop strategies to deal with them. The ability to be friendly and approachable will most certainly enable you to fit into any team.
- Be prepared to invest in yourself. Unless you are prepared to take the time and effort to develop yourself, you are unlikely to succeed, as someone else will not do this for you. This investment is likely to enable career progression and increased job satisfaction. You will be looking at a career in dentistry spanning several decades. You will not be able to undertake every course that you want to in the first few years, otherwise you will be in significant debt. Plan your development.
- Have a 5-year career plan. This does not need to be definite as things will naturally change and evolve over time, both in terms of your professional life and personal life; however, by having a plan you have something to work towards and it gives you direction in your career. Be flexible and prepared to change as the situation changes.

Chapter 1

Dental Foundation Training

Introduction to Dental Foundation Training

- Finally finishing dental school marks the first major milestone in your dental career path. The next, which is almost a mandatory requirement for UK graduates, is completion of Dental Foundation Training (DFT).
- Individual clinical experience will vary at the point of graduation; however, DFT should provide an environment to build on and develop the basic knowledge and skills achieved at undergraduate level.
- The overall aim of DFT is to work towards becoming an independent, safe practitioner in the general dental service or to act as a basis for further training. Training will not only be directed at providing safe clinical care to a high standard in an efficient manner, but also to introduce aspects of practice management and further practical elements of clinical governance.
- The practitioner should be familiar with all parts of primary dental care and DFT should mark the starting point of lifelong learning.
- DFT has a curriculum to which the training is mapped.[1] This is subject to regular review, however, and so the aim of this handbook is for the contents to be as contemporaneous as possible, covering the significant aspects of the curriculum that are likely to be subject to only subtle or minimal changes in the future.
- Each individual scheme will have some degree of variation in terms of the educational content as will each practice in terms of the set-up, number and types of staff, patient demographics, and dental health needs.
- Your dental principal and the practice are likely to have been established for some time and therefore wherever you are located, you should be in a position to gain valuable insight and wisdom from someone who has seen and overcome many of the challenges that you will face, so try to make the most of it!

---

1 www.copdend.org

National recruitment

Recruitment to DFT is now undertaken on a national basis and all applicants seeking a post have to apply though the same application process in England, Wales, and Northern Ireland. Scotland runs a separate recruitment process for its Dental Vocational Training placements. Historically, individual candidates applied to specific practices for jobs and the decision was left to the practice concerned. There have been many reasons for a move to a national recruitment scheme including:

- A fairer process, with each applicant having the same application/ interview experience
- Less time needed to be taken away from undergraduate studies. By having a single application process, fewer interviews are required and so students no longer have to take as much time off
- The assessment centres are located regionally, minimizing travel burdens
- Recruitment to schemes can be based on a consistent and uniform process ensuring places are allocated fairly and on merit.

The process of recruitment can encompass the following steps; however, it can vary according to the individual situation:

- Online application form.
- Situational judgement test (SJT).
- Assessment centre.
- Scheme preference.
- Final allocation of places.

It is important to read the latest information provided at each recruitment round as the process is subject to change. The information provided here is purely for guidance and may not reflect the exact situation at each recruitment round. The specific details can also vary. For example, recruitment may be completely online or use only an SJT (NB: for the 2023 DFT National Recruitment Selection a SJT only will be used. Applicants will not be asked to undertake a communication station and the SJT will account for 100% of the overall assessment score).[1]

Online application form

This is used for the provision of contact details and eligibility assessment. It is not used for the purpose of selection.

Assessment centre

- The *first stage* involves completion of a SJT.[1]
- The SJT contributes 75% to the overall score. Its purpose is to assess non-clinical/non-academic skills such as professionalism, decision-making, patient-centred care, coping under pressure, and critical thinking.
- The SJT consists of answering 56 questions by either:
  - selecting one or more correct answers
  - ranking the answers (e.g. from the most important to least important, from the action with the highest priority to the lowest priority).

1 www.copdend.org

- The *second stage* consists of one panel with two assessors. This lasts for 10 minutes and there is 5 minutes of preparation time.
- Panel: assessment of clinical and communication skills including role play. Examples of situations of who you might be asked to manage include the following:
  - A patient attends the practice as an emergency with avulsed teeth.
  - A patient arrives at the practice complaining that her veneers have fallen out after they were cemented recently by an associate at the practice. She has an important family function in 2 days. On trying in, you can see that they do not fit, and the patient is not happy.
  - An emergency patient arrives who is in pain and you are already running late for your routine appointments. A second patient who the receptionist feels is more serious also arrives. How do you manage the situation?
  - A patient reporting dental trauma attends the practice.
  - A patient arrives with a severe episode of pericoronitis from a lower wisdom tooth which you feel is beyond your competence to extract.
- The panel contributes the remaining 25% of the score.

Tips on managing these scenarios
- When dealing with emergencies think about:
  - checking for danger then 'ABCDE' (Airway, Breathing, Circulation, Disability, Exposure)
  - get help when appropriate. Avoid managing by yourself wherever possible.
- When dealing with issues surrounding patient safety, think about the specific details that need to be covered and discussed including the following[2]:
  - Find out as much about the immediate situation as possible from nurses or other members of staff who may know the person concerned.
  - Identify if any patients are at risk, have been put at risk, or have already suffered harm.
  - What action you intend to take bearing in mind the safety of yourself and others.
  - Make sure you involve others and avoid trying to manage by yourself—this could include other associates, the principal managers, defence organizations, or even the General Dental Council (GDC).
  - When appropriate, provide support to the colleague concerned.
- If trying to make a difficult decision, think about the options from the lowest risk to the highest risk and deferring the decision where possible.
- Take a look at the websites or periodicals of your defence organization. They will often have various cases that have been discussed and possible solutions.

Scheme preferences
Following the assessment centre stage, decisions must be made about which schemes the Dental Foundation (DF) trainee is prepared to train in, and their order of preference.

2 Picard O, Wood D, Yuen S. (2013). *Medical Interview. A Comprehensive Guide to CT, ST, Registrar Interview Skills* (2nd ed). ISC Medical.

The schemes need to be ranked from the highest down to the lowest preference. Not all schemes need to be considered; however, limiting the number of preferences may mean that you are not allocated a post at all. The highest-scoring candidate will be allocated their first-choice scheme, as would the second-highest-scoring candidate and so on until it reaches a point where a candidate's first-choice scheme is full. At that point they would be allocated their second choice provided that it is not full, or their third choice until they are allocated a scheme or run out of preferences.

Allocation to a practice within the scheme

When selecting practices, consider the following:

- Look at the practice website—most if not all will have one. You can find out about the location, opening hours, number of dentists and possibly nurses, availability of a hygienist or therapist, and parking facilities.
- Are there dentists there with any special skills or interests that may interest you, such as orthodontics, implants, oral surgery, and dentists with enhanced skills or specialists?
- Identify exactly where the practice is and whether the commute is acceptable, balancing this with the opportunities the practice may bring.
- Where do you see yourself in 5 years' time and how do you feel your time in that practice will contribute to that?
- Are you aware of others who have been trainees at that practice and what their thoughts are of the practice and the trainer?
- Also consider what you are able to offer the practice. Do you live/plan to live locally and so would be unlikely to have punctuality affected by adverse weather or transport difficulties? Can you be available at short notice? Are there any interests you may have in common with the staff?
- On practice websites there are likely to be profiles of the dentists—do you feel you could get on with them on a personal level as well as professionally? Although not a vital requirement, it may be of interest on a social level.

Questions to consider asking when selecting practices

It may not be possible to contact the practice to ask questions, but the following may be things to think about if it is available on the practice website:

- Who will be providing the nursing support—are there trainee dental nurses or an experienced qualified nurse?
- Are there extra duties that the nurses are competent to do (oral health/radiology qualifications etc.)? Are the nurses fluent in the use of the practice management software?
- What is the range of treatments that are carried out regularly? What are the patient demographics, such as families, older adults, or is the practice located in a central area and see more working adults? Is it in a highly deprived area with high dental needs? Is there much opportunity to provide advanced elements of care such as endodontics or is it mainly routine, urgent, and preventative care, or a mix?
- What additional skills can be gained?
- What is the procedure for annual leave? Does this need to be coordinated with the nurse(s) and are there times when leave must be taken or cannot be taken?

- What is the educational supervisor's expectation of their trainee from the outset?
- How many patients would you expect the DF trainee to see from the first day? Appointment time flexibility?
- What are the educational supervisor's outside interests (sports, hobbies, etc.)?
- What has the current DF trainee gained from the post?
- Are there any areas that the current DF trainee has found difficult to gain experience in and how has this been addressed?
- What is the educational supervisor's clinical commitment at the practice?

Allocation of places

There are occasions when a candidate is unsuccessful at the final exams of the dental degree and, therefore, they may have to relinquish their post. The post may then be reallocated.

The practice team

Introduction to the practice team

The environment that you will be moving into will be very different to that of a dental school. The roles of the common members of the primary dental team will be explained in this section, including:

- Principal
- DF educational supervisor
- Associate dental practitioner
- DF trainee
- Dental hygienist or therapist
- Practice manager
- Treatment coordinator
- Oral health educator
- Registered dental nurse
- Trainee dental nurse
- Receptionist
- Domestic staff.

Some of those staff members may play multiple roles.

Principal

The principal, in most cases, will be a dentist who owns the practice. They will ultimately be responsible for the overall management of the practice and to ensure that it is running smoothly as a business. In some cases, there may be a dental care professional who owns the practice. In many corporate bodies there may be an equivalent clinical lead who will have similar duties to a principal dentist. The dental corporate practices rely more heavily on practice managers and regional managers for the day-to-day running of the practice, with implementation of the business decisions from higher management within the company.

DF educational supervisor

The DF educational supervisor will be a dentist who has the responsibility to both the DF trainee and the regional health education board (deanery) for training in the practice. Their role will be to act as a mentor to the DF trainee, establishing the educational agreement, providing training, and monitoring progress and development through workplace-based assessments. They will also provide tutorials each week and will be part of the regional teaching programme organized by the deanery. The educational supervisor historically would have been the principal dentist; however, increasingly there are many associates who are undertaking these training roles.

Associate dental practitioner

An associate of the practice is usually a self-employed dentist who provides a range of general dental services and has an agreement with the principal to deliver certain services. This may specify service requirements privately, on the National Health Service (NHS), and on private capitation schemes. As with all dentists, the range of services they provide may be general or they may have developed areas of specific interest and may only provide these areas of dentistry. Unless the associate dentist is part of the

DF educational supervisor team, they will not have any obligations to the DF trainee but may be able to provide informal advice and assistance.

DF trainee

Although most practices will only have one DF trainee, some employ two at the same time. Where DF trainees are part of a longitudinal scheme (2-year programme of Joint Dental Foundation Core Training (JDFCT)), there may be two trainees, but operating on different weeks. In some cases, you will both share the same set of patients and one or both of you may be delivering different parts of the same plan; alternatively, you may end up seeing each other's patients at different times of the year for the recall appointment. This can have its natural difficulties—one DF trainee may not agree with the other's treatment plan, or a mistake carried out by one DF trainee may be noticed by the other. The benefit of this sharing of patients is peer review of treatment provided. Many practices overcome some of these problems by allocating each patient to one DF trainee, whom they complete their courses of treatment with. Either way there is a likelihood that at some stage you may be required to see each other's patients for one reason or another, or even see an associate's patient in an emergency.

It is therefore important to keep good relations with the other dentists and keep a professional attitude when dealing with patients who have been treated by colleagues.

Dental hygienist/therapist

In some cases, you may have a dental hygienist or therapist present in the practice. Discuss carefully with your DF educational supervisor and/or principal about your decisions to delegate work to them. In many cases the cost of employing the hygienist or therapist may be met in part or full by the referring associate. They may employ the hygienist or therapist to allow better use of the skills of dental care professionals in the team, enabling the associate dentist to carry out other work which may be deemed more profitable and therefore it becomes more cost-effective to delegate some work to the dental care professional.

As a DF trainee, any patients you treat would be for the purpose of training rather than to meet financial or activity targets. It may be deemed inappropriate to therefore delegate work to a hygienist or therapist as there is educational gain in treating these patients yourself.

If you are in the position where you can refer patients, ensure that your prescriptions are well written and specify exactly what needs to be performed. Appropriate referrals are another area of development need so take this time to develop your skills in appropriate referral and use of the wider dental team. Dental hygienists and therapists are now able to see patients without the need for a prescription (direct access); however, not all dental care professionals wish to provide this access and may still require a prescription.

Practice manager

The practice manager is a required role and is often officially recognized by the Care Quality Commission (CQC) as the person responsible for running the dental service, in some cases it is the principle that is recognised by the CQC.

The role of the practice manager can vary; however, it will most likely include payroll, staffing, health and safety, compliance with infection prevention, CQC, Control of Substances Hazardous to Health (COSHH) regulations, Reporting of Injuries, Diseases and Dangerous Occurrences Regulations (RIDDOR), implementation and maintenance of practice policies, and dealing with complaints. Their work may also cross over with that of the principal. The practice manager may have a background in dentistry as a dental care professional or this role may be provided by the principal, a partner in the practice, another dentist, head nurse, or a non-clinical member of staff.

Treatment coordinator

Sometimes termed practice coordinators, treatment coordinators are often dental nurses who have undergone additional training. Their duties usually include welcoming new patients to the practice, discussing treatment options with patients prior to and after they have seen a clinician, answering questions, and possibly managing complaints. Their role can be vital in managing patient expectations and facilitating an effective patient journey. Not all practices will have a treatment coordinator, but if your practice does, it is a useful experience to shadow them to better understand the effective communication required to ensure patients understand their options and how others explain treatment options.

Oral health educator

This is often one of the dental nurses who has completed additional training in oral health education. Their role can vary but can include recording of plaque indices, providing oral hygiene instruction, and diet advice. The benefits of such a practitioner are that the time required for important preventative advice can be provided by delegation to another member of the dental team, ensuring the dentist's time can be managed effectively.

Registered dental nurse

Effective dental care requires coordinated treatment by the dentist with assistance from dental nurses. Registered dental nurses make up one of the largest groups of dental care professionals on the GDC register and are the ones the DF trainee, and any dentist for that matter, needs to develop a good professional relationship with for effective team working. They are there to provide chair-side assistance for the effective provision of four-handed dentistry, ensuring high standards of infection control, patient management, and organization of the day list. They will often know the practice very well and may have worked with previous DF trainees so will have experience of the abilities of a DF trainee as a 'new beginner'. They may also know the patients very well and so may have a good rapport with them.

Trainee dental nurses

Trainee dental nurses would normally be on a registered training programme such as a National Vocational Qualification, National Certificate, or other approved qualification leading to registration with the GDC. As a significant part of their training, they will be required to carry out chairside experience. In general, overall responsibility lies with the dentist, even when working with qualified dental nurses; however, there is almost absolute responsibility on the dentist when working with trainees as they are not registered with the GDC.

Receptionist

Dental reception teams may be made up of a variety of members, some of whom may be non-clinical and others with a dental background or management background. The reception teams are vital to the effective management of the clinical day, through organizing patient bookings/cancellations, emergency telephone triage, and payments; often managing patient expectations; and being the initial point of contact at the practice.

It is important to bear in mind that the receptionist may have limited privileges to patient information. While they may be able to book patients in and arrange further appointments, they may not have the right to certain information such as the type of exemption from NHS dental charges, this may have to be discussed in the surgery. Patients may not be happy to discuss confidential information with the receptionist in front of a full waiting room. In the course of their work, receptionists may have access to sensitive information. It is therefore vital that they have training in patient confidentiality and data protection.

The reception team may have a great deal of experience in dealing with patients and managing triage of emergencies. It is useful to understand their background and knowledge to enable effective management of patients, particularly emergency calls. Good communication between the reception team and clinical team is needed and establishing your role at the start of your training is useful, advising them of your needs with time compared to the other dentists in the practice.

Domestic staff

Most practices will employ domestic staff to clear away general waste and maintain hygiene of any sanitary facilities in the practice. They may only be present after the practice closes and so you may never get the opportunity to meet them. They are the reason why the practice always looks presentable even though there may have been >100 people using it the previous day. Ensure that infection prevention protocols have been followed and all sharps are disposed of in the correct manner prior to domestic cleaning. Ensure all confidential patient information is put away and computers are logged off. Most of this is common sense.

Dealing with difficulties

Difficulties will occur at many stages with different people. Examples are:
- With patients
- With nurses/dental care professionals
- With other dentists.

It may be advisable to get your educational supervisor involved when certain difficulties are occurring; however, there are some tips on managing some of the difficulties that can arise.

Difficulty with patients

- Communication is often one of the main causes of difficulties with patients. Effective communication at a patient level is essential to develop to ensure good patient management.
- The initial response is to identify the difficulty the patient has. There may be nothing wrong with any treatment or care that you have provided or there may very well be a simple complication. Early effective management when investigating the concern and communicating with the patient is essential.
- An apology is usually adequate to resolve most situations. It is not admitting any wrongdoing, but merely acknowledging the patient's dissatisfaction and addressing their concerns.
- Should this fail, another effective way of managing the situation would be to use active listening. Prior to giving any response to the patient, allow them to vent their frustrations, listen carefully to what they say, then allow a pause. Repeat back to them their concerns showing that you have acknowledged what they have actually said and ask if that summarizes their concerns. Use empathy in both verbal and non-verbal language.
- If they have further concerns, then allow them to finish and then pause again, before repeating back what they have said using a summary and what they said previously and ask again if that summarizes their concerns.
- Once the patient has had time to discuss their concerns, only then state your side clearly and give a very straight and precise account of your position and what you feel is the best way forwards, explaining very clearly what you can or cannot achieve. Do not do this before repeating back what the patient has said as it is important for the patient to feel listened to, before they are willing to listen back.
- Find out how the patient then feels about the situation and what they want to do next.
- If they make an unreasonable request, then start the process again, repeating back what they have said to show you acknowledge what their request is, and then again state your position very clearly about what you cannot do and what can be done and then ask again how they wish to progress. Try to repeat this process until there is an understanding of the best way forward for both parties.
- If in doubt, ask for a second opinion from your educational supervisor.

Difficulty with colleagues

When dealing with colleagues, particularly new ones, if relationships start to break down, it is important to address the problem in a timely manner with effective communication, opening a dialogue between the parties involved to enable a solution. It is beyond the scope of this text to address all issues related to difficulties with colleagues, but here are some strategies of management:

- Be clear in your own mind as to what you feel the problem is, and how you are going to approach it, as well as what has happened as a result.
- When stating what has gone wrong/the problem, be mindful of their perceptions of the issue. For example, rather than saying 'You were rude', state what the colleague said and how it made you or others feel.
- State the result of their action and how it has affected others in a non-confrontational manner.
- It may be appropriate to ask the colleague how discussing this information has made them feel and how they may wish to address the concern. The importance of this is to develop their awareness of the issue affecting others and to enable them to create their own solution.
- If they divert the problem or discuss unrelated issues, then make it clear that the other issues would need to be dealt with separately and bring the discussion back to the original point.

Difficulty with other dentists

When there are concerns about patient safety with other dentists then use the method described previously (➔ Tips on managing these scenarios).

Other sources of advice in dealing with difficulties

- DF educational supervisor.
- Practice manager.
- Other associate dentists in the practice.
- If you work in a corporate, then the clinical director.
- Other DF trainees.
- Training programme director.
- Associate dental dean.
- Postgraduate dental dean or lead employer.
- Your defence indemnity provider.
- GDC.

Tutorials, study days, and appraisals

Tutorials and study days are protected time and form part of the educational training.

Tutorials

Tutorials are different to study days in that they are run by the educational supervisor within the practice.

Requirements are as follows:
- One hour of protected time during normal working hours.
- A patient may be present for the purpose of the tutorial; however, the tutorial should not be used to complete additional service with no specific educational goal.
- They can be used to gain one-to-one teaching on specific clinical skills such as tooth extraction or crown preparation if a patient is present.
- If there are specific procedures that you wish to gain experience of, you can inform your educational supervisor and they may be able to identify a suitable case from their own patient base if one cannot be found from your own patient base.
- In order to get the most out of a tutorial, it is important to be organized prior to the tutorial, having read relevant background information.
- Look at your personal development plan (PDP) and identify areas of deficiency where you may wish to develop your skills or knowledge and that may not be already covered elsewhere in your programme study days.
- Identify how you need to meet this particular need. Tutorials are useful for something that can be achieved in 1 hour in a practice environment where it falls within the realm of general dental practice.
- At the start of your training year, it would be worth listing some topics within your PDP to give your educational supervisor a basis on which to develop the tutorial programme. Your educational supervisor will already have some ideas on areas in which to provide tutorials, but it is worth tailoring your learning to your specific individual needs.

Examples of tutorial sessions and how to organize:
- Surgical removal of a tooth:
  - Identify the patient prior to the session and inform your educational supervisor.
  - Ensure any necessary background reading has been undertaken, particularly around vital structures and basic anatomy, and that this is understood.
  - Prior to the arrival of the patient talk through the procedure with your educational supervisor.
  - Make sure you are familiar with any equipment required.
- Didactic tutorial session:
  - Identify what you want to learn prior to the session.
  - List a set of aims and objectives.
  - Keep this realistic as you will only have 1 hour.
  - Keep the list focused and relevant to your particular practice.
  - Limit the objectives to ensure sufficient time is available for each objective to be met.

- Give your aims and objectives to your educational supervisor in advance. Ensure you have done sufficient reading in advance.
- The Educational Supervisor may have some material they wish to find to assist you. Give them the time to prepare so that you can get the most of the tutorial.
- Possible tutorial activities/topics:
  - Professionalism activities: Appraisals, Clinical Audit, Critical decision making, GDC, Duty of candour, difficult interactions, patient safety, medical emergency management, Confidentiality, consent and complaints, Equality, diversity and ethics.
  - Management topics: contracts, legal elements of a practice, General Data Protection Regulation, Health and Safety Infection control and radiography, safeguarding.

At the end of the tutorial, it is worth spending some time reflecting on what has been gained and document this reflection in your portfolio.

Study days

Common features of study days:
- Usually, there are 30 study days throughout the training year.
- There is a lot of variation between individual schemes; however, the purpose is to meet the aims of the DFT curriculum.
- Study days are regarded as working days therefore attendance is mandatory and forms part of the competencies for the Annual Review of Competence Progression (ARCP).
- They include all the trainees within the DFT scheme in that area and usually take the form of small group teaching.
- They can be combined with other schemes. This can allow for certain activities which may not have been possible in smaller groups.
- They may take the form of a teaching session run by the training programme director for your scheme or attendance of a local, regional, or national conference. On occasions, international events may be funded.
- Annual leave is often not permitted during these study days.
- At the start of locally arranged study days, there is usually a debrief for trainees to share and discuss their week of training.
- Travel expenses for attendance at such study days are funded provided they are reasonable and are within the accepted limits.
- Most study days contribute to verifiable continuing professional development (CPD); however, it is important to remember that no CPD contributes to the GDC CPD scheme in the first year of registration.

Topics covered during the study days could typically include:
- Medical emergencies
- Cross-infection control
- Radiology and radiation protection
- Communication skills
- Law and ethics
- Clinical governance
- Treatment planning
- Tips and techniques

- Restorative dentistry
- Oral surgery
- Paediatric dentistry
- Orthodontics
- Case presentations
- Key skills
- Trade exhibitions
- Attendance at national conferences or other professional societies.

Review

Reviews will typically occur at the start, midpoint (interim), and end of the training year. They generally include clinical skills, professionalism, leadership and management, and communication.

The first review would normally include an educational agreement which is usually a standard document that needs to be completed.

Clinical skills
- Provide your logbook of the number and types of procedures that you have completed by the end of your undergraduate training.
- Try to gauge which areas you feel confident/competent in, and areas in which you feel that you require further development.
- It is important to be honest at this stage, as most graduates will be relatively inexperienced at most procedures but will feel more comfortable with certain procedures. It is important to identify areas that you feel you need to gain more experience of early in your training so that they can be addressed quickly.
- As training progresses the experience in all clinical domains needs to be recorded and used as part of the interim and final reviews

Professionalism
- Ethics and law.
- Dealing with other staff professionally.
- Dealing with patients professionally.
- Ensuring own conduct is in line with what is expected of a dental professional.

Leadership and management
- Time management.
- Legal aspects of practice including health and safety.
- Understanding the business of dentistry and financial implications.
- Managing the staff.

Communication
- Patient communication and building rapport.
- Written communication to laboratory staff and prescriptions to dental care professionals.
- Verbal communication with staff.
- Communication with the family of patients where appropriate.

Aim to address most of these, although some aspects may be new and so will only be identified at the interim review. The benefit of the interim review is that it still leaves time to develop these areas.

Practice management

There will always be someone within the practice who undertakes the management of the practice; however, as a dentist, it is beneficial to understand how to manage a practice. This extends from practice policies to regulation management and staffing.

Practice policies

The practice will have a number of policies in place which you will be encouraged to become familiar with and sign these policies to confirm your reading and understanding. They will often serve as an excellent guide, particularly when facing difficulties. They may have been formed using a template created by a dental organization, or one the practice has created.

Examples of practice policies
- Complaints procedure.
- Cross-infection control policy.
- Hand hygiene policy.
- Inoculation injury policy.
- Surgery routine protocol.
- Radiography equipment local rules.
- Health and safety policy.
- Patient confidentiality policy.

Appointments

Timing of appointments is crucial and great care is needed to ensure that sufficient time is allowed for each patient. Allowing insufficient time for a patient can create undue pressure, and lead to the need for additional appointments, running late, or even the temptation to reduce quality. Allowing overly generous time for an appointment can lead to a lack of training and experience. At the start of the training year, it is wise to allow more time than you think you will need but discuss this with your educational supervisor as they will be able to advise. This will give you the opportunity to identify the amount of turnover time required, such as time for writing of contemporaneous notes, decontamination, and setting up for the next patient. Running late can also become a source of complaints and often has a knock-on effect for the next appointments of the day.

Practice regulation

While many general dental practices may be small businesses, it is under the scrutiny of many regulations. There are several bodies that have been charged with the responsibility of ensuring that such regulations are met including the GDC, NHS, CQC, and the Health and Safety Executive (HSE).

General Dental Council

The purpose of the GDC is to protect patients and regulate the dental team. As a body, it registers individual dentists and dental care professionals who then are entitled to practise dentistry in the UK. The regulatory focus is on individual professionals rather than the practice as a whole. Nonetheless, it may share information with other bodies if issues were to arise or refer complaints accordingly. There may be some crossover, for example, proof of training in the use of radiography equipment may be part of the CPD requirement and the Ionising Radiation (Medical Exposure) Regulations 2017 (IRMER).[1]

Care Quality Commission

The CQC registers the site that provides the dental service, such as the dental practice, and holds the name of the practice manager.

The function of the CQC is to 'Register. Monitor, inspect and rate. Enforce. Independent Voice'.

- As far as dental practices are concerned, it bases its inspections on five questions, asking if the practice is:
  - safe
  - effective
  - caring
  - responsive
  - well led.
- It makes two main types of inspection:
  - Comprehensive: 10% of practices are inspected, which is announced and 2 weeks' notice is given. All five criteria are inspected and it takes place over 1 day.
  - Focused: unannounced inspection in response to a complaint or raised concern and may involve other parties. Not all of the criteria are looked at.[2]

Health and Safety Executive

The HSE is the body responsible for ensuring the many health and safety regulations are being met. It is able to enter dental practices, access any necessary areas, and interview any employee if there is a health and safety issue that needs to be addressed. If it feels a breach of the regulations has occurred, then it is able to issue a notice to improve or even prohibit certain activities. It is also able to take away or alter items which it considers may be of harm and could also prosecute the practice.

More details are provided in → Key skills portfolio. The following is a list of regulations affecting dental practices:

- Workplace (Health, Safety and Welfare) Regulations 1992.
- Manual Handling Operations Regulations 1992.
- Electricity at Work Regulations 1989.
- Regulatory Reform (Fire Safety) Order 2005.
- Health and Safety (First Aid) Regulations 1981.
- Reporting of Injuries, Diseases and Dangerous Occurrences Regulations 1995.
- Ionisation Radiation Regulations 2017.
- IRMER
- Control of Substances Hazardous to Health Regulations 2002.
- Health and Safety (Sharp Instruments in Health Care) Regulations 2013.[3]

1 www.gdc-uk.org
2 www.cqc.org.uk
3 www.hse.gov.uk

Infection control
While not within NHS regulations, there are technical documents such as 'Decontamination in primary care dental practices' (Health Technical Memorandum (HTM) 01-05) which state essential and best practice standards. Details of this document is beyond the scope of this text.[4]

Financial matters

Introduction to financial matters
- As a DF trainee, this may be your first substantial employed position. It is important to know that any quoted salary or pay is subject to a range of deductions including income tax, National Insurance Contributions (NICs), statutory levy, and pension contributions.
- The following information in this section has been sourced from His Majesty's Revenue and Customs (HMRC).[5]
- For further advice on financial matters, we suggest the use of a financial advisor who will be able to guide you in this area.
- In a fully employed position (a trainee in DFT or Dental Core Training (DCT)), it is your employer that will make the arrangements for income tax to be deducted at source through pay as you earn (PAYE) as well as NICs, statutory levy, pension contributions through superannuation, and any student loan repayments. Your employer may be either the practice owner or a lead employer who employs all the trainees in your region.
- If you are self-employed (such as an associate or practice principal) you would be expected to complete your own tax return (Self-Assessment), detailing your turnover and expenditure and submit these to HMRC.
- Submissions to HMRC can be:
  - paper (deadline 31 October)
  - online (deadline, 31 January).
- HMRC will calculate the tax you owe and advise you of deadlines to pay. Or this can be conducted through an accountant.
- There are two payment deadlines for self-assessment:
  - 31 January (payment on account and balancing payment).
  - 31 July (payment on account).
- The 'balancing payment' addresses any shortfalls in the two 'payment on account' predictions of your tax for a specific financial year.
- 'Payments on account' are advance payments towards your tax bill if you are self-employed. Each payment is half your previous year's tax bill.
- Caution is needed if there are significant changes in your income as this will affect payments on account. If your income is going to be less in a particular year, you can request that HMRC reduces the payment on account.
- Self-Assessment tax returns can be completed by yourself or your accountant.
- If you have complex tax affairs or are operating under a limited company, or you feel this is out of your remit, then it may be prudent to use the services of an accountant to help manage this.
- An accountant can provide useful advice on your tax planning and hopefully ensure that you are tax efficient.

4 🔗 www.gov.uk/government/publications/decontamination-in-primary-care-dental-practices
5 HMRC. Money and tax. 🔗 https://www.gov.uk/browse/tax

- As a general rule, an accountant would suggest that you save around 33–35% of your self-employed income for tax, although this will depend on your earnings.
- Failure to pay the appropriate tax may result in significant financial penalties. Failure to declare your tax liabilities may result in a criminal conviction. Therefore, it is important to understand this topic and arrange the appropriate advice.
- Information provided is only a guide and is based on the 2021–2022 financial year. Should there be any doubt over your financial matters you should consider speaking to an accountant or financial advisor.

Income tax

Personal allowance

- The standard personal allowance is £12,570, which is the amount you can earn up to before having to pay income tax.
- The personal allowance drops by £1 for every £2 income above £100,000.
- You may also receive a personal allowance on any savings interest depending on your income from other earnings.

Income tax following personal allowances

- For every £1 of income beyond the personal allowance up to £50,270, 20% basic income tax would have to be paid.
- As an example, if £12,670 of income was generated, this results in £100 beyond the standard personal allowance of £12,570, therefore 20% of the £100 needs to be paid in income tax resulting in an income tax payment of £20.
- Beyond £50,270 a higher rate of income tax of 40% would have to be paid. So, £12,570–£50,270 is subject to 20p income tax per £1 and every £1 above £50,270 would be subject to 40p income tax for every £1 earned up to £150,000.
- Every £1 earned above £150,000 would be subject to 45% income tax.

National Insurance Contributions

Introduction to National Insurance

- Generally, NICs are compulsory if you are earning >£184 per week as an employee.
- If you earn between £120 and £184 per week you may not have to pay NICs but it may be registered as if you have made such payments.
- Payment of class 1, 2, and 3 contributions entitles you to some contribution-based benefits.
- Class 1 NICs need to be paid by employed persons.
- Class 2 and class 4 NICs need to be paid by the self-employed.
- Class 3 NICs are voluntary payments to fill any gaps in your National Insurance record.
- Failure to pay a sufficient number of years of NICs may limit entitlements to contribution-based benefits such as a State Pension.

Class 1 NICs

- Paid by employees, usually by direct deduction from salary.
- For earning from £184 to £967 per week it is usually 12%. Earnings above this are deducted at 2%.
- Will normally be encountered during DFT and DCT.

Class 2 NICs
- Paid for by self-employed persons, only if trading profits are >£6515 per year.
- Flat rate of £3.05 per week.
- If you work as an associate following DFT, you are likely to pay this through your self-assessment.

Class 3 NICs
- If there are gaps in your National Insurance record and you wish to claim a State Pension, this is something you may need to consider.

Class 4 NICs
- Paid for by self-employed persons, only if trading profits are >£9569 per year.
- For profits between £9569 and £50,270, 9% is usually payable. Every £1 above this is subject to 2% NICs.

Claiming expenses
- As an employee you may be able to reduce your taxable income by informing HMRC of certain expenditures required to do your job. Such expenditures may extend to payment of the annual retention fee to the GDC, indemnity fees, memberships of professional bodies, and laundry of uniforms. You should consult an accountant if you are unsure what you may be able to claim.
- As a self-employed person there may be further expenses you may be able to claim as part of doing your job.

Statutory levy
- Payment for Local Dental Committee work.

Student loan repayment
- If you took a student loan to assist you financially during your studies, you would typically have accumulated interest at the Retail Price Index (RPI) with an addition of 3% per year.[6]
- Following graduation, the interest rate would depend on annual gross income. Based on the 2021 rates this would be[6]:
  - RPI + 3% for those with an annual gross income >£49,130.
  - equal to RPI rate if gross annual income is >£27,295
  - tapered for those with a gross annual income between £27,295 and £49,130.
- Repayments would typically be 9% of earning >£27,295.
- After 30 years following the first year of repayment, the remaining amount may get written off.[6]
- Repayments are made by your employer, on your behalf, through salary deductions or through HMRC Self-Assessment.

NHS Pension Scheme
The benefits of the NHS Pension Scheme have changed over the years with different member benefits depending on when you started in the scheme. This section will only cover the most recent pension scheme, the 2015 scheme, because as recent graduates you are most likely to be in this scheme.[7]

6 🔗 https://www.gov.uk/browse/education/student-finance

7 🔗 www.nhsbsa.nhs.uk/nhs-pensions

- The NHS pension is optional, but you are automatically enrolled into the pension as an NHS worker, but you can opt out of paying into this pension. We would suggest consultation with a financial advisor regarding this.
- Deductions for your pension are via superannuation (company pension scheme) and will be deducted at source (your employer).
- Superannuation payments are not subject to tax, effectively a tax-free reduction in your earnings, but tax is payable when you receive your pension at the appropriate level.
- The 2015 scheme is a career average revalued earnings (CARE) scheme based on a proportion of pensionable earnings in each year of membership.
- 2015 scheme benefits:
  - Pension worth 1/54th of each year of pensionable earnings, revalued at the beginning of each following scheme year in line with a rate set by the Treasury plus 1.5% while in active membership.
  - Lump sum may be an option with exchange of part of the pension up to 25%.
  - Benefits received at State Pension age or age 65.
  - Early retirement option at 55. Pension value reduced.
  - Ill health retirement benefits.
  - Death benefits (the higher of): 2× last 12 months of pensionable service or 2× revalued pensionable earnings up to 10 years earlier.
  - Life assurance and family benefits:
    - Adult dependent pension for spouse/civil partner/nominated partner.
    - Child dependant pension (if no adult).
- You can access your Annual Benefit Statement (ABS) through the online Total Rewards Statement.[8]
- *Lifetime allowance* is the maximum tax-free pension saving in your lifetime. This is currently £1.03 million. Over this amount you will be subject to tax charges.
- *Annual allowance* is the maximum amount of growth in your pension savings that you can receive tax relief on. Currently this is £40,000. This may be tapered if you earn >£150,000.

Advice on your pension and savings can be invaluable for your future retirement planning. Discussions at this early stage in your career will prepare you for your future.

8 www.nhsbsa.nhs.uk/total-reward-statements

Teledentistry

Introduction

- The concept of telecommunications in healthcare is not a new one. For example, patients having telephone consultations with their general medical practitioner (GMP).
- Better technology, including smart phones and better internet connections, has vastly improved the quality and capability of these services.
- Virtual consultations, remote prescribing, webinars, conferences, and viva examinations are all commonplace.

Virtual consultations

Preparation

- The quality of the connection may well be limited by the technology the patient uses; however, where possible, make sure any equipment or internet connection is good at the practice.
- If possible, try to establish in advance if the patient wants a video or telephone consultation. There are still many in society who are not able to use the technology for video consultations. Where video consultations occur, ensure the patient is given clear and full joining instructions.
- Ensure that the patient details are checked prior to starting the consultation; this information therefore needs to be readily available.
- If any consultations are being recorded, then ensure patients give consent for this and transfer the recording to the patient's electronic notes.
- Even if the consultation is not directly recorded, but clinical notes are being taken, consent for this would also be needed.
- Try and hold the consultation in a neutral room with little background noise or where you cannot be easily disturbed.
- Be aware of your own health and safety in carrying out such consultations. Avoid bending your neck to hold a phone handset with your head and shoulder. Consider a headset/earpiece.

Conducting the consultation

Establishing an emergency

It is not easy to determine if an emergency (such as spreading infections or abscesses) is occurring[1]; however, there are some things that can be assessed virtually:

- Take a history including pain history to identify the site, severity, radiation, type of pain, onset, and exacerbating and relieving factors.
- *Airway*: is the patient's airway compromised? If a patient is able to speak clearly over the phone, the airway is likely to be patent. However, if a patient complains of difficulty breathing, cannot speak clearly, or is distressed this may imply partial airway obstruction which may proceed to total airway obstruction. Dental infections can contribute to swelling and airway compromise.

---

1 Resuscitation Council UK (2021). *Advanced Life Support* (8th ed). Resuscitation Council UK.

- *Breathing*: breathing should be quiet and usually inaudible over the phone. Listen for respiratory effort and distress over the phone. The most important element of assessing the breathing is the respiratory rate (number of breaths per minute). If the respiratory rate is >20–25 then this indicates a patient could suddenly deteriorate. If you can hear more than one breath every 3 seconds then this should be worrying. Trauma resulting in swallowed or inhaled tooth fragments, restorations, or orthodontic components require emergency investigation.
- *Circulation*: this can be difficult to assess virtually. Reduced mental state can imply poor central perfusion. Feeling faint or syncope can imply hypotension, possibly due to blood loss. Dental or facial trauma can result in blood loss. If this causes hypotension, it may imply hypovolaemic shock which is an emergency. Jaw pain can also be a sign of angina. Jaw pain on exertion which is relieved with rest may well be stable angina; however, spontaneous pain could well be an acute coronary syndrome. Likewise, if the patient expresses shortness of breath, or chest pain, then these can be important and require immediate escalation to the emergency services.
- *Disability*: there are limits to determining disability virtually. Disability may be identified if the phone consultation is being taken on behalf of the patient or by video consultation. If possible, examine pupil size (this can be difficult even with high quality video). Use the AVPU scale (Alert, responds to Verbal stimuli, Painful stimuli, or is Unresponsive) to assess consciousness. Low blood glucose could be indicated by feeling faint. Where dental trauma has occurred, and consciousness has been impaired, this may imply other head injury which may be an emergency.
- *Exposure*: this can be assessed using video calls, the patient could send photos, or by taking details over the phone. Identify where the trauma has occurred, and if there are other injuries. In the event of infection, identify any facial swelling or high temperature.

Establishing urgency

In an emergency situation, the patient should be directed immediately to the local emergency department. If it is not an emergency, then the level of urgency needs to be determined.[2]

Factors to consider when determining the urgency and need for an urgent appointment:
- Trauma: complex fracture of a permanent tooth involving the pulp, avulsion of a permanent tooth, displacement of a permanent or primary tooth affecting the occlusion.
- Soft tissue: presence of an ulcer for >2 weeks.
- Haemorrhage: moderate bleeding that has failed to stop.
- Pain: severe pain preventing sleep or eating.
- Infection: spreading infection without affecting the airway.

2 Scottish Dental Clinical Effectiveness Programme (2020). Management of acute dental problems during COVID-19 pandemic. ✂ https://www.sdcep.org.uk/media/ttndnxyr/20-04-30-sdcep-covid-guide-survey-results.pdf

Remote management
- Only do so if it is safe and sufficient information has been provided from the consultation to do so.[3]
- Get consent from the patient to share information with others (such as the GMP) if necessary and for any proposed remote management.
- Direct patients to other appropriate services if necessary.
- An option for declining treatment should be given. Where remote treatment is offered, a review should also occur even if this is a telephone review.

Possible options for remote management
- Advice: this can include the use of analgesia such as paracetamol or ibuprofen, the use of off-the-shelf mouth rinses such as benzydamine or chlorhexidine, or the use of off-the-shelf temporary cements to manage cavities or de-bonded restorations.
- Remote prescribing: prescribing analgesia or mouthwashes may be indicated. Prescribing antibiotics may also be helpful where there is a suspicion of spreading infection.
- An antibiotic prescription should not be made for the management of pain nor should it be made as a result of patient pressure. In such situations, the following should be clearly communicated to the patient:
  - Prescribing antibiotics may not help the patient's situation.
  - Relief of the patient's symptoms can occur in the absence of antibiotics and even if the patient has had improvement of symptoms in the past, there is a good chance that this would have occurred even in the absence of taking the antibiotics.
  - The more antibiotics that are taken, the less effective they become.

Remote consultations for elective care
- A great deal of information can be gathered by carrying out a consultation for elective care.
- Establish the patient's main concerns.
- Establish a full medical and social history including occupation, smoking, and how they came to hear about the specific dental service.
- A full dental history including their attitude to dental services and what treatment they have had in the past.
- An important element would be to identify the patient's ideas, expectations, and concerns.
- The benefit of doing this prior to a physical consultation is that it would be easier to establish rapport with the patient at the outset and to gauge a patient's expectations so that they can be respectfully managed. There would not be many circumstances where it would be in the patient's best interests to provide elective remote management without a physical consultation.

3 Academy of Medical Royal Colleges, Faculty of Pain Medicine, General Medical Council, et al. (2019). High level principles for good practice in remote consultations and prescribing. ℘ https://www.nmc.org.uk/globalassets/sitedocuments/other-publications/high-level-principles-for-remote-prescribing-.pdf

Webinars and conferences

- These are becoming increasingly common as they enable a wider audience to participate without the need for lengthy journeys to attend. They can often be fitted around existing work commitments and recordings can be available to view later in many cases.
- There are limits in terms of networking, and where there are sponsors, it would not be possible to try products or equipment on the day.

Examinations

- Viva examinations and Objective Structured Clinical Examinations (OSCEs) can be conducted online and have now been used by several providers including the Royal Colleges with great success.
- There may be remedial requirements in place if there are any disconnection issues for either party to ensure the integrity of the examination.
- There will be a requirement on candidate visibility. Recordings may be scrutinized and checked at a later stage.

Commissioning

- It is beyond the remit of this handbook to fully discuss commissioning and its arrangements; however, the flow of finance can be an important point and may come up during training. Due to complexities, only the arrangements for England will be mentioned.
- The overall leadership (England) lies with the Secretary of State for Health and Social Care who is above the Department of Health, which distributes finances to the NHS Commissioning Board, Public Health England, and Health Watch (there are separate arrangements across the other UK nations):
  - Health Watch: looks at things from the patient perspective.
  - UK Health Security Agency: responsible for protecting the population from chemical, biological, nuclear and radiological incidents and other health threats.
  - NHS Commissioning Board/NHS England: distributes finances to regional offices, which then distribute to the Integrated Care Systems and the other part of the funding they retain to commission other services.
- Clinical Commissioning Groups are responsible for funding routine elective services including community health and ambulance contracts. This would include things like gall bladder removal. CCGs are being phased out.
- Local area teams are involved with commissioning more specialized services and highly specialized services. These include specialist cancer, radiotherapy, specialist dentistry, neurology, and cardiac surgery.
- Local area teams also commission primary care dental services and primary medical services, even though they are not specialist services.
- It is important to note that it is the local area team that manages virtually all dental services rather than the Clinical Commissioning Groups.
- Integrated Care Boards may take over commissioning from the Clinical Commissioning Groups and control NHS resources for their local population. Local area teams and Clinical Commissioning Groups are being phased out.
- Integrated Care Partnerships may design integrated care plans to provide guidance for local decision-making and would incorporate local governments, NHS bodies, and other various agencies.

Key skills portfolio

- The key skills portfolio is a collection of evidence and reflective summaries to demonstrate that the DF trainee understands how to provide quality care in a safe environment.
- While it is not compulsory to complete in all schemes it is worth bearing in mind the content of the key skills portfolio as it goes well with good clinical governance.
- It is not meant to be a set of extensive essays on clinical governance and regulations, rather how the workplace meets that framework and the evidence to prove it.
- The fundamental areas that are addressed are:
  - medical emergencies
  - infection control
  - radiation and ionization protection
  - health and safety
  - record keeping
  - teamwork
  - law and ethics
  - prevention and dental public health.
- It is recommended that medical emergencies, infection control, and radiation and ionization protection are completed, and a further two other areas are also covered.
- Evidence can include anonymized patient records, photos, completed and valid documents or completed forms, certificates, and logbooks.
- Links should be made between each of the areas where appropriate; for example, consignment notes for waste disposal would feature in both infection control and health and safety therefore the evidence can be linked to both of these key skills.
- Examples of the various issues within each key skill are listed and ought to be discussed in the portfolio with relevant evidence.
- You can use this as an opportunity to learn about the standards and goals of your future desired career. For example, if you want to work in general dental services than record keeping, health and safety, and teamwork may be best. If you want a career in public health, than prevention and dental public health with teamwork or law and ethics may be better areas to focus on.
- The purpose of the key skills portfolio may seem like an additional unnecessary burden particularly at the start of your professional career; however, this is the ideal opportunity to gain real insight into what is needed to run a professional dental service beyond the role of the clinician and can be very helpful when going out and working as an associate or even when becoming a principal as you would have a comprehensive record of the policies, procedures, and documents required for effective management of the practice.
- Each of the key skills will be discussed and examples provided of what is needed. This is not an exhaustive list but will certainly help as a starting point and should be geared to your workplace.

This section is summarized from Faculty of Dental Surgery (FDS) and Faculty of General Dental Practice (UK) (FGDP(UK)) (2010). *MJDF Portfolio Guide*. London: FDS and FGDP(UK). Please note that FDS and FGDP(UK) no longer use this guide and that the advice it contains may be out of date. For up-to-date guidance, please visit the College of General Dentistry website at ✏ www.fgdp.org.uk or https://cgdent.uk/

Medical emergencies

Describe and explain details regarding management of medical emergencies with respect to:
- Education, CPD, and training
- How medical histories are taken and recorded
- How medical emergencies occur
- How you recognize the common signs and symptoms of medical emergencies
- How you treat medical emergencies
- Managing a collapsed patient
- What drugs and equipment used to manage medical emergencies
- How the drugs and equipment are maintained
- How to use the defibrillator
- How to administer emergency drugs.

Evidence includes:
- CPD certificates for medical emergencies and basic life support
- Audits of medical histories
- Practice protocols on medical emergencies
- Algorithms used and where they are located
- Photos of the location and contents of resuscitation equipment and drugs
- Signed checklist of the contents and expiry dates of any drugs and equipment
- Picture and position of the defibrillator.

Reflect on
- What has been learnt on medical emergency training courses and what deficiencies were identified and how have they been remedied?
- How medical histories are risk assessed (e.g. using the American Society of Anesthesiologists (ASA) scale).
- A recent management of a patient who was showing signs or symptoms of a medical emergency. What went well, what could be improved?
- What is the staff knowledge on the administration of emergency drugs?
- Should a medical emergency occur, how would the management of it occur? What was the outcome of a timed exercise?

Infection control

The following infection control issues in your workplace need to be explained:
- Management in the work environment.
- Staff training including any induction training.
- Personal protective equipment.
- How handwashing is carried out.

- How the surgery design facilitates infection control.
- How universal precautions are undertaken.
- Aerosol problems.
- Contamination of water lines.
- Instrument decontamination including reprocessing.
- Pre-sterilization disinfection and inspection.
- Storage and dating instruments.
- Decontamination of work surfaces.
- Cleaning of the waiting room and other facilities.
- Single-use items.
- Management of clinical waste.
- Current infection control guidelines.
- Immunization of staff.
- Inoculation injuries management.
- Decontamination of laboratory work.
- Relationship between infection control and health and safety.
- Management of aerosol-generating procedures.

Examples of evidence:
- Protocol for infection control/infection control policy.
- Waste disposal policy.
- Waste transfer notes.
- Waste consignment note.
- Virology reports confirming immunity.
- Sharp safety policy.
- Hand washing protocol.
- Laboratory prescription.
- Photographs of surgery layout.
- Protocols for decontamination.
- Staff training/induction/CPD certificates in infection control.
- Fit testing of respiratory protective equipment.
- Anonymized incident forms.
- Audits.

Reflection
- How well current procedures are maintained in cross-infection control.
- How these procedures could be improved.

Radiation and ionization protection
The following issues relating to radiography and radiation protection in your workplace need to be explained:
- What type of equipment you have in the practice that emits ionizing radiation and the details of such equipment.
- What are the local rules including the details of the legal person, radiation protection supervisor, and medical physicist; and equipment details including make, model, and location?
- How is the equipment maintained?
- Understanding and awareness of the Ionising Radiation Regulations and IRMER.
- What training have staff completed?
- Describe the controlled zone.

- Need for dosimetry badges?
- Selection criteria for taking radiographs.
- How the dosages are limited.
- How radiographs are interpreted.
- Health and safety concerns for radiographs.
- Quality system for radiography.
- How a selection of your radiographs conforms to current legislation.

Examples of evidence:
- Inventory.
- Local rules.
- Examples of a range of radiographs with interpretation and findings.
- Staff training or CPD certificates in radiography.
- Quality assurance protocol used.
- Service documents for any radiographic equipment used.
- Equipment service report.
- Staff training log.
- Diagram of the controlled zone.

Reflection
- Comment on the training that staff have completed and how staff are adequately protected.
- Comment on the criteria used for radiography in the workplace.
- Comment on the quality assurance programme in the workplace.

Health and safety

The following issues concerning health and safety should be discussed:
- Define a risk and a hazard.
- How would you undergo a risk assessment?
- Where are the risk assessments documented and kept?
- Training that staff undergo for health and safety and any induction training.
- Describe the health and safety policy of the practice.
- Where is the health and safety poster displayed?
- Is there any employer liability insurance—if so, what are the details and where is the certificate displayed?
- How does the workplace conform to the each of the regulations as listed by the HSE?
- How is the equipment checked for safety?
- What kind of personal protective equipment is used?
- For any autoclaves—how is the equipment checked?
- What protection is there from radiation?
- How is waste disposed of?
- How are exposures to hazardous substances prevented or controlled?
- What kind of assessments are undertaken for hazardous substances?

Examples of evidence:
- Copies of risk assessments.
- Induction checklists.
- Health and safety policy.
- Health and safety poster.
- Employer liability insurance certificate.
- Evacuation procedure.

- Fire extinguisher types and locations.
- Fire safety certificate.
- Fire risk assessment.
- Fire equipment service report.
- Emergency first aid at work certificate.
- Incident form.
- Pressure vessel inspection certificate.
- Complaints policy.

Reflection
- What could be improved in the accessibility or number of risk assessments to make them more useful?
- Are there any areas that could be improved to conform to health and safety?
- How do clinical governance issues relate to health and safety?
- What are your complaints procedures like?

Record keeping

Commentary on the following should be carried out:
- Could the notes be clearly understood by another dentist?
- If the notes are handwritten, are they in indelible ink, dated (and timed if appropriate), signed, and is the name of the clinician clear?
- Are all details including history, clinical information, treatment details, discussions, and outcomes clear?
- Should you need to defend your actions, could you do so based on the documentation in the clinical notes?
- What process do you use to obtain valid consent?
- What methods are there to ensure security of the clinical records?
- How does the management of the data conform to legal requirements?
- Are the referral letters succinct but provide sufficient information to allow the referred practitioner to easily prioritize and understand the purpose of the referral?

Evidence
- Anonymized copies of patient notes showing examples of a range of procedures including history, examination, investigations and reporting, diagnosis, treatment planning, methods of obtaining consent, and provision of routine dental procedures.
- Anonymized referral letters.
- Anonymized consent forms.
- Anonymized medical history forms.
- Audits for clinical records.

Reflection
- How your record keeping conforms to GDC standards.
- Are there areas that you feel you could improve on?
- If you use templates for computerized systems, are there features you could change?

Team working

Commentary on the following:
- Who are the various members of your practice team, both clinical and non-clinical?

- What skills do each of the clinical team have?
- Are there additional non-clinical skills that either the clinical or non-clinical team members have that may contribute to good clinical governance such as emergency first aid at work, complaints manger, and so on?
- How do you decide what CPD you need to carry out (e.g. PDP)?
- How do you log any learning that you and other team members complete?
- Does all the educational activity align to one of the principles of the GDC standards for dental professionals?
- What duties are delegated to non-clinical staff members such as receptionists?
- Do any dental care professionals carry out duties under direct access and if so, how do they refer patients on if they believe the treatment is beyond their scope?
- How do dentists delegate tasks to dental care professions?
- Is there any diversity and equality training?

Evidence
- CPD logs.
- Prescriptions to dental care professionals.
- Policy on the required information on referrals to dental care professionals.
- Workplace staff lists and roles with descriptions of responsibility.
- Staff training policy including mandatory training if applicable.
- Policies on equal opportunities.
- Any references to meetings where team training was discussed.

Reflection
- How do you think the system of PDPs could be improved?
- Comment on how core or common training in areas such as medical emergencies happens. What common areas do you think are better to train as a practice and which areas are better trained as individuals?
- Comment on the quality of communication between team members— are the prescriptions and referral letters clear and contain sufficient detail?

Law and ethics

Comment on the following:
- What steps are taken to protect patient confidentiality?
- What is the process of obtaining valid consent?
- How is the consent process documented?
- How does obtaining consent compare to what is expected from the GDC standard for dental professionals?
- What are the local safeguarding policies for children and vulnerable adults?
- What is your safeguarding training?
- How do you handle complaints?
- What are the conditions required for a claim of negligence to be proved?

Evidence
- Show notes and consent forms to prove how the consent process occurs.
- Certificates for courses attended on patient confidentiality, consent, and safeguarding.
- Practice patient confidentiality policy.
- Practice complaints policy.
- Complaints logbook entries.
- Patient information leaflets.
- How patient expectations are met and documented to prevent medico-legal issues from arising.

Reflection
- How well do you think the policies work?
- How do you manage situations that need to be escalated, for example, children believed to be subject to domestic violence or abuse, or patients who are seeking compensation or making unreasonable demands?
- Where communication difficulties have arisen, what has been done well and what could have worked better in hindsight? What would you do different next time?

Prevention and dental public health

Comment on the following:
- What methods do you use to detect behaviour that is likely to cause deterioration of oral health in terms of caries, periodontal disease, tooth wear, and soft tissue changes (e.g. how do you identify the patient's oral hygiene routine and smoking status)?
- What do you understand by primary, secondary, and tertiary prevention?
- What kind of advice do you provide to patients to prevent deterioration of oral health and how is this advice delivered (e.g. oral hygiene instruction, dietary advice, and smoking cessation)?
- What kinds of preventative interventions do you undertake and how do you decide when and whom to provide this to (e.g. fissure sealants, fluoride varnish, and high-fluoride toothpaste)?
- What is your understanding of interim care management appointments?
- How do you carry out an oral health assessment and review?
- What dental health indices are you aware of and can you use this as part of a dental public health programme such as DMFT or basic periodontal examination (BPE)?
- How do you identify high-risk individuals?
- How do you decide on your recall interval?
- What oral health educational activities are you aware of at a practice, community, or national level?
- What common links are you aware of between oral and non-oral conditions?

Evidence
- Patient notes on how you detect and record behaviours likely to deteriorate or cause oral health disease in terms of caries, periodontal disease, tooth wear and soft tissue changes.

- Patient notes on how you have provided preventative advice to manage any behaviours likely to cause deterioration of oral health.
- Patient notes on any preventative interventions taken and why they were appropriate for that patient.
- Patient notes showing evidence of taking BPE scores or decayed, missing, and filled teeth (DMFT) scores and the implications of the score for that patient.
- Evidence of carrying out an oral health assessment.
- Show how you have placed a patient into a risk category and what treatment options are available to them.
- Show how preventative measures have resulted in an improvement at oral health review.
- Referrals for oral cancer under the urgent 2-week arrangement.
- Any activities carried out with relation to 'Oral Health' month and 'Mouth Cancer Awareness' week.

Reflection

- What preventative measures work well? What ones need improvement? How would you change this (e.g. use of mouth models or computer animations for oral hygiene instructions, use of oral health educators)?
- How have national programmes helped—are there additional activities you could use?

The Dental Foundation educational supervisor

Introduction to the educational supervisor

In DFT, the educational supervisor (formally known as the trainer) will be one of the dentists within the practice who has been appointed to be the trainer. They will be the mentor of the trainee for the period of the training year and will usually have a number of years' experience as a general dental practitioner (GDP).

Prioritization, escalation, and responsibility

- The educational supervisor should be the first person to approach if there are difficulties or if advice is required.
- It is important to know that working as a DF trainee is not like dental school and the educational supervisor does not take over the role of the undergraduate supervisor (or clinical tutor or demonstrator). As a DF trainee you are a fully registered dentist and therefore are professionally accountable for your actions. Therefore, there is no expectation that the educational supervisor needs to check each and every case or stage and so the onus is on the DF trainee to seek advice when appropriate.
- The educational supervisor is there to assist and advise as necessary. At the start of the year, they are likely to need to assist and advise more than at the end of the year and will plan their time accordingly. They will be working at the same time as you, treating their patients, so it is important to establish early how they wish to supervise you.
- It is therefore important to identify which patients need to be seen immediately, which patients need only advice, and which patients can be sent home and discussed at the end of the session or rebooked.
- In all cases, patient safety and care must be the priority.

Responsibilities of the educational supervisor

- Take the DF trainee as an employee and provide the same employment rights as any other employee in a similar position.[1] DF trainees are not associates and are not self-employed.
- Identify the DF trainee's strengths and weakness and monitor progress.
- Provide the DF trainee with guidance on clinical and administrative matters.
- Allow the DF trainee to attend any set study days and not permit leave or other activities that could distract from this.
- Conduct tutorials in work time.

1 ✆ www.copdend.org

Regional variation

While the aims and objectives of DFT are consistent with the delivery of the curriculum, there can be considerable variation in the delivery of the programme.

- Depending on the geographic location of the practices, there may be a relatively long distance to the study venues. For that reason, the study days may be clustered into a 1-week block of teaching every couple of months, or these may be delivered as virtual sessions.
- Individual speakers will vary. There may be certain speakers who will rotate around several schemes and many schemes will be invited to certain national events; however, in most cases there will be different speakers.
- While the core topics will remain the same and the remaining topics covered will aim to fulfil the requirements of the DF curriculum, the topics chosen to explore further can vary considerably.
- Every practice must be able to provide appropriate patients to ensure that a wide range of general dentistry can be experienced by the trainee; however, depending on the geographic location, socioeconomic status among the local population, age, and general dental health needs will affect the type of experience gained.
- Those on longitudinal programmes have their training spread over 2 years and will have the benefit of experience in hospitals or community settings and general practice. This is usually provided with trainees rotating to their placements on a weekly basis or this may be provided in blocks or placements in different settings.
- The individual expertise and special interests of the educational supervisor may give individuals exposure to different techniques or skills.
- Certain practices may have access to dental hygienists, therapists, and technicians, so some work may be delegated to them, developing the dental team; however, this can vary, and you may be expected to provide all of the treatment yourself as part of building your experience.

Overseas qualified dentists

For those who qualified outside of the European Economic Area, the primary dental qualification may not be eligible for registration with the GDC in the UK. For those individuals there are several routes which could be considered for entry onto the GDC register.

Exempt person

This route is for those wishing to pursue an enforceable community right to access the profession under the Dentists Act 1984 as amended. There are relevant directives which govern the rules surrounding this and legal advice should be sought if going down this route.

Temporary registration

- This is registration granted for specific purposes in a hospital or dental school.[1] Generally, it is not accepted for private or general practice.
- To be eligible, the primary dental degree has to be eligible by the UK national agency for international qualifications and skills (ENIC).[2]
- Once confirmation is gained from ENIC, a post has to be identified.
- Posts (otherwise known for the purpose of temporary registration as direction) generally have to be under the supervision of a dental consultant.
- Posts or direction that are generally considered suitable are:
  - DCT posts
  - specialty trainee posts
  - teaching posts—considered on individual circumstances
  - research posts—considered on individual circumstances.
- The details of the specific direction need to be passed on to the GDC for consideration to grant temporary registration for this purpose.
- Once granted, an individual may not go on to practise outside of the direction, for example, in general practice.
- Time carrying out clinical work in terms of treating patients may contribute towards the 1600 hours required for application of the Licence in Dental Surgery or Overseas Registration Examination; however, simply completing several years under temporary registration does not allow for full registration.

Overseas Registration Examination

You should consult the GDC website for specific up-to-date information regarding the current regulations and requirements[3]:
- Minimum of 1600 hours providing personal dental treatment to patients inclusive of treatment provided during undergraduate studies.
- International English Language Testing System (IELTS) result of no less than 7.0 overall and no less than 6.5 in any section.
- Certificate of current professional status to confirm that the candidate is of good standing.
- Certified copy of primary dental degree.

1 www.gdc-uk.org/registration/join-the-register/temporary-registration

2 www.enic.org.uk

3 https://www.gdc-uk.org/registration/overseas-registration-exam

- The exam itself consists of two parts—parts 1 and 2.
  - Part 1: the format of the exam is in single best answer and extended matched questions. There are two papers: 1 and 2. Paper 1 focuses on applied dental sciences and human disease. Paper 2 focuses on clinical dentistry, ethics, and health and safety.
  - Part 2: this is the practical element of the examination. There are several sections to this:
    o An operative test on a manikin: these test the ability to perform specific procedures, typically restorative preparations on plastic teeth.
    o A diagnostic and treatment planning exercise: this is with a patient actor from whom you can take a history, but not examine; several other artefacts such as clinical photos, study models, and radiographs; and other special investigations such as vitality tests may need to be requested as they become available. From this you would be expected to make a diagnosis and treatment plan and explain this.
    o Medical emergency test: this would involve an oral viva of different medical emergencies and demonstration of basic life support on a manikin.
  - OSCE: this consists of multiple stations each consisting of a well-defined task over a set period. This can test a range of skills, not just technical ones including communication skills, history taking, giving explanations, denture design, suturing, radiographic interpretation, and so on. It can cover any aspect of the curriculum. This will last for 2 hours and 30 minutes.

Licence in Dental Surgery of the Royal College of Surgeons of England (RCS England)

- This is another qualification offered by RCS England,[4] which can allow registration by the GDC.
- The exact regulations should be checked with the RCS England website, but the general requirements stand as:
  - minimum of 1600 hours providing personal dental treatment to patients inclusive of undergraduate studies
  - health declaration
  - IELTS result of no less than 7.0 and no less than 6.5 in any section.
  - certificate of current professional status to confirm that the candidate is of good standing.
- Part 1 is a written exam consisting of single best answer and extended matched answer questions.
- Part 2—there are several parts to this:
  - An OSCE of 20 stations of which 16 are examined and four are rest. It is 2 hours in duration with five minutes per station and an additional minute for reading a large range of tasks can be allocated including practical, communication, and professional skills demonstration.

- A dental manikin test is a 3-hour test which would typically involve the preparation of the restoration of teeth; however, it may also include any of the preoperative and postoperative tasks including documentation, infection control procedures, and communication with laboratories.
- There is an unseen case examination consisting of four cases in which a history is taken from a patient actor for which 10 minutes is allowed. Several artefacts will be provided such as clinical photos, study models, and radiographs. A further 10 minutes is provided to prepare; following this, a further 10 minutes will be given to the discussion with the patient for a procedure or management and discussion. Notes will also be made and if there are causes for concern, this can lead to a fail mark, even if the minimum pass mark has been met or exceeded. Comments of concern can relate to a behaviour or attitude which may be considered incompatible with being a dental professional and so may lead to failure.

Right to work in the UK

Being eligible for temporary registration or being successful at the Overseas Registration Examination or Licence in Dental Surgery does not allow the right to work in the UK. This is the role of Home Office and Immigration departments, and has to be applied for separately.

Performer's List Validation by Experience

Performers List Validation by Experience

There are those who may have graduated outside the European Economic Area who may be eligible to practise dentistry in the UK, although they may not have completed the formal DFT. In order to be eligible for a full performer number, an individual may be required to undergo Performer List Validation by Experience, which involves producing evidence and reflective commentary where appropriate. The following would usually be expected[1]:

- Summary documents:
  - Curriculum vitae (CV).
  - PDP.
  - Record of CPD.
  - Employment contract.
  - Two clinical references from NHS dentist colleagues.
  - Recorded attendance at staff training and practice meetings.
  - Experience of NHS dentistry and a log of procedures showing a wide range of treatment for NHS patients.
- Courses to attend:
  - GDC requirements.
  - NHS induction.
  - NHS complaints management.
  - NHS regulations.
  - CPR training.
  - Clinical elements of the PDP.
  - IRMER training.
  - Health and safety and COSHH course.
  - Prescribing drugs and drug interactions.
  - Record keeping.
  - Child safeguarding level 2.
- Copies of policies and procedures relating to your workplace:
  - NHS complaints policy.
  - Drug prescribing protocol.
  - Infection control policy.
  - Health and safety policy.
  - COSHH policy.
  - Emergency drug policy.
  - Child safeguarding policy.
- Anonymized patient notes/anonymized correspondence:
  - Patient complaint and response.
  - Referral letters.
  - Notes showing appropriate prescribing.
- Work-based assessments and feedback:
  - Patient satisfaction survey.
  - Multisource feedback.
  - Appraisal.
  - Case-based discussions.

---

1 UK Committee of Postgraduate Dental Deans and Directors (COPDEND) (2020). Performers List Validation by Experience (Version 5). ℘ https://www.copdend.org/eea-overseas-dentists/plve-documents/

- Dental evaluation of procedures.
- Audit of clinical records.
- Other clinical audits or evidence of peer review.
- Reflective commentary on the following:
  - Recent training completed.
  - Any CPD completed in the training year.
  - Understanding of GDC requirements.
  - Understanding of the NHS complaints management.
  - Understanding of good record keeping.
  - Understanding of the drugs and drug interactions.
  - Understanding of HTM 01-05.[2]
  - Understanding of health and safety in relation to general dental practice.
  - Understanding of COSHH in relation to general dental practice.
  - Understanding of employment and contract law.
  - Understanding medical emergencies.
  - Understanding of child safeguarding.
  - Clinical experience.

This is by no means a definitive list. Depending on where the assessment is carried out, some or all of the courses may be locally delivered and there may be very specific courses that must be attended.

Similarly, there may be flexibility in this, and the cost may have to be met by the candidate.

The number and types of work-based assessments would also vary and there may be additional requirements on top of these or certain activities may require external quality control or verification.

Career opportunities in general dental practice

- There are many career opportunities in general dental practice, far greater than ever before and this is only set to increase, with a greater emphasis on the desire for care to be provided in the community and primary care services.
- The traditional model of general dental care being delivered in practice and specialist care in hospitals, particularly under the NHS, is showing a steady change with greater commissioning of specialist services within primary care.
- One of the aims of NHS commissioning is the delivery of care based on complexity, identifying practitioners with the appropriate skills for the required services. Within England, NHS England[1] has published commissioning guides, detailing the level of care appropriate for each service commissioned. These have been divided into three levels:
  - Level 1 services are allocated as routine, preventative, and urgent care.
  - Level 2 consists of moderate difficulty treatment.
  - Level 3 is aligned to those cases with more of a specialist nature.
- Levels 1 and 2 should be managed in general practice by general dentists or dentists with enhanced skills. Level 3a cases should be provided by specialists and level 3b cases that require either multidisciplinary care, consultant-led treatment, or general anaesthesia services would be managed in hospital.
- This creates a vast opportunity for general practitioners who may wish to increase their skills and diversify their base by providing additional services.

College of General Dentistry

- This was formerly a faculty of RCS England but became an independent college in 2021.[2] The purpose this college is to cater for primary dental care practitioners and support members of the primary dental care team including dental care professionals in terms of training and promoting high standards in primary dental services.
- To be eligible for membership, a dentist must complete any postgraduate diploma or higher qualification related to dentistry. Traditionally this would have been one of the membership exams of one of the Royal Colleges.

Training
- The provision of courses includes postgraduate diplomas, certificates, and short courses.
- Such courses include restorative dentistry, implant dentistry, and leadership and management as well as other practice management topics.

---

1 www.england.nhs.uk
2 www.cgdent.uk

Publications and guidelines
- There is access to certain publications.
- There are several guidelines produced in areas such as radiography, record keeping, and antibiotic prescribing.

Fellowship
- Fellowship can be gained by either equivalence or through experience.
- Fellowship by equivalence can be gained by demonstrating an existing fellowship with a recognised organisation.
- Fellowship by experience involves providing evidence or reflective accounts of professional development in a minimum of three of the following domains: clinical, leadership, teaching, research, law and ethics.
- For the latest requirements see the college website.

Dentists with enhanced skills

- Formally known as dentist with special interest, although this term is still frequently used.
- This is an appointment or job role rather than a transferable title. This is different from a specialist who is on the specialist register.
- The need for such practitioners will vary from place to place and the individual skills needed will also vary.
- The role of a dentist with enhanced skills in one location may be very different to the role of a dentist with enhanced skills in another location depending on the local commissioning requirements.
- For example, a dentist with enhanced skills in minor oral surgery may have the skills and experience for extraction of wisdom teeth, but not for the exposure of canine teeth. A contract may be granted for only removing wisdom teeth in this case.
- The requirements will also be set locally. Previously having the appointment in one area does not make an individual eligible in another.
- Criteria used would typically involve relevant experience, postgraduate qualifications, and references. There may be a requirement for certain CPD activity membership of specific societies or other activity including clinical audit.
- Typical areas for dentists with enhanced skills to work in include:
  - periodontics
  - endodontics
  - minor oral surgery
  - special care dentistry
  - paediatric dentistry
  - orthodontics
  - conscious sedation
  - prison dentistry.
- They are not restricted to the definitions of specialties of the GDC, but more to the service need requirements.
- To be eligible, a job first needs to be found and then approval locally that the skills and knowledge required can be verified to carry out the job.

- The commissioning of these would be different to normal contract terms as treatment would need to be through a referral and specific acceptance criteria may have to be met to provide treatment.

Salaried dental services

- These are generally in the community dental services where dentists are employed either as a dental officer, senior dental officer, or clinical director (➔ Application for NHS appointments).
- The community services are generally focused on the delivery of special care dentistry and paediatric dentistry, although there are a number of community dental services that provide oral surgery and general dental services.
- General dental services may be provided in access centres where the provision of general dental services may be low.
- In these situations, the dentist would provide normal general dental services and patients would see the dentist as their primary dental care provider and be expected to pay normal patient charges if they are not exempt.
- The dentist would be salaried for their services and employed with normal employment rights and paid according to a national scale.
- There may be opportunities to progress to a senior dental officer or clinical director; however, this will often be based on service need and when a vacancy arises and may require additional skills or qualifications.

Opportunities to work abroad

- Healthcare professionals, such as dentists, are often in great demand to work anywhere in the world. Opportunities are dependent on the individual nation's dental programme and the number of dentists trained for their population. Certain countries find rural locations more difficult to recruit in and therefore greater opportunities may be available in these locations around the world.
- However, unlike many other jobs, dentists are generally one of the more heavily regulated professions and each nation will have its own rules on the regulation of dentists.
- Applications to register may take a considerable amount of time as proof will be required of your current training and primary dental qualification, as well as a certificate of professional status or good standing from an existing dental regulator.
- Other documents that may be required include references and statements from recognized institutions to ensure that the individual has the appropriate work experience related to that of a registered dentist.
- Every country will have its own set of rules and what they will accept. Some countries will accept a primary dental degree issued in the UK, while others will require further examinations or may not accept the qualification at all. This is all subject to change and usually decided by the dental regulator of each country.
- Even if you are eligible to register with another dental regulator in a different country to practise dentistry, it does not often give you the right to work there.

- The right to work is often completely different and decided by immigration, customs, or the border control authority. A specific visa allowing work may be required and these are decided by each individual country. Countries often have very different criteria for issuing such visas and they can even discriminate on protected characteristics such as age.

Dental officer for the armed forces

- There are a number of opportunities available for those wishing to work as dental officers for the Army, Royal Air Force, and Navy.
- It is possible to sign up prior to graduation and eligible candidates may be entitled to financial support through their studies.
- By signing up during studies, the student will be subject to military law, although during undergraduate studies there may be only a minimal requirement for them to participate in any particular activity or service need. However, upon graduation there will be a minimum time period required to serve wherever the individual is commissioned—this could be at any given base around the world.

Role of a dental officer

- The predominant role will be as a clinician.
- There is officer training involved and so there is some degree of leading and managing a team. The role of the officer is different from that of a soldier.
- It is possible to move up the ranks, although the officer training given as a dental officer will be different to that of other officers as the main role will be a clinical one.

Selection

- It is worth checking the individual website for advice on what is involved in the current recruitment process.
- It is important to start preparing early as there are fitness levels that need to be reached and there are a limited number of panels throughout the year. At least 12 months should be allowed for the application process.
- A candidate submits an application with completion of a medical questionnaire. It is worth noting that some conditions would render an application unsuccessful even if the medical condition would otherwise be acceptable to a civilian role.
- An up-to-date CV would need to be submitted.
- Interview with a career's advisor.
- Full medical examination and relevant investigations.
- Briefing with the selection board.
- Attend Main Board with Officer Selection.
- Dental Selection Board.
- Professionally qualified officers training.

Development

- There are often a large number of benefits and unique training opportunities available as a dental officer.
- There is an equivalent of the DFT, which is transferrable outside of the armed forces for the purposes of a performer number.[1]

1 ℘ www.army.mod.uk

Chapter 2

Dental Core Training

Purpose of Dental Core Training

- DCT[1] is a period of postgraduate training that enables the new DF trainee or GDP to develop their skills further in a variety of hospital or community settings. The training at this level varies from 1 to 3 years with multiple endpoints but can lead to applying for specialty training.
- DCT is not a statutory requirement but exists to enable further training and career development.
- It provides experience of working in different settings to DFT, providing greater experience in a range of disciplines across multiple healthcare settings.
- It enables working in a supportive environment with continued supervision from multiple supervisors. A range of supervisors will be available to gain knowledge and experience from, enabling acquisition of new skills.
- It enables development of competence and working towards independence.
- Working in hospital or community settings enables management of more complex levels of care within multidisciplinary teams.
- It will enable continued experience of clinical governance.
- It aims to develop leadership skills.

Dental Core Training Year 1 (DCT1)

- This is aimed at development of the skilled generalist.

Dental Core Training Year 2 (DCT2)

- This is aimed at development of (or readiness for) specialist skills.

Dental Core Training Year 3 (DCT3)

- This is aimed at the enhancement of specialist skills which may enable further progression into specialty training.

- The supportive environment of a DCT post will enable the trainee to develop their career aspirations.
- Provides the opportunities to develop their portfolio with study days aimed at their level, and presentations at local/regional/national meetings.
- There are now more posts available across several specialties and a greater number of run-through posts, combining DCT1 and DCT2 in more of a general professional training programme.
- There are also posts available combining DFT and DCT known as JDFCT posts. These tend to rotate trainees between primary care dental practice and a hospital-based discipline.
- DCT posts are available in a range of dental specialties with some posts providing experience in several specialties such as:
  - oral and maxillofacial surgery
  - oral surgery
  - orthodontics
  - paediatric dentistry

1 COPDEND. ⅋ www.copdend.org

- special care dentistry
- restorative dentistry
- oral medicine
- oral and maxillofacial pathology
- oral and maxillofacial radiology.

Application and recruitment

Although recruitment processes are subject to change, the most recent process (2022) is described in this text to give readers a basis on which the recruitment process has been completed. For up-to-date information on recruitment, see the COPDEND website (www.copdend.org.uk).

Essential criteria for applying for DCT1

- Bachelor of Dental Surgery (BDS) degree or equivalent.
- Eligible to work in the UK.
- Evidence of at least 12 months of postgraduate clinical experience at the time of starting the post.
- Fit to practise.

Essential criteria for applying for DCT2

- BDS or equivalent.
- Eligible to work in the UK.
- Evidence of completion of UK DCT1 post or equivalent at the time of starting the post.
- Evidence of at least 24 months of postgraduate clinical experience at the time of starting the post.
- Fit to practise.

Essential criteria for applying for DCT3

- BDS or equivalent.
- Eligible to work in the UK.
- Evidence of completion of UK DCT2 post or equivalent at the time of starting the post.
- Evidence of at least 36 months of postgraduate clinical experience at the time of starting the post.
- Fit to practise.

Application process

This is a national recruitment process for all posts within the UK (Health Education England (HEE), NHS Education for Scotland (NES), Northern Ireland Medical and Dental Training Agency (NIMDTA), and Health Education and Improvement Wales (HEIW)). The process follows several stages:

- Online application form to determine eligibility for the role applied for (longlisting).
- SJT:
  - Computer-based assessment.
  - 60 questions.
  - Accounts for 33% of overall score.
  - Questions based around coping with pressure; critical thinking, appraisal, and decision-making; patient-centred care; and professionalism.
- Preferences of posts.

- Interview:
  - Applicants will be presented with a number of scenarios prior to the interview.
  - Based on two of the scenarios (one clinical and one clinical governance, quality improvement, and professional skills).
  - Forms 67% of the overall score (33.5% per scenario).
- Ranking of applicants and offers of posts.

Dental Core Training curriculum

- The curriculum for DCT defines the outcomes of training[1]
- DCT is reliant on the trainee driving their own training against the objectives of the curriculum. Trainees need to be proactive to ensure successful training progression. Although trainees will be supported by a number of clinical and educational supervisors and training programme directors (TPDs), the ultimate responsibility for satisfactory completion rests with the individual trainee.
- Trainees should refer to the curriculum as a guide to the mandatory outcomes that are expected and the competences that are required for satisfactory completion.
- It is a requirement that the DCT year is completed satisfactorily to enable progression to the next stage of training. Failing to satisfactorily complete will result in the next post being unavailable to you.

Study days

- As part of training, each DCT will have a range of mandatory study days provided to deliver the curriculum. These mandatory study days will cover a wide range of DCT competencies.
- You will also have local training in your unit which will deliver more specialty-specific training useful for your current post.
- As part of your contract, you have 30 days of study leave per year (full-time equivalent). The majority of this study time will be used up by mandatory study days and local teaching. Any additional study will need to be approved by your educational supervisor and TPD, based on the curriculum delivery matrix, which gives detailed information on courses that will be considered for leave and funding. There has to be a clear purpose for any course of study, applicable to your career development, particularly within your current DCT role. This must be contained within your PDP, following a clear discussion with your educational supervisor as to the reasons why you wish to pursue this training and how it will benefit your current role and career aspirations.
- It may be worth considering self-funding any additional training which is not contained within your curriculum delivery matrix, yet you feel would be beneficial to any future role.

Starting your Dental Core Training post

- The change from working in a dental practice as a DFT to working in larger hospital teams or community settings for your DCT role can be quite a dramatic difference. The DCT supervisors are aware of this significant difference and are there to assist the transition to your new role.
- It is often possible to gain shadowing opportunities of the current DCTs prior to you starting your role so that you have a greater insight into the new role, and this is important particularly in the transition to an oral and maxillofacial surgery (OMFS) DCT post with on-call commitments which will not have been experienced as part of DFT.
- At the start of each DCT post, there will be a period of induction to:
  - introduce you to the department and to meet your fellow DCTs
  - any mandatory Trust level induction and human resources processes
  - provide essential computer training and introduce the computer systems in place
  - introduce the TPD and educational supervisor and an overview of the DCT role and responsibilities
  - provide a clinical induction.
- Trainees are supported by a number of clinical and educational supervisors to enable trainee-led learning. They will introduce you to the requirements of the role and the workplace-based learning opportunities.

Assigned educational supervisor meetings

As a minimum, there should be three meetings with your assigned educational supervisor, although any number of meetings are possible:
- Initial: 3 months into post enabling assessment of the PDP and progress achieved.
- 6 months: prior to Interim Review of Competence Progression (IRCP).
- 10 months: prior to Final Review of Competence Progression (FRCP).

Initial assigned educational supervisor meeting

It is advisable to meet with your assigned educational supervisor within the first 2 weeks of your post. This meeting should include:
- An introduction
- The educational agreement
- PDP with Specific, Measurable, Attainable, Relevant, and Timely (SMART) objectives and to discuss career and training aspirations
- Introduction to the electronic portfolio (ePortfolio)
- Discussion of the competencies required (contained within the curriculum) and how these competencies are assessed.

Competence assessment

- Competence is assessed through a range of evidence provided within the ePortfolio.
- This is formally assessed by the TPD and associate dental deans at:
  - IRCP
  - FRCP.
- Clinical supervisors and assigned educational supervisors will complete reports for the above assessment periods. This report will be based on observations throughout the placement, including the assessments of the supervised learning events (SLEs) or workplace-based assessments (WBAs). It will also include assessments of clinical logbooks, participation in quality improvement processes, research, teaching, multisource feedback, and patient feedback.
- The evidence for competence progression needs to be uploaded into the ePortfolio. If it is not contained within the ePortfolio, there is no evidence that this happened, and competence progression cannot be assured.

Evidence required for Final Review of Competence Progression

- Educational portfolio.
- Structured educational supervisor report contained within the ePortfolio.
- Trainee assessment form.
- Clinical activity log.
- Audit activity.
- Evidence of completed SLEs.
- Teaching and research involvement.
- PDP.
- CPD log.
- Multisource feedback.
- Patient feedback.

Detailed information with be provided from your Deanery/TPD as to the requirements and the specific location of evidence within the portfolio to assist the panel in determining competence progression. It is important to follow this information as failure to upload the relevant information in the required areas will lead to failure to progress.

Further reading
℗ www.copdend.org.uk

Chapter 3

Paediatric dentistry

Introduction to paediatric dentistry

Paediatric dentistry refers to the provision of oral healthcare for infants, children, and young people up until the age of 16 years. It is not a technique-limited specialty and therefore a holistic approach to care is required.

Key aims

- Promote a lifelong positive approach to oral healthcare for the children and their families.
- Instigate evidence-based preventive care from an early stage.
- Maintain healthy primary and permanent dentitions.
- Where disease does occur, identify it early and provide the appropriate management.
- Make accurate diagnoses and formulate treatment plans that address all of the child's needs.
- Use techniques to deliver care in a way in which the child will find acceptable.
- Provide effective, evidence-based restorative techniques.
- Work as part of multidisciplinary teams to provide accessible, high-quality care.

History taking

- Use a structured approach which involves the child and the accompanying adult.
- The purpose is to gain information and to establish a rapport with the patient.
- Introduce yourself and establish who is accompanying the child. Children may attend without the person with parental responsibility which will have implications for the consent process (⊖ Consent).
- Referral source:
  - Determine who has referred the patient and establish the reason for the referral.
- Presenting complaint:
  - Firstly, where possible, establish what the child's concerns are and then ask the parent (e.g. toothache, swelling, appearance of the teeth, or dental trauma) as patient and parental concerns may differ.
  - Obtaining a clear pain history from younger children or those with special needs can be difficult. Questions such as 'Do your teeth hurt you when you eat or when you are trying to sleep?' can be of use. For those with communication difficulties, altered behaviour particularly at night or during mealtimes may indicate dental symptoms.
  - Ask whether analgesia has been needed and if so, what regimen has been followed and establish its effectiveness.
- History of presenting complaint:
  - Document when the concern arose.
  - In cases with a history of pain/swelling, ask how many episodes have been experienced and enquire about antibiotic usage.
  - Have the symptoms changed over time?
  - Are symptoms worsening or improving?
  - Aim to determine whether any pulpitis present is reversible or irreversible (Table 3.1).

Table 3.1 Symptoms suggestive of reversible and irreversible pulpitis

Reversible pulpitis	Irreversible pulpitis
Short-lasting pain that stops when stimulus is removed	Long-lasting (can be constant and throbbing) pain that requires analgesia
Precipitated by sweet, cold, or hot stimuli	Aggravated by hot stimuli and may be relieved by cold stimuli
Mainly occurs when eating	Symptoms often worse at night and can disturb sleep
	May follow symptoms of reversible pulpitis that were not appropriately managed

- In trauma cases, it is important to document when the trauma occurred and whether any other care has already been sought. For avulsion cases, the total extra-alveolar and extra-alveolar dry time needs to be documented, along with any storage media that may have been used. These factors will impact the prognosis of the traumatized tooth/teeth (⊙ Dental trauma).
- Medical history:
  - Use of a proforma is encouraged but this should be supplemented with additional questions. For example, who the patient sees for the management of their condition (GMP/paediatrician/respiratory team) and how often they are reviewed, medications and how often they are used, and any acute hospital admissions.
  - Childhood diseases and previous medical treatment.
  - Where allergies are disclosed, establish the nature of the allergic reaction (e.g. rash or facial swelling).
  - Experience of general anaesthesia (GA) and any complications.
- Dental history:
  - Attendance history.
  - History of preventive or restorative care.
  - Establish previous experience of local anasthesia (LA) and how the child responded.
  - Ask whether the patient has experienced any dental trauma in the past.
  - Oral hygiene practices (⊙ Prevention).
  - Ask about dietary practices (e.g. any history of drinking milk from a bottle during the night). For older children, find out what they like to drink and whether they snack between mealtimes.
  - Pacifier/digit habits should be identified.
- Social history:
  - The social history is a useful way to find out more about the child and helps to develop a strong rapport.
  - Ask how old the patient is and whether they have any siblings. If so, document the name and ages of the siblings.
  - Establish who else lives at home.

- Determine what school they attend—this is important as school nurses may become involved in the patient's care, particularly in cases where there are safeguarding concerns.

Examination

Extraoral examination

- Assess the general appearance of the child:
  - Do they look well? Are they unkempt?
  - Do they appear small/underweight for their age? If any growth/ weight concerns are suspected, plot the child's height and weight on a growth chart. A referral to a paediatrician is indicated where there are parental concerns about the child's development, or if the child is plotted below the 0.4th/above the 99.6th centiles on a growth chart.
  - Know your local safeguarding procedure in case of any concerns.
- Examine the skin for colour, dryness, and lesions which could indicate systemic disease (e.g. café-au-lait spots).
- Assess the ectodermal structures:
  - Hair and eyebrows.
  - Nails.
  - Thin/sparse hair and/or nail abnormalities may suggest an ectodermal disorder such as ectodermal dysplasia.
- Feel for submandibular and cervical lymphadenopathy:
  - Where identified, note location and texture of lymph nodes (soft/ firm, mobile/fixed, tender/non-tender).
  - Lymphadenopathy associated with dental infections—lymph nodes are usually soft and tender. Where the pattern of lymphadenopathy is unusual (e.g. lymph nodes are of a firm consistency, there are multiple enlarged lymph nodes, or where systemic symptoms such as fatigue and weight loss are reported), an urgent referral for a paediatric medical assessment is indicated.
- For patients attending with facial swellings:
  - Note the site and texture of the swelling (soft/hard, diffuse/well localized).
  - Take the child's temperature. Pyrexia: >37.5°C.
  - Note any trismus. Where present, make an urgent referral to OMFS.
- For patients presenting with a history of significant trauma:
  - Establish whether the child may have suffered a head injury (e.g. by asking whether there has been any loss/reduced level of consciousness, any nausea or vomiting, or any behaviour change). Where the presence of a head injury cannot be excluded, an ambulance or urgent A&E referral is indicated.
  - Palpate the facial skeleton and condyles to exclude facial fractures.
  - Determine whether there is any facial dysaesthesia/paraesthesia that may indicate a facial fracture.
- Note skeletal pattern and any facial asymmetry:
  - Record whether lips are incompetent at rest.
  - Frankfort mandibular plane angle.
- Palpate the temporomandibular joints and examine their mobility:
  - Note restrictions and deviations during movement.

Intraoral examination
- Adopt a systematic approach.
- Complete a full charting:
  - Teeth should be clean and dry.
  - Asymmetric eruption of teeth/abnormalities in the eruption sequence may warrant further investigation (➔ Chronology of dental development).
  - Note caries, staining, altered morphology, enamel defects, and tooth surface loss.
  - Where anomalies such as enamel defects are identified, note whether they are generalized, localized, or could represent a chronological disturbance (➔ Enamel defects).
  - Carefully examine the buccal aspects of first permanent molars (FPMs) and palatal aspects of upper permanent incisors for the presence of pits/grooves. Pits/grooves should be fissure sealed.
- Examine the soft tissues:
  - Fully describe the appearance, size, and location of any abnormalities.
  - Note prominent frenula.
- Palpate any swellings.
- Assess the quality of the saliva.
- Assess the oral hygiene and gingival health:
  - From 7 years of age, record a simplified BPE score using the six index teeth upper right (UR) 6, UR1, upper left (UL) 6, lower left (LL) 6, LL1, and lower right (LR) 6[1] (Box 3.1).
  - NB: for immunocompromised patients, the neutrophil count should be >1000 mm³ for periodontal probing.

Box 3.1 BPE codes

- 0: healthy.
- 1: bleeding on probing.
- 2: calculus or plaque retention factor.
- 3: shallow pocket (4 mm or 5 mm).
- 4: deep pocket (≥6 mm).
- *: if furcation present.

NB: for 7–11-year-olds, only use codes 0–2 due to the risk of false pockets in the mixed dentition.

- Examine the occlusion:
  - Palpate for the unerupted maxillary permanent canines between the ages of 9 and 10 years.
  - Increased overjet with incompetent lips is associated with an increased risk of dental trauma. Provide a mouth guard for sports and consider orthodontic referral if appropriate.
  - For orthodontic assessment, see ➔ Orthodontics.

Radiographic examination

In paediatric dentistry, the following radiographic techniques may be indicated:
• Bitewing (BW) radiographs:
  • Essential adjunct to clinical examination for approximal and occlusal caries (Box 3.2).
  • Should be taken at the initial consultation for children with closed posterior contacts who are able to tolerate BWs.
  • Can also be used to assess for presence of inter-radicular radiolucencies indicative of non-vital pulp tissue.

Box 3.2 BW intervals according to caries risk

• *High risk*: 6-monthly BWs until no new or active lesions are apparent and the child has entered another risk category.[2]
• *Moderate risk*: annual BWs until no new or active lesions are apparent and the child has entered another risk category.
• *Low risk*: in the mixed dentition, BWs should be taken at 12–18-monthly intervals and ~2-year intervals in the permanent dentition. More extended intervals may be appropriate following caries-risk assessment.

  • Intervals between subsequent BWs should be determined according to the child's caries risk assessment.
• Periapical (PA) radiographs:
  • To assess for periapical pathology.
  • Following dental trauma.
  • During endodontic treatment.
• Occlusal radiographs:
  • To assist with localizing teeth or root fractures by applying parallax.
  • Where the tooth being localized moves in the same direction as the tube shift, the tooth is positioned palatally/lingually and vice versa ('SLOB: Same (direction) = Lingual; Opposite (direction) = Buccal').
• Dental panoramic tomography (DPT):
  • To assess the developing dentition (e.g. to determine the presence/absence of teeth, establish dental age).
  • Presence of multiple carious teeth requiring extraction.
  • Where a lesion/tooth cannot be imaged by intraoral techniques.
• Cone-beam computed tomography (CBCT):
  • To supplement plain films (e.g. to localize supernumerary teeth ($) and determine their relation to adjacent structures).
• Soft tissue films:
  • To exclude the presence of unaccounted tooth fragments or foreign bodies following trauma.

Additional special tests
• Percussion:
  • Where teeth are tender to percussion, a diagnosis of acute apical/inter-radicular periodontitis should be suspected.
  • Teeth may also be tender to percussion following dental trauma when an injury to the periodontal ligament (PDL) has been sustained.

---

2 ℘ www.fgdp.org.uk/guidance-standards/selection-criteria-dental-radiography

- Sensibility tests:
  - Electric pulp test and ethyl chloride.
  - Record the outcome in terms of consistency (consistent or inconsistent), response (positive or negative), and, where appropriate, grade the response (normal, i.e. compared to control tooth; hypersensitive; or delayed).
- Mobility.
- Temporary tooth separation for interproximal caries diagnosis.
- Transillumination:
  - Dark may indicate pulp necrosis.
  - Yellow may indicate pulp obliteration.
  - Fibreoptic transillumination for caries diagnosis—technique sensitive and BWs will detect more approximal lesions than fibreoptic transillumination. Therefore, recommended as an adjunct to BWs but not an alternative.
- Electrical caries diagnosis methods:
  - Different systems currently under development (e.g. CarieScan®).
- Laser fluorescence methods:
  - Detects fluorescence from bacterial by-products (e.g. DIAGNOdent™ and DIAGNOdent™ pen).
  - False positives can be a problem.
- Quantitative laser fluorescence:
  - Identifies caries as intensity of fluorescence decreases in carious lesions when compared to sound tissue.
- Identify signs of a non-vital primary molar (Box 3.3).
- Consider obtaining clinical photographs which can be particularly useful following traumatic injuries.

Box 3.3 Signs of a non-vital primary molar

- Chronic sinus or swelling.
- Alveolar tenderness.
- Tenderness to percussion.
- Non-physiological mobility.
- Inter-radicular radiolucency on radiographic examination.

Diagnosis

A list of diagnoses should follow the clinical and radiographic examination and incorporate the results of any specialist tests. The following factors should be considered:

Caries and caries risk assessment

The carious teeth should be recorded along with a caries risk assessment (i.e. increased or low). The most important caries predictive factors are previous caries experience, socioeconomic background (caries is more common in lower socioeconomic groups), and the clinical judgement of healthcare workers.[3] Dietary habits, exposure to fluoride, oral hygiene, salivary flow rates, and medical history should also be considered.

3 ♪ www.sdcep.org.uk/published-guidance/caries-in-children/

Hard tissues

In addition to caries, any defects of enamel and dentine should be clearly noted along with any additional abnormalities.

Pulp pathology

When children present with a history of toothache, the history and examination should help to determine the presence and nature of pulpitis. Pulp pathology such as pulp polyps and chronic/acute inter-radicular or periapical periodontitis should be also noted.

Soft tissues

Any signs of infection, ulceration, swelling, or pigmented lesions.

Gingival/periodontal condition

Interpret the findings of the simplified BPE and radiographic examinations to include diagnoses of localized/generalized gingivitis and/or periodontal conditions (➔ Periodontal disease in children).

Behaviour

Include an assessment of the child's cooperative ability (➔ Behaviour) and whether the child is dentally anxious.

Developing dentition

Any orthodontic concerns should be noted (➔ Orthodontics).

Management strategies for carious primary teeth

- Although carious primary teeth may remain asymptomatic until exfoliation, ~1/3 of primary molars that develop caries with pulp involvement by age 3 will become symptomatic.[1] Furthermore, 6% of carious primary molar teeth presenting without pulpal involvement after 8 years of age will become symptomatic.[1]
- Therefore, it is important to assess the risk of pain and/or sepsis prior to exfoliation by considering:
  - extent of lesion
  - site of lesion
  - caries risk
  - caries attack rate
  - patient's dental age
  - patient's cooperative ability
  - parental/carer motivation and cooperation with prevention.
- There will usually be more than one approach which could be adopted; therefore, the clinician should use their clinical judgement to determine the most suitable management strategy. The management options should also be discussed with the person with parental responsibility and the child.

Management options

All children and young adults should receive appropriate preventative advice and intervention according to their risk (➔ Prevention).

Intensive prevention, no caries removal

- Indications:
  - Motivated families.
  - Low risk of pain and/or sepsis prior to exfoliation.
  - Non-cavitated/cavitated lesions.
  - Children lacking cooperative ability.
- Contraindications:
  - Signs and symptoms of pain and/or sepsis.
  - Children at risk of infection (e.g. immunocompromised patients, patients at increased risk of infective endocarditis).
  - High risk of pain and/or sepsis prior to exfoliation.
  - High caries attack rate.
- Parent/carers should be advised of the risk of pain and infection should caries progress.

Intensive prevention, no caries removal, make lesions self-cleansing

- Indications:
  - Motivated families.
  - Cavitated lesions.

1 Levine R (2002). *Br Dent J* 193, 99.

- Low risk of pain and/or sepsis prior to exfoliation.
- Children lacking cooperative ability for operative intervention.
- Contraindications:
  - Signs and symptoms of pain and/or sepsis, high caries attack rate.
  - Children at risk of infection (e.g. immunocompromised patients, patients at increased risk of infective endocarditis).
  - High risk of pain and/or sepsis prior to exfoliation.
  - High caries attack rate.

No caries removal, seal with fissure sealant

- Indications[2]:
  - Motivated families.
  - Non-cavitated occlusal lesions.
  - Low risk of pain and/or sepsis prior to exfoliation.
- Contraindications:
  - Signs and symptoms of pain and/or sepsis.
  - Children at risk of infection (e.g. immunocompromised patients, patients at increased risk of infective endocarditis).
  - High risk of pain and/or sepsis prior to exfoliation.
  - High caries attack rate.

No caries removal, seal with preformed metal crown (PMC) via Hall technique

- Indications:
  - Non-cavitated/cavitated posterior lesions in primary molars.
  - Pulp involvement excluded.
  - Low risk of pain and/or sepsis prior to exfoliation.
  - Hypomineralized primary molar teeth.
- Contraindications:
  - Signs and symptoms of pain and/or sepsis.
  - Children at risk of infection (e.g. immunocompromised patients, patients at increased risk of infective endocarditis).
  - High risk of pain and/or sepsis prior to exfoliation.
- For procedure, see ⊃ Paediatric restorative techniques for the carious primary dentition.

Partial caries removal, seal with restoration

- Indications:
  - Non-cavitated/cavitated lesions.
  - Low risk of pain and/or sepsis prior to exfoliation.
- Contraindications:
  - Unrestorable tooth.
  - Signs and symptoms of pain and/or sepsis.
  - Children at risk of infection (e.g. immunocompromised patients, patients at increased risk of infective endocarditis).
- For procedure, see ⊃ Paediatric restorative techniques for the carious primary dentition.

2 Smallridge J (2010). Int J Paed Dent 20 (Suppl 1), 3.

Complete caries removal, seal with restoration

- Indications:
  - Cavitated/non-cavitated occlusal lesions.
  - Approximal lesions.
  - Anterior lesions.
- Contraindications:
  - Unrestorable tooth.
  - Signs and symptoms of pain and/or sepsis.
  - Tooth close to exfoliation.
- For procedure, see ➔ Paediatric restorative techniques for the carious primary dentition.

Extraction

- Indications:
  - Unrestorable tooth.
  - Signs and symptoms of pain and/or sepsis.
- Contraindications:
  - Patients with bleeding tendencies.
- Premature extraction of primary molar teeth often results in mesial migration of the teeth distal to the extraction site resulting in an increased risk of crowding in the permanent dentition.

All children received best-practice prevention

Evidence

While there are studies looking at different caries management approaches for primary teeth, often the follow-up periods are short, and the studies are deemed to be at high risk of bias.[3] The FiCTION (Filling in Children's Teeth: Indicated Or Not?) trial compared the clinical effectiveness of conventional restorations and biological management (sealing in caries) with prevention alone in a three-armed primary care-based patient-randomized controlled trial.[4,5] All children received best-practice prevention. The conclusion was that there was no evidence of an overall difference in the clinical outcomes of the approaches when applied in primary care. However, it should be noted that BW radiographs were not routinely taken at baseline and, therefore, pulpal involvement could not have been excluded. In addition, there was a low use of PMCs in the biological management group.

3 Ricketts D (2013). *Cochrane Database of Sys Rev* 3, CD003808.

4 Maguire A (2020). *Health Technol Assess* 24, 1.

5 FiCTION trial: ℘ https://research.ncl.ac.uk/fictiontrial/

Treatment planning

Treatment planning

- Once the treatment needs have been established, the available management options (along with their risks and benefits) should be discussed with the person with parental responsibility and the child.
- The treatment plan will be dependent upon the cooperative ability of the child and the child's dental needs:
  - The plan for a child who requires a GA for treatment will differ from a child who will accept dental treatment without pharmacological behaviour management techniques.
- Treatment planning can be completed in two stages:
  - List the child's treatment needs by referring back to the diagnoses and considering the restorability of the teeth.
  - Order the treatment required visit by visit ensuring all preventive and restorative needs are addressed.
- Where patients present with symptoms, initial management should be focused on diagnosing and managing the child's symptoms (e.g. with a sedative dressing to allow a period of acclimatization prior to definitive management). For pre-cooperative children, consider specialist referral for pharmacological behavioural management techniques (◐ Pharmacological behaviour management techniques).
- The recall intervals for clinical and radiographic examinations should be included in the treatment plan.

Key considerations

Primary dentition
- Determine the restorability of the teeth and consider whether extractions are indicated:
  - Where multiple extractions are indicated in a young child, a referral to specialist services to consider providing dental care under GA may be required.
- Where extraction of primary teeth is indicated, consider the need for a balancing extraction:
  - A balancing extraction is the extraction of a contralateral tooth in the same arch to prevent a midline shift.
- Potential consequences of early loss of primary teeth:
  - Space loss (Es > Ds).
  - Loss >3 years before natural exfoliation can delay eruption of permanent tooth by up to 6 months.
  - Risk of midline shift with unbalanced loss of Cs and Ds.
- Ensure parent/carer is aware of all the management options along with their risks and benefits.

Mixed dentition
- For children with caries affecting the primary dentition, the initial approach should be to prevent caries in the permanent dentition prior to managing the carious primary teeth (unless the child is experiencing acute dental symptoms). Placement of fissure sealants on FPMs also aids acclimatization.
- Where there is considerable pathology associated with FPMs in paediatric patients, the long-term prognosis of the tooth/teeth should be considered. A referral for a specialist opinion may be indicated.

- Indications for the extraction of FPMs:
  - Extensive caries or unrestorable tooth.
  - Multi-surface hypomineralized enamel defects in molar–incisor hypomineralization (MIH) cases.
  - Severe episode of infection requiring immediate emergency management.
  - As part of an orthodontic treatment plan.
  - Balancing extraction of an upper FPM following loss of the lower FPM.
- Contraindications to the extraction of FPMs:
  - Hypodontia cases (unless FPM deemed unrestorable).
  - Spaced dentition (unless FPM deemed unrestorable).
  - Patients with generalized developmental dental defects where the second permanent molar is likely to have a similar prognosis (unless FPM deemed unrestorable).
- Considerations relating to the extraction of FPMs of poor prognosis[1]:
  - Obtain a DPT to confirm presence of all permanent teeth and determine the child's dental age.
  - Consider the ideal timing for the extractions to take place. For example, the ideal timing for the extraction of a lower FPM where there is a class I molar relationship with no/mild crowding is dental age 8.5–9.5 years when the bifurcation of the lowers of the lower second molars are starting to calcify. The timing of the extraction of upper FPMs is less critical due to the increased tendency for mesial drift in the maxilla.
  - Consider the need for balancing and compensating extractions (compensation: extraction of the same tooth in the opposing arch undertaken to maintain the buccal segment relationship). *Extraction of an upper FPM does not necessarily require a compensating extraction of the lower FPM.*
  - Orthodontic input regarding the timing and extraction pattern may be required (➔ First molars of poor prognosis).

Permanent dentition

- Once in the permanent dentition, balancing and compensating extractions are usually not indicated. However, a referral for an orthodontic opinion may be prudent in cases where treatment is to be provided under GA.

Treatment planning for LA

- Non-pharmacological behavioural management techniques should be used from the outset to promote a positive attitude towards dentistry (➔ Non-pharmacological behavioural management techniques).
- An acclimatization visit may be useful in order to introduce the child to the dental environment and to gain a better understanding of their cooperative ability. A dental prophylaxis or placement of fissure sealants on sound teeth can provide a useful introduction to dentistry. Where children struggle to accept fissure sealants, it is likely that further treatment under LA will not be successful. Identifying this at an

---

1 Cobourne M (2014). *Br Dent J* 217, 643.

early stage is beneficial as alternative management approaches can be considered.
- Ideally each appointment should include a preventive and restorative component.
- Where LA is used, quadrant dentistry should be performed where possible to avoid the need for repeated LA administration in the same area.
- The first quadrant should ideally be in the maxilla as maxillary analgesia can usually be provided more easily.
- An example of a treatment plan for a paediatric patient is shown in Table 3.2.
- The recall interval will depend upon the child's caries risk status and preventative regimen. Often for children at increased risk of caries, a recall interval of 3 months is indicated. Otherwise, an interval of 6 months may be sufficient.

Table 3.2 Example treatment plan for a paediatric dental patient

Visit	Examination/operative treatment	Prevention
1	Examination, treatment planning	Provide diet sheet Fluoride varnish (2.26%)
2	Sedative dressing 75	Collect diet sheet, plaque free score, tooth brushing instruction, fissure sealants
3	Restoration of 52, 51, 61, 62	Diet analysis, oral hygiene review
4	Restoration of 54 under LA	Plaque free score
5	Pulpotomy and PMC 85 and restoration 84 under LA	Fissure seal 74 Fluoride varnish (2.26%)
6	Extraction 75 under LA	Diet and oral hygiene review
7	Review 3 months	Fluoride varnish (2.26%) Diet and oral hygiene review

Treatment planning for GA
- Often formulated in specialist services.
- Due to the risks associated with the provision of a GA (➔ General anaesthesia), treatment planning becomes more radical for children receiving dental care under GA.
- Every effort should be made to reduce the need for repeat dental GAs and therefore all dental disease should be diagnosed accurately and addressed in the treatment plan.

- The treatment plan often involves more dental extractions and a greater use of restorative techniques with the highest success rates (e.g. PMCs for primary molars) in order to minimize the risk of the child requiring a second GA for dental treatment.
- Any child receiving dental care under GA requires intensive prevention (➲ Prevention) which should be provided in primary care.
- Clinicians referring children for treatment under GA should clearly justify the use of GA in the referral letter but understand that the ultimate decision on whether a GA is appropriate lies with the GA service provider.[2]

2 Adewale L (2011). Guidelines for the management of children referred for dental extractions under general anaesthesia. ✆ www.bspd.co.uk

Behaviour

Dental fear and anxiety

- Dental anxiety has been defined as a 'non-specific feeling of apprehension'[1] whereas dental fear is the response to a specific stimulus. Dental phobia is when the fear response is out of proportion to the degree of threat posed.
- Dental anxiety is common in children and young adults. Prevalence: 23.9%.[2]
- Aetiology is multifactorial:
  - Factors relating to the child: age, sex, temperament, past dental history, past medical history.
  - External factors: parental anxiety, socioeconomic status, dentist's management techniques and manner.
- Consequences of dental anxiety include:
  - behaviour management problems
  - increased caries levels
  - increased need for GAs
  - poor dental attendance.

Classifying children's behaviour

Behaviour can be classified as cooperative, potentially cooperative, or lacking cooperative ability such as very young children (pre-cooperative) or those with significant developmental delay. Other commonly used classifications include the Frankl and Houpt scales:

- Frankl behaviour rating scale:
  - Definitely positive (++): good rapport with dentist.
  - Positive (+): acceptance of treatment but cautious.
  - Negative (−): reluctant to accept treatment.
  - Definitely negative (−−): refusal of treatment, crying.
- Houpt behaviour rating scale:
  - 1: treatment aborted.
  - 2: poor: treatment interrupted; only partial treatment completed.
  - 3: fair: treatment interrupted but eventually completed.
  - 4: good: difficult but all treatment performed.
  - 5: very good: some limited crying or movement.
  - 6: excellent: no crying or movement.
- Factors that may influence a child's behaviour in the dental setting:
  - Level of dental anxiety.
  - Child's awareness of a dental problem.
  - Parental presence.
  - Parenting styles.
  - Dental staff and environment.

1 Klingberg G (2008). *Eur Arch Paediatr Dent* 9 (Suppl 1), 11.
2 Grisolia B (2021). *Int J Paediatr Dent* 31, 168.

Non-pharmacological behaviour management techniques (NPBMTs)

NPBMTs are suitable for cooperative and potentially cooperative children. The management strategies involve behaviour shaping often achieved by combining several techniques[3]:

- Non-verbal communication:
  - Child-friendly, welcoming environment.
- Tell–show–do:
  - Requires effective, age-appropriate communication, that is, use of 'childrenese' (Box 3.4).
  - Used to introduce and familiarize children to procedures.
  - Tell the child what you are planning to do. For example, the 'tell' stage for a prophy could involve saying 'I am going to clean your teeth with my buzzy brush'. The 'show' stage could involve demonstrating the use of the prophy brush on your finger and then theirs before performing a prophy on their anterior teeth during the 'do' stage.

Box 3.4 Examples of 'childrenese'

- Probe: 'tooth tickler'
- Slow-speed handpiece: 'buzzy brush'
- High-speed handpiece: 'whizzy brush'
- Topical anaesthetic: 'magic jelly'
- LA: 'sleepy juice'
- Rubber dam: 'rubber raincoat'
- Forceps: 'silver fingers'

- Positive reinforcement:
  - Strengthens a pattern of behaviour.
  - Examples of positive reinforcers: verbal praise, stickers, toys.
  - More effective when given directly after good behaviour or when specifically linked to a positive aspect of the child's behaviour.
- Modelling:
  - Demonstration of the procedure on a model (either live or by video/photographs) who is displaying the appropriate behaviour.
  - Most effective when the model is a similar age to the patient and is praised for their behaviour.
- Distraction:
  - Used to divert the child's attention, for example, pulling the lip during LA or counting techniques.
- Enhancing control:
  - Use of stop signals, for example, asking the child to raise one of their hands.
- Systematic desensitization:

---

3 Campbell C (2011). Clinical guidelines in paediatric dentistry. Update of non-pharmacological be-haviour management. ⬧ www.bspd.co.uk

- Constructing a hierarchy of anxiety-provoking stimuli and gradually exposing the child to the hierarchy while utilizing relaxation techniques.
- Voice control:
  - Controlled alteration of tone or pace.
  - May not be acceptable to all parents.
- Negative reinforcement:
  - The strengthening of a pattern of behaviour by removing a stimulus which the patient perceives as unpleasant (a negative reinforcer) as soon as the required behaviour is shown.
  - Includes selective exclusion of the parents, hand-over-mouth techniques, restraint, and flooding.
  - In the UK, hand-over-mouth techniques, restraint, and flooding are not widely accepted and therefore are not recommended.
  - The GDC do not support the use of physical restraint in dealing with difficult patients other than in the most exceptional circumstances.
- Clinical holding:
  - May be used in exceptional circumstances, for example, where the patient's behaviour poses a risk to themselves or others, and there are not any alternative options available.
  - Requires a risk assessment, training as well as clear procedures and policies.[4]

Pharmacological behaviour management techniques

Conscious sedation
- Fundamental part of pain and anxiety management in paediatric dentistry.
- Definition: 'a technique in which the use of a drug or drugs produces a state of depression of the CNS [central nervous system] enabling treatment to be carried out, but during which verbal contact with the patient is maintained throughout the period of sedation. The drugs and techniques used to provide conscious sedation for dental treatment should carry a margin of safety wide enough to render loss of consciousness unlikely'.[5]
- Should not be regarded as a substitute for effective NPBMTs and LA techniques.
- Main techniques in paediatric dentistry:
  - Inhalation sedation with nitrous oxide and oxygen.
  - Intravenous (IV) sedation.
  - Oral sedation.
- Less commonly used techniques:
  - Nasal sedation.
  - Rectal sedation.
- Written patient information and instructions should be provided in advance of the procedure.

---

4 Allen Y (2016). British Society of Paediatric Dentistry: a policy document on the use of clinical holding in the dental care of children. ℑ www.bspd.co.uk

5 Dental Faculties of the Royal Colleges of Surgeons and the Royal College of Anaesthetists (2020). Standards for conscious sedation in the provision of dental care (V1.1). Report of the Intercollegiate Advisory Committee for Sedation in Dentistry. ℑ www.rcseng.ac.uk

- Written informed consent should be obtained prior to treatment.
- All members of the team must have undertaken validated training and have demonstrated that they are competent in the sedation technique.[5]
- All team members should be trained in life support skills.[5]
- Polypharmacy techniques are not advocated in paediatric dentistry.

Inhalation sedation with nitrous oxide and oxygen
- Indications:
  - Children >4 years old with sufficient understanding of planned procedure and sufficient cooperative ability.
  - Unable to manage treatment with NPBMT and LA due to mild–moderate dental anxiety.
  - Pronounced gag reflex.
  - Difficulties achieving LA (e.g. hypomineralized teeth).
- Contraindications:
  - Pre-cooperative children/patients lacking cooperative ability.
  - Patients unable to breathe through their nose (e.g. upper respiratory tract infections).
  - First trimester of pregnancy.
  - Patients who have received bleomycin chemotherapy or methotrexate.
  - Patients with psychotic disorders.
  - Otitis media (nitrous oxide causes pressure volume effects).
  - Severe muscular depression.
- Advantages:
  - Non-invasive.
  - Titration enables optimal level of sedation which can be altered.
  - Rapid absorption and onset within 2–3 minutes.
  - Rapid elimination and complete recovery within 5 minutes.
  - Weak analgesic effect.
  - Minimal impairment of reflexes.
  - Minimal effect on cardiovascular and respiratory systems.
- Disadvantages:
  - Requires cooperation from patient to wear nasal hood.
  - Nitrous oxide needs to be continuously administered throughout procedure and nasal hood can impede access to anterior maxillary teeth.
  - Lacks potency.
  - Requires continuous use of semi-hypnotic suggestion.
  - Potential for nitrous oxide pollution.
- Risks:
  - Nausea and vomiting (1–10%).
  - Diffusion hypoxia.
  - Pressure volume effects.
  - Oversedation.
  - Malignant hyperthermia.
- Procedure:
  - Should only be carried out by appropriately trained, competent practitioners.
  - Requires use of semi-hypnotic suggestion and relaxation techniques.
  - Continuous clinical monitoring ± pulse oximetry.

- Safe discharge by ensuring all vital signs are normal and that the child is discharged to a responsible adult.
- Success: >90%.[6]

IV sedation

- Involves IV injection of benzodiazepine (commonly midazolam).
- Indications:
  - >12 years old with sufficient understanding of procedure and emotional stability.
  - Complex oral needs.
  - Unable to manage treatment with NPBMT and LA.
  - Mild–moderate dental anxiety.
  - ASA I (or mild ASA II).
- Contraindications:
  - Severe behavioural problems.
  - Hypersensitivity to benzodiazepines.
  - Patients at risk of respiratory depression.
  - Obstructive sleep apnoea.
  - Hepatic dysfunction.
  - Myasthenia gravis.
  - Acute closed-angle glaucoma.
  - Pregnancy and breastfeeding.
- Advantages:
  - Immediate onset.
  - Ability to titrate.
  - Site of administration distant from operator site.
  - Less reliant on semi-hypnotic suggestion.
  - Good amnesia.
  - No pollution/chronic exposure risk.
- Disadvantages:
  - Requires cannulation for IV access.
  - Risk of respiratory depression.
  - No analgesic effect.
  - Effects can vary.
  - Narrow margin of safety reported in younger patients.
- Risks:
  - Nausea and vomiting.
  - Confusion.
  - Oversedation.
  - Sexual fantasy.
  - Respiratory depression.
  - Cardiovascular depression.
  - Mortality.
- Procedure:
  - Sedative agent given in small increments (usually 0.1 mg for paediatric patients) and titrated according to the effect.
  - Clinical monitoring, pulse oximetry, and blood pressure monitoring.
  - Safe discharge by ensuring all vital signs are normal and that the child is discharged to a responsible adult.

6 Foley J (2005). *Eur J Paed Dent* 6, 121.

Oral sedation

- Agent usually midazolam.
- Requires specialized training and must be carried out by practitioners who are competent in IV sedation.
- Indications:
  - Pre-cooperative children requiring short procedure.
  - Mild–moderate anxiety.
  - Can be used as a pre-medication.
- Contraindications:
  - Outside hospital environment.
  - Sleep apnoea.
  - Increased body mass index (BMI).
  - Allergy/hypersensitivity.
  - Concurrent medication with benzodiazepine or other CNS depressant.
- Advantages:
  - Non-invasive and low cost.
- Disadvantages:
  - Compliance needed.
  - Disagreeable taste.
  - Effects can be unpredictable.
  - Inability to titrate and alter level of sedation.
  - Variable onset.
  - Short duration of action.
- Risks:
  - Nausea and vomiting.
  - Confusion.
  - Oversedation.
  - Respiratory depression.
  - Cardiovascular depression.
  - Mortality.
- Procedure: 0.5–0.75 mg/kg midazolam given 30 minutes prior to treatment.
- Monitoring and discharge arrangements are as for IV sedation.
- High failure rate: ~10–40%.[7]

General anaesthesia

- Written informed consent should be obtained prior to treatment.
  - Alternative management options along with their risks and benefits must be discussed prior to a GA referral.
  - Discuss the risks of GA.
  - Warn about possible waiting times.
- GA must be carried out in a hospital setting with adequate critical care facilities.
- Considerations for GA:
  - Cooperative ability of the child.
  - Previous attempts and response to treatment.
  - Degree of surgical trauma anticipated.
  - Complexity of the planned procedure.
  - Medical history.

7 Day P (2006). *Eur Arch Paed Dent* 7, 228.

- Indications:
  - Pre-cooperative children/patients lacking cooperative ability.
  - Extensive treatment need (e.g. multiple extractions/difficult procedures).
  - Acute conditions requiring emergency management.
  - Failure of treatment under LA and conscious sedation.
  - Treatment is not possible without GA.
  - Patients with medical conditions best managed under GA (e.g. bleeding disorders, allergy to LA).
- Contraindications[8]:
  - Orthodontic extraction of sound permanent premolar teeth in healthy child.
  - Patient/carer preference except where alternative techniques have been tried.
  - Children at increased risk of GA (e.g. sickle cell disease, cystic fibrosis).
- Advantages:
  - All treatment carried out at one appointment.
  - NPBMT not required.
  - Can be more cost-effective is extensive treatment is required.
  - May aid control of complications (e.g. post-extraction bleeding).
- Disadvantages:
  - Increased morbidity.
  - Increased risk of mortality.
  - More radical treatment planning needed.
  - No learning experience/acclimatization for patient.
  - Long waiting times.
  - Inequalities in access to GA services.
  - Increased cost and resources.
  - Can be a traumatic experience for child and family.
- Risks:
  - Nausea and vomiting (~24%).
  - Sore throat.
  - Shivering.
  - Headache.
  - Tiredness.
  - Confusion.
  - Breathing problems.
  - Mortality.
- Preparation:
  - Written patient information and instructions should be provided in advance of the procedure.
  - The child and parent/guardian should be allowed sufficient time to ask any questions they may have.
  - Starving instructions on the day of the GA should be clearly stated verbally and in writing. The child should not have anything to eat

---

8 Davies C (2008). UK National Clinical Guidelines in Paediatric Dentistry. Guideline for the use of general anaesthesia in paediatric dentistry. ℘ www.rcseng.ac.uk.

for 6 hours before the GA. Clear fluids are allowed up until 2 hours before the GA.
- Discharge:
  - Shared responsibility of the dental and anaesthetic team.
  - Verbal and written postoperative instructions should be provided.
  - Advice on mouth care and analgesia should be given.
  - Arrangements for dental follow-up should be agreed.

Prevention

Oral hygiene

Key points:
- Tooth brushing with a fluoride toothpaste should start as soon as the first tooth erupts.
- Parents/carers should brush their child's teeth until they are able to tie their own shoelaces/button up a shirt.
- Teeth should be brushed last thing at night and on at least one other occasion during the day.
- After tooth brushing, excess toothpaste should be spat out. No rinsing, eating, or drinking should take place within 30 minutes after tooth brushing.
- Plaque disclosure and tooth brushing instruction should be provided by the dental team:
  - Disclosing tablets are a useful adjunct to oral hygiene at home.
  - Parents can monitor progress and identify areas where cleaning needs to improve.
- Parents should be shown how to brush partially erupted molars from the side to ensure that the bristles contact the occlusal surfaces of the teeth.
- Advice and instruction on interdental plaque control can start from 12 years of age.

Fluoride

- For toothpaste concentrations, see Table 3.3.
- Children with special medical, social, or dental needs and patients with fixed appliances should be regarded as high priority for dental prevention.

Table 3.3 Toothpaste concentrations according to age and risk/priority category of patient

Age (years)	Risk/priority category	Concentration
<3	Standard	Smear of toothpaste of no less than 1000 parts per million of fluoride (ppmF)
3–6	Standard	Pea-sized amount of toothpaste containing >1000 ppmF
>7	Standard	1350–1500 ppmF
0–6	Increased risk/high priority	Smear (<3 years)/pea-sized (3–6 years) amount, 1350–1500 ppmF
>10	Increased risk/high priority	Prescribe 2800 ppmF
>16	Increased risk/high priority	Prescribe 2800 ppmF or 5000 ppmF

- Fluoride varnish (2.2% NaF) applications:
  - Biannual for all children from 3 years of age.
  - Children aged 0–6 years regarded as high caries risk/high priority: apply varnish two or more times per year.
  - Dispense no more than 0.25 mL for primary dentition, 0.4 mL for mixed dentition, and 0.75 mL for permanent dentition.
  - Contraindications: allergy to constituents, known sensitivity to colophony/resin, multiple allergies, severe asthmatics, ulcerative gingivitis/stomatitis, large open intraoral lesions, or allergy to sticking plaster.
- Silver diamine fluoride (38%)[1]:
  - Contains 44800 ppm fluoride concentration.
  - Licensed for de-sensitization, but off-label for caries management.
  - Can cause dark staining of treated carious lesion.
  - Potassium iodide solutions can be used to reduce the staining.
  - Bactericidal effect and remineralization effects, occludes dentinal tubules, and inhibits the enzymes that cause collagen degradation.
  - May improve the bond of glass ionomer (GI) cement.
  - Need protection of the soft tissue whether that is rubber dam or petroleum jelly.
  - Apply for 1 minute and then keep protected for a further 3 minutes to allow it to set. Remove any excess with a cotton pellet.
  - Review in 4 weeks to assess arrested carious lesion and restore or consider reapplication of the silver diamine fluoride in 6 months.
- Daily fluoride (0.05%) mouth rinses can be used at a separate time to tooth brushing from 8 years of age (providing the child can rinse and spit out safely).
- Probable toxic dose of fluoride = 5 mg/kg body weight. Where this level of fluoride is ingested, seek immediate medical advice.

Fissure sealants

- High caries risk/high-priority patients should have their permanent molars sealed with resin-based sealant.
- Good isolation is important for retention.
- Indications for the fissure sealing of FPMs:
  - Children with special needs.
  - Children with caries affecting the primary dentition.
  - Where there is occlusal caries affecting one FPM, the remaining FPMs should be fissure sealed.
  - Deep fissures/buccal pits should be sealed.
- Procedure for resin sealants:
  - Clean tooth (e.g. wipe with gauze, use dry toothbrush or bristle brush).
  - Isolate with cotton wool rolls, mirror, and saliva ejector (or rubber dam if other restorative treatment under LA is being carried out in the same quadrant).
  - Etch with 37% phosphoric acid for 30 seconds.
  - Wash and dry the tooth.

1 Seifo N (2020). Br Dent J 228, 75.

- Where possible, use of bonding agent prior to placement of sealant is encouraged.
- Apply sealant with thymosin or excavator flowing the resin into the fissures and any buccal grooves or pits.
- Light cure.
- Check retention and integrity of sealant with a probe.
- In children lacking cooperative ability for resin-based fissure sealants, GI sealants can be used until cooperation permits the placement of resin-based sealants. GI sealants have poorer retention rates and therefore should be used as a temporary measure until resin sealants can be placed.
- Procedure for GI sealant:
  - Clean tooth as above.
  - Isolate.
  - Place small amount of GI (e.g. Fuji Triage™) on one fingertip and petroleum jelly on the adjacent fingertip.
  - Apply GI from the fingertip to the tooth surface to be sealed and keep finger firmly in place until GI starts to set.
  - Cover GI sealant with petroleum jelly before moisture contamination occurs.
  - Should be closely monitored for integrity and topped up with additional resin/GI as needed.

Diet

Key messages:
- From 6 months, infants should be encouraged to drink from a free-flow cup.
- Bottle-feeding should be discouraged from 12 months.
- Sugar should not be added to food or drinks.
- Reduce the amount and the frequency of intake of sugary food to no more than four occasions in 1 day.
- Encourage sugar-free snacks such as carrot sticks, peppers, plain breadsticks, and a small amount of cheese.
- Only drink milk or water between meals.
- Investigate dietary habits with a 4-day diet diary for high caries risk/high-priority children and provide advice in line with the 'eat well' plate.
- Ensure any medications are sugar-free, where possible.

Regular dental reviews

The recall interval will depend upon the child's caries risk status and preventative regimen. Often for children at increased risk of caries, a recall interval of 3 months is indicated. Otherwise, an interval of 6 months may be sufficient.

Operative techniques

Local analgesia

- Common source of fear in patients.
- Administering LA to children is also a source of anxiety for dentists.
- LA should be routinely used for conventional restorative techniques in all age groups.
- Preparing the child:
  - NPBMTs should be used throughout (➲ Non-pharmacological behaviour management techniques).
  - Explain the procedure to the child using terms they understand.
  - Avoid use of the word 'injection' as this is often associated with negative experiences. Childrenese terms such as 'sleepy juice' are preferable.
  - Explain that the 'sleepy juice' will put the gum and tooth to sleep.
  - Explain how it feels (e.g. 'tingling', 'fat', and 'fuzzy') but that it will return to normal after a couple of hours. In young children with limited understanding of time periods, it is useful to give a specific event (e.g. 'Your cheek and your tooth will wake up before lunchtime').
- To assist LA delivery:
  - Always use topical analgesia.
  - Dry the mucosa first.
  - Use a small amount of topical analgesic directly at the site of LA.
  - Use of the saliva ejector may be required to prevent saliva washing the topical analgesic away.
  - Topical analgesic will take at least 2–3 minutes to work. Additional small amounts of topical may be required during this time.
  - Remember topical only affects the superficial mucosa and therefore the first drops of LA should be deposited slowly and *superficially* at first.
  - Pull mucosa taut.
  - Establish a rest for the barrel of the syringe (e.g. against lower lip).
  - Just as needle is going to enter the mucosa, pull mucosa over the needle tip and rotate the barrel to ease needle penetration.
  - Inject slowly and talk to the child throughout LA delivery.
  - Use distraction techniques (e.g. counting to ten while delivering LA).
  - Use positive reinforcement (e.g. verbal praise).
- Postoperative advice:
  - Warn parent/guardian and child about the risk of self-inflicted trauma to the anaesthetized tissues.
  - Advise that the child should avoid eating or drinking anything too hot until the LA has worn off.
  - Tell the child that everything will wake up after a few hours. For young children it is helpful to give an indication of when this might be (e.g. before lunch/teatime).
- Commonly used LAs:
  - 2% lidocaine with 1:80,000 adrenaline.
  - 3% prilocaine with felypressin.
  - 4% articaine with 1:100,000 adrenaline. There is some evidence that 4% articaine given via infiltration is more effective at achieving

analgesia in the FPM region when compared to lidocaine for routine dental procedures.[1] *Articaine should not be used in children <4 years* (no safety data available) or *for block techniques* (due to the risk of prolonged analgesia).
* For maximum doses, see Box 3.5.
* During the administration of LA, continue to use non-pharmacological behaviour management techniques (→ Non-pharmacological behaviour management techniques). The most useful techniques during LA are:
  * Tell–show–do using childrenese terms.
  * Distraction, such as pulling the lip taut during needle penetration, counting techniques.
  * Positive reinforcement with verbal praise and encouragement.
  * Systematic desensitization may be required for particularly anxious children.

Box 3.5 Maximum doses of LA
* 2% lidocaine and 1:80,000 adrenaline: 4.4 mg/kg.
  * Equates to 1/10th of 2.2 mL cartridge per kg.
* 3% prilocaine with felypressin: 6.6 mg/kg.
  * Equates to 1/10th of 2.2 mL cartridge per kg.
* 4% articaine and 1:100,000 adrenaline: 7 mg/kg.
  * Equates to 1.75 mL for a child weighing 10 kg, 2.6 mL for child weighing 15 kg, and 3.5 mL for child weighing 20 kg.

'Rule of 10'
Pulpal analgesia can reliably be achieved with infiltration techniques when the sum of the tooth number (i.e. D = 4, E = 5) and the age of the child does not exceed 10.

Specific techniques

Infiltrations
* Most routinely used technique.
* A 30-gauge 1 cm needle can be used.

Intrapapillary injection
* Provides suitable palatal/lingual analgesia for rubber dam clamp, matrix band, and conventional PMC placement.
* A 30-gauge 1 cm needle can be used.
* Procedure:
  * Following buccal infiltration, penetrate the mesial and distal interdental papillae to a depth of 1–2 mm holding the barrel of the syringe parallel to the occlusal plane and perpendicular to the line of the arch.
  * Inject slowly and advance the needle into the tissue to a depth of a few millimetres while continuing to deposit LA.
  * Check for blanching of the palate indicating analgesia of the gingival cuff.

1 Katyal V (2010). *J Dent* 38, 307.

Indirect palatal injection
- For more profound palatal analgesia (e.g. prior to extraction of a primary maxillary molar).
- A 30-gauge 2 cm needle can be used.
- Procedure:
  - Similar to intrapapillary injection but needle is angled slightly upwards and advanced through the interdental papilla to a greater depth enabling LA to be deposited beneath the palatal mucosa.
  - Can be supplemented with a direct palatal infiltration.

Direct palatal injection
- Once indirect palatal analgesia has been achieved, a direct palatal infiltration can be performed.
- A 30-gauge needle can be used.

Intraligamentary injection
- An intraligamental syringe with a 30-gauge 1 cm needle should be used.
- Procedure:
  - Introduce needle into the interproximal periodontal sulcus and gently advance into the periodontal space until bony resistance is felt.
  - Should only be placed mesially and distally (i.e. not buccally or lingually) to avoid damaging the permanent successor.
  - Inject LA under steady pressure.
  - If no back-pressure is felt, withdraw needle and reinsert it at a slightly different site.
  - 0.4–0.6 mL of LA should be deposited mesially and distally.
- Contraindications:
  - Immunocompromised patients.
  - Patients who are at increased risk of infective endocarditis.
  - Acute periodontal inflammation present.

Inferior alveolar block
- For small children, a 30-gauge 2 cm needle can be used, otherwise a 27-gauge 3 cm needle is recommended.
- Due to the downward and forward growth pattern of the mandible, the mandibular foramen in children lies relatively lower and deeper along the ascending ramus to that in adults.
- Procedure:
  - Following topical analgesia, encourage the child to open their mouth as wide as possible.
  - Palpate external oblique ridge with your thumb and tauten the mucosa.
  - Insert needle at level of the occlusal plane midway between the external oblique ridge and pterygomandibular raphe by approaching from the opposite side of the mouth.
  - Immediately inject a small amount of LA *slowly* and then gently advance the needle with slow injection and aspiration until the bone of the ramus is felt.
  - Withdraw needle by 1 mm then deposit the remainder of the LA.
- *Block techniques are contraindicated* in patients with bleeding disorders unless appropriate haematological cover has been arranged.

Failure of LA

- Operator factors:
  - Poor technique.
  - Insufficient LA administered.
- Patient factors:
  - Psychogenic.
  - Anatomical variation.
  - Infection.
  - Pulpitis.
  - Hypomineralized teeth.

Adjuncts to LA

There are a number of different LA delivery devices available. Computerized delivery devices administer LA at a slow, fixed rate and often have additional benefits such as a more child-friendly appearance.

Rubber dam

- Useful adjunct to paediatric restorative care.
- Can be referred to as a 'tooth raincoat'.
- Advantages:
  - Improved access.
  - Retraction and protection of soft tissues.
  - Moisture control.
  - Contamination-free field.
  - Increased patient comfort (water, tastes).
  - Protects the airway (e.g. during cementation of conventional PMCs).
  - Cross infection (reduced microbial contamination of aerosol with use of high-speed handpiece and 3-in-1 syringe).
  - Aid to patient management.
- Disadvantages:
  - Clamp placement requires buccal and lingual/palatal analgesia (achieved by firstly performing a buccal infiltration then intrapapillary infiltrations).
  - Patients who are unable to breathe through their nose.
  - Can complicate matrix band placement unless sectional matrix bands are used.
- Range of clamps available (Table 3.4):
  - Wingless clamps are advised for paediatric patients.

Table 3.4 Recommended rubber dam clamps

Tooth	Recommended clamp
Partially erupted primary molar	AW
Erupted primary molar	DW
Partially erupted permanent molar	FW
Erupted permanent molar	BW or FW
Permanent incisors	212 clamp

- Procedure for molar teeth:
  - Floss should be tied to the clamp.
  - Punch five to seven holes in the central region of the rubber dam sheet to create a trough (use non-latex sheets for patients with latex allergies).
  - Apply the clamp ('raincoat button') first with the floss lying buccal to the clamp.
  - Once the clamp is secure (test by applying finger pressure), the rubber dam sheet should be placed over the distal aspect of the clamp.
  - Apply the frame ('coat hanger').
  - Stretch the trough forward to isolate all the required teeth in the quadrant.
- Procedure for anterior teeth:
  - Dry dam can be used and stabilized with widgets.
  - Where some gingival retraction is required, anterior clamps (e.g. 212 clamp) can be used following administration of buccal and intrapapillary LA. These clamps can be aggressive and therefore should not be used in cases where the tooth structure is severely compromised or if the tooth has very immature root development.
- Saliva/water can accumulate beneath the rubber dam sheet and therefore the narrow aspirator may be used intermittently behind the rubber dam.

Restorative techniques for the primary dentition

- The morphology of primary molar teeth differs from permanent molar teeth in the following ways:
  - Crowns are more bulbous.
  - Narrower occlusal table.
  - Thinner enamel and dentine.
  - Wide dentinal tubules.
  - Splayed roots.
  - Relatively large pulp space.
  - Porous pulpal floor with accessory canals.
  - Prominent cervical constriction.
- Anatomical differences mean that caries in the primary dentition progresses rapidly and leads to inflammation in the pulp sooner than for permanent teeth. Pulpal inflammation quickly becomes irreversible.
- The indications for restoration and extraction are shown in Table 3.5.

Table 3.5 Indications for restoration and extraction of primary teeth

	Indications for restoration	Indications for extraction
Medical factors	Patients at risk of an extraction (e.g. bleeding disorders)	Extensive caries in patients at risk of infection (e.g. patients at increased risk of infective endocarditis, immunocompromised patients)
Dental factors	Restorable tooth	Unrestorable tooth
	To prevent space loss following early loss of primary teeth	Presence of pathology (e.g. extensive internal resorption or facial swelling requiring emergency treatment)
	Hypodontia	Tooth close to exfoliation (<1/3 root remaining)
	Adhere to preventative advice	Balancing/compensating extractions
Social factors	Regular dental attender	Irregular attender
	Compliant patient	Poor compliance
	Function and aesthetics	

Techniques without removal of caries

No caries removal and seal in caries

Rationale: seal carious lesion from oral environment to slow or arrest progression:

- Fissure sealants can be used over non-cavitated pit or fissure caries.
- For more extensive lesions, use of Hall technique is more appropriate.

Hall technique
- Involves sealing caries into primary molars using a PMC without the use of LA.
- Indications:
  - Hypomineralized primary molars.
  - Class I and II lesions with restorable crowns.
  - Pulp involvement excluded.
  - Patients lacking cooperative ability for conventional techniques.
- Contraindications:
  - Signs/symptoms of irreversible pulpitis or loss of vitality.
  - Unrestorable crown.
  - Children at increased risk of infection (e.g. immunocompromised patients, those at increased risk of infective endocarditis).
  - Tooth close to exfoliation.
- Advantages:
  - Does not require use of LA.
  - Full coverage restoration providing effective coronal seal.
- Disadvantages:
  - Requires careful case selection.
  - Requires a degree of cooperation from the child.
  - Child can experience discomfort.
  - Some families have aesthetic concerns with the use of silver PMCs.
- Preparation:
  - Advise the child and parent/guardian what to expect.
  - Tell the child they will need to help by biting the crown into place.
  - Explain that the cement ('special tooth glue') won't taste very nice but that the taste will go away.
  - Warn that there may be some discomfort postoperatively and the child's 'bite' may be temporarily altered for 1–2 weeks (an anterior open bite following cementation is common).
- Procedure[1]:
  - Placement of separators mesially and distally to the tooth to be crowned for 5–7 days prior to cementation may facilitate fitting of the crown by temporarily separating the teeth.
  - Remove separators prior to fitting crown.
  - Protect airway with gauze and consider keeping the child sat upright in the dental chair.
  - Select PMC and perform trial fit taking care not to fully seat the crown as it may be difficult to remove.
  - Load crown with glass ionomer cement (GIC).
  - Fit the crown and remove excess cement.
  - Check the fit and if adequate, encourage patient to bite on a cotton wool roll as hard as they can to fully seat the crown (playing a 'tug-of-war' with the cotton wool roll at this stage encourages the child to continue biting and provides some distraction from any discomfort/taste of the cement). If fit is poor, quickly remove crown using excavator prior to cement setting.

1 Evans D (2010). The Hall technique: a minimal intervention, child centred approach to managing the carious primary molar. A users manual. ℘ https://heeoe.hee.nhs.uk/sites/default/files/1311845532_nqvh_the_hall_technique_manual.pdf

- Remove excess cement and check occlusion (an anterior open bit of up to 2 mm is acceptable). Adjust crown if necessary.
- Clinical and radiographic review as indicated by patient's caries risk assessment.
- Success: 92% (minimum follow-up of 48 months).[2]

Partial caries removal and restoration

- Rationale: to remove sufficient caries and obtain an effective coronal seal to prevent progression of caries left at base of the cavity.
- Indications:
  - Arrested, carious lesions affecting primary incisors.
  - Class I and II lesions with restorable crowns.
  - Pulp involvement excluded.
  - Patients lacking cooperative ability for conventional techniques.
- Contraindications:
  - Signs/symptoms of irreversible pulpitis or loss of vitality.
  - Unrestorable crown.
  - Children at increased risk of infection (e.g. immunocompromised patients, those at increased risk of infective endocarditis).
- Advantages:
  - Minimally invasive and therefore reduced risk of pulp exposure.
  - Does not require use of LA.
- Disadvantages:
  - Limited evidence for effectiveness.
  - Requires careful case selection.
  - If marginal seal is lost, caries will progress increasing risk of symptoms.
- Procedure:
  - If needed, gain access to caries using high-speed handpiece (take care not to encroach upon sound dentine which could be painful for the child).
  - Remove superficial caries and caries at the amelodental junction with sharp excavator or rose head bur in slow handpiece avoiding a pulp exposure.
  - Place adhesive restoration.
  - For posterior teeth place fissure seal over restoration and sound occlusal fissures.
  - Close clinical and radiographic review.
- Success[3]:
  - Class I cavities: ~79% (30-month follow-up).
  - Class II cavities: ~ 51% (30-month follow-up).

Techniques with complete caries removal

Strip crowns for primary incisors
- Indications:
  - Extensive or multi-surface caries.
  - Developmental enamel defects.
  - Fractured incisors.

2 Innes N (2011). *J Dent Res* 90, 1405.

3 Lo E (2001). *Int J Paed Dent* 11, 3.

- Amelogenesis imperfecta.
- Dentinogenesis imperfecta.
- Discoloured incisors.
- Procedure:
  - Preoperative sectional silicone putty impression could be taken at an earlier visit to obtain study model upon which the crown forms could be trimmed to minimize chairside time.
  - LA should be used unless minimal use of handpieces is anticipated (e.g. the incisors are spaced removing the need for interproximal reduction and the carious lesion is shallow) and minimal manipulation of the gingival tissues will take place.
  - Remove caries with a rose head bur in a slow handpiece.
  - Incisal 1 mm reduction with high-speed diamond bur.
  - Mesial and distal slices with high-speed tapered diamond bur.
  - Fit the trimmed crown forms and check the occlusion. A common cause of failure of strip crowns is loss of the crown due to occlusal error.
  - Etch entire tooth with 37% phosphoric acid, wash and dry tooth.
  - Apply bonding agent to entire tooth surface, gentle air dry to evaporate solvent, then cure.
  - Where discoloration is present, use of a thin layer of opaque composite over the discoloured tooth tissue is advised.
  - Fill crown form with composite taking care not to overfill the crown form by hollowing out composite in the middle of the crown form. Overfilling the crown increases the risk of the crown form splitting when it is seated.
  - Seat the crown forms, one at a time, on the prepared teeth.
  - Remove excess composite at the margins with a probe.
  - Cure composite from labial and palatal aspect.
  - Remove crown form by using small excavator at the margin. Where is it difficult to remove the crown form, use a coarse soft-flex disc to remove the incisal edge of the crown form then lift the remaining crown form away with a small excavator.
  - Smooth and polish composite crowns.
  - Check the occlusion and adjust length of crowns as needed.

Plastic restorations: class II restorations
- Indications:
  - Small one- or two-surface carious lesions where >50% marginal ridge is intact and pulp involvement excluded.
- Procedure:
  - Administer LA and place rubber dam.
  - Access through marginal ridge with jet 330 bur avoiding iatrogenic damage to adjacent tooth.
  - Walls of cavity should be parallel to the external tooth surface.
  - Following caries removal, place matrix band and wedge to achieve correct adaptation of matrix band.
  - Etch and bond prepared cavity and entire occlusal surface.
  - Place definitive composite restoration then fissure seal over top of restoration and sound occlusal surface (NB: avoid GIC for class II cavities due to high failure rate).
  - Where rubber dam is not used, consider use of amalgam.

Conventional PMCs
- Success of PMCs > plastic restorations.
- Indications:
  - Primary molars requiring multi-surface restorations.
  - Restoration of primary molars in high caries risk cases.
  - Following pulp therapy.
  - Restoration of primary molars with developmental defects (e.g. amelogenesis imperfecta (AI), dentinogenesis imperfecta (DI), or hypomineralized second primary molar).
  - Molars with extensive tooth surface loss.
- Contraindications:
  - Child lacking cooperative ability to allow safe placement.
- Procedure:
  - Following LA and rubber dam placement. Remove caries if present.
  - Reduce occlusal height by 1 mm using high-speed diamond bur.
  - Using a high-speed tapered tungsten carbide or diamond bur, perform mesial and distal slices ensuring the contacts have been cleared so that no ledges are left. Ledges will prevent the PMC from fully seating. Round any sharp edges.
  - Select a crown and perform trial fit. Crowns should be placed from the palatal/lingual aspect first then rotated to the buccal aspect to fully seat. Ideally, the crown should 'snap' on to the tooth.
  - When the crown is loose or does not snap on to the tooth, a smaller size should be tried. Crimping pliers may be needed to bend in the crown margins to improve the fit. *The margins of PMCs for primary molars should not be adjusted with scissors.*
  - Once happy with the fit, the PMC should be cemented with GIC. Apply pressure on the occlusal aspect of the crown to ensure the crown is fully seated as the cement starts to set.
  - Remove the excess around the edges of the crown with a probe and use floss interproximally.
- Tip: if struggling to find a well-fitting crown for a lower first primary molar, use contralateral upper first primary molar crown instead (i.e. fit PMC for URD on LLD and vice versa).
- Success: 70–98%.[4]

Pulp therapy

Indirect pulp cap
- Performed to arrest caries and encourage remineralization of carious dentine to allow pulp healing.[5]
- Careful tooth selection required.
- Indications:
  - Restorable tooth.
  - Absence of signs or symptoms of irreversible pulpitis/loss of vitality.
- Contraindications:
  - Unrestorable tooth.
  - Spontaneous pain/signs of loss of vitality (e.g. chronic sinus/ interradicular radiolucency upon radiographic examination).

4 Attari N (2006). *Eur Arch Paed Dent* 7, 58.

5 Rodd HD (2006). *Int J Paediatr Dent* 16 (Suppl 1), 15.

- Immunocompromised children or those at risk of infection (e.g. increased risk of infective endocarditis).
- Procedure:
  - Caries removal under LA and rubber dam.
  - Removal of all caries at enamel–dentine junction.
  - Careful removal of soft deep caries using hand excavator (or large rose head bur) taking care to avoid a pulpal exposure.
  - Placement of non-setting calcium hydroxide (NSCH) plus resin-modified GIC/mineral trioxide aggregate (MTA)/other biocompatible material GIC base prior to restoration (ideally PMC for primary molars).
- Success rates: >90% at 3 years:
  - Cavitated occlusal caries > cavitated proximal caries.
  - Second primary molars > first primary molars.
  - PMC > plastic restoration.

Direct pulp cap

Not recommended for primary molars due to low success rates.

Pulpotomy

- Vital pulp procedure.
- Involves removal of the coronal pulp tissue leaving vital, non-inflamed radicular pulp *in situ*.
- Indications:
  - Large proximal carious lesions with ≥1/3 marginal ridge breakdown.
  - Carious/mechanical exposure of vital pulp.
  - No history of spontaneous pain.
  - No history or signs of infection (abscess or sinus tract).
  - Haemostasis of radicular pulp stumps achieved.
  - Cases where extractions should be minimized where possible (e.g. children with bleeding disorders).
- Contraindications:
  - Children at increased risk of infective endocarditis.
  - Children who are immunocompromised (e.g. those undergoing chemotherapy).
- Procedure:
  - Administer LA and place rubber dam.
  - Remove caries and access the pulp chamber with a high-speed non-end cutting bur (e.g. flat fissure diamond bur).
  - Remove the entire roof of the pulp chamber taking care not to move the bur any deeper to avoid perforating the floor of the pulp chamber.
  - Remove the coronal pulp with a sharp large excavator or slow-speed handpiece with a large rose head bur.
  - Apply the medicament as follows:
  - For ferric sulphate (FeSO$_4$) pulpotomy: apply FeSO$_4$ to the radicular pulp stumps with a cotton pledget for 15 seconds. Remove cotton pledget and ensure haemostasis has occurred. Rinse and dry then restore pulp chamber (e.g. with zinc oxide eugenol cement/Biodentine™) ensuring it is well condensed over the pulp stumps.

- For MTA pulpotomy technique: apply cotton pledget soaked in saline on to radicular pulp stumps with pressure for a maximum of 60 seconds. Ensure haemostasis prior to applying MTA paste to radicular pulp stumps and at least 1 mm beyond the amelodentinal junction. Restore pulp chamber with zinc oxide eugenol cement/GIC/Biodentine™.
- *Where the pulp is hyperaemic or where haemostasis is not easily achieved, a decision regarding whether the radicular pulp tissue is irreversibly inflamed needs to be made. In this case, extraction or pulpectomy is indicated.*
- Place coronal restoration (ideally PMC).
- Success:
  - >90% at 2 years.
  - No clear evidence to suggest superiority of either MTA or FeSO$_4$.[6]

Pulpectomy
- Non-vital pulp procedure.
- Performed to remove irreversibly inflamed/necrotic pulp prior to cleaning and filling the root canals with a suitable resorbable material.
- Indications:
  - Non-vital tooth/irreversible pulpitis.
  - Good patient compliance.
  - Restorable tooth.
  - >2/3 root length remaining.
- Contraindications:
  - Unrestorable tooth.
  - Extensively carious dentition.
  - Advanced pathological root resorption.
  - Children at risk of infection.
  - Child lacking cooperative ability for whom treatment under LA is not possible.
- Procedure:
  - Preoperative radiograph showing entire root length and apices.
  - LA and rubber dam.
  - Remove caries and roof of pulp chamber and any remains of coronal pulp tissue.
  - Note whether radicular pulp is bleeding or necrotic (usually requires a two-stage procedure).
  - Identify root canals.
  - Irrigate with normal saline (0.9%), chlorhexidine solution (0.4%), or sodium hypochlorite (0.1%).
  - Estimate working lengths of root canals keeping 2 mm short of the radiographic apex.
  - Insert small files (less than size 30) into canals and gently file canal walls.
  - If infection present, dress root canals with NSCH and temporize (two-stage procedure).
  - If canals can be dried with paper points, fill canals with iodoform paste (e.g. Vitapex®) or NSCH.

6 Smail-Faugeron V (2014). *Cochrane Database Syst Rev* 8, CD003220.

- • Place definitive restoration (ideally PMC).
- • Take postoperative periapical.
- Clinical and radiographic review. Where pathology persists, extraction is indicated.
- Success rate: 86% at 3 years.

Paediatric restorative techniques for the permanent dentition

Hypomineralized FPMs

- Composite is the restorative material of choice for hypomineralized FPMs where a plastic restoration is indicated.
- Indications:
  - Well-demarcated enamel defects confined to one or two surfaces.
  - Supragingival margins.
- Contraindications:
  - Extensive multi-surface defects.
  - Non-demarcated defects.
- Procedure:
  - Under LA and rubber dam.
  - Caries removal.
  - Two different approaches to the removal of hypomineralized enamel have been reported: (1) removal of all defective enamel, and (2) removal of porous enamel with slow-speed rose head bur until resistance to the bur is felt (less destructive approach).
  - Etch and bond entire tooth surface.
  - Reduced bond strengths to hypomineralized enamel have been reported and therefore some advocate the use of two layers of bond for hypomineralized teeth.
  - Incremental restoration with composite.
  - Fissure seal over restoration and any sound fissures and grooves.
  - Check occlusion.
- Close clinical and radiographic review paying particular attention to the margins of the restoration.

Onlays

- Indications:
  - Amelogenesis imperfecta.
  - Dentinogenesis imperfecta.
  - Selected cases of hypomineralized enamel (MIH).
  - Teeth deemed of good long-term prognosis.
- Contraindications:
  - Cases where a full coverage restoration/extraction is preferable.
- Procedure:
  - Silicone impression (light-bodied silicone around the tooth and heavy-bodied silicone placed in impression tray) taken then cast metal onlays constructed.
  - Often, no tooth preparation is carried out in order to conserve the remaining tooth tissue.
  - Cementation of onlay with resin cement under LA and rubber dam to ensure moisture control.
  - Inevitably causes a transient anterior open bite due to the absence of occlusal reduction.

Preformed metal crowns

- PMCs for permanent molar teeth may be indicated in the following situations:
  - Moderate to severely hypomineralized FPMs where their extraction is contraindicated (e.g. developmentally absent second premolars).
  - Amelogenesis imperfecta.
  - Dentinogenesis imperfecta.
  - Following root canal treatment of permanent molars in children.
- Contraindications:
  - Tooth unrestorable.
  - Extensive defects in FPMs where all permanent teeth are present, and patient's dental age is around the ideal time for planned loss of FPMs.
- Procedure:
  - Under LA and rubber dam.
  - Remove caries and hypomineralized enamel until resistance with slow-speed rose head bur is felt.
  - Occlusal reduction 1 mm (unless occlusal height is already reduced, e.g. through post-eruptive breakdown (PEB)).
  - Mesial and distal interproximal slices.
  - Choose appropriately sized PMC and trim ~1 mm around the cervical margin of PMC using Bebe scissors.
  - Trial fit and trim PMC further as required.
  - Check occlusion.
  - Remove PMC and smooth sharp edges with stone in a slow-speed straight handpiece. Margins of PMC may need to be crimped inwards.
  - Re-check fit of PMC.
  - Cement PMC with GIC.
  - Check occlusion and adjust if needed.

Pulp cap therapy

Indirect pulp cap
For procedure, see ⬧ Pulp therapy.

Direct pulp cap
- Indications:
  - Small carious exposures.
  - Asymptomatic teeth.
  - No history of swelling.
  - Haemostasis achieved at exposure site.
  - No radiographic signs of PA pathology.
- Contraindications:
  - Crown unrestorable.
  - Immunocompromised patients or those at increased risk of infection (e.g. increased risk of infective endocarditis).
  - Where extraction would be preferable (e.g. to address any orthodontic concerns).

- Procedure:
  - Under LA and rubber dam, if pulp exposure occurs, place NSCH plus GIC/MTA/other biocompatible material on exposure prior to definitive restoration.
- Close clinical and radiographic monitoring for signs and symptoms of loss of vitality.

Partial pulpotomy following trauma

- Not to be confused with the pulpotomy technique for carious primary molar teeth (➔ Chapter 10).

Pulpectomy (root canal treatment)

- Where apical development is complete, root canal treatment for permanent teeth in paediatric patients is as for adult patients.
- For the management of non-vital immature permanent incisors, see ➔ Management of the non-vital immature permanent incisor.

Management of the immature non-vital central incisor

Definition

An immature tooth is one in which the apex is open, that is, a size 60 gutta-percha (GP) point can be passed through the apex without resistance.

Classification

According to the shape of the open apices:
- Tapering walls.
- Parallel walls.
- Divergent root canals.

Management

Referral to specialist as management can be challenging due to the thinness of the dentine walls, the size of the apex, and the cooperative ability of the child.

Calcium hydroxide apexification

- Less commonly used as prolonged use of calcium hydroxide within root canals increases the risk of root fractures.[1,2]
- Involves placement of intracanal NSCH dressing after pulp extirpation and chemo-mechanical cleansing of the root canal. NSCH dressing is changed every 3 months (or sooner if a defect within the dressing is noted following radiographic examination) until an apical barrier is detected with the gentle use of a paper point.
- Mean time of barrier detection reported as 43.3 weeks.[3]
- Disadvantages:
  - Multiple visits.
  - No qualitative increase in root dimensions.
  - Increased risk of root fracture (40% risk of cervical root fracture after 4 years of follow-up).[1]

Apical plug

- Involves the placement of an MTA/Biodentine™ plug at the apex.
- Advantages:
  - Reduced number of visits.
  - Good biocompatibility.
- Disadvantages:
  - Can be technically demanding.
  - Care is needed to minimize MTA being deposited along the root canal walls as the high pH of MTA will denature proteins and increase the risk of root fracture.
  - Potential cost implications.

---

1 Cvek M (1992). *Endod Dent Traumatol* 8, 45.

2 Rosenberg B (2007). *Dent Traumatol* 23, 26.

3 Kinirons M (2001). *Int J Paediatr Dent* 11, 447.

GP apical plug

- Some advocate the use of a GP apical plug in immature teeth with tapering walls to avoid the risk of MTA being smeared onto the walls of the root canal during the placement of an MTA plug.
- Not a well-documented technique.

Regenerative endodontic therapy

- Aim is to achieve continued root development and deposition of dentine and cementum.
- Procedure involves pulp extirpation and placement of antibiotic paste (metronidazole and ciprofloxacin) within the root canal until there is resolution of infection. Second stage involves instrumentation beyond the apex under LA to induce formation of a blood clot in the canal prior to placement of MTA, GI, then composite.
- Previously, a triple antibiotic paste was used (metronidazole, ciprofloxacin, and minocycline) but minocycline has since been omitted as a result of discoloration of the crown.
- Further studies are required.

Dental developmental anomalies

Abnormalities of tooth number

Hypodontia

See ➔ Hypodontia.

Supernumerary teeth ($)

Definition

- Presence of teeth additional to the normal series.

Aetiology

- Multifactorial with a strong genetic component.

Prevalence

- Primary dentition: 0.3–0.6%.
- Permanent dentition: 1–3.5%.
- Affects maxilla > mandible by 9:1 ratio.
- Males > females.

Classification according to morphology

- Conical (peg-shaped):
  - Most common $ (~75%).
  - Often presents as a mesiodens in the anterior maxilla.
  - May erupt spontaneously.
  - Can cause rotation/displacement of upper permanent incisors but rarely delays their eruption.
- Tuberculate (~12%):
  - Barrel shaped, possess more than one cusp.
  - Commonly found palatal to upper central incisors.
  - Associated with delayed/failure of eruption of the incisors.
- Supplemental (~7%):
  - Resembles a tooth.
  - Often occurs at the end of a series (e.g. additional lateral incisors, second premolar, or a fourth molar).
  - Majority of $ in the primary dentition are supplemental.
- Odontome (~6%):
  - Not universally accepted as a $.
  - Tumour of odontogenic origin which can be classified according to their degree of morpho-differentiation.
  - *Complex*: diffuse mass of disorganized dental tissue.
  - *Compound*: some anatomical similarities to a normal tooth. Denticles may be seen.

Classification according to position

- Mesiodens: between the upper central incisors.
- Distomolar: distal to the arch.
- Paramolar: adjacent to the molar teeth.

Management

- Often a multidisciplinary approach is required.
- Exact management depends upon the type of $ and its effects.
- May involve extraction of the $ or close clinical and radiographic monitoring (Table 3.6).

Table 3.6 Indication for removal and monitoring of supernumerary teeth

Indications for extraction	Indications for monitoring
Delayed/altered eruption of incisor	Satisfactory eruption of adjacent teeth
Pathology associated with $, e.g. cyst	No associated pathology
Active orthodontic alignment of incisor close to $	No active orthodontic treatment planned
$ would compromise alveolar bone grafting in cleft patients	$ would not compromise any future surgical procedures
$ would affect placement of implants when indicated	$ asymptomatic
Following spontaneous eruption of $	High risk of damage to adjacent teeth during surgical removal

Associated dental anomalies
- ~50% of cases of $ in primary dentition also have $ affecting permanent dentition.

Commonly associated conditions
- Cleidocranial dysplasia.
- Cleft lip and palate.
- Gardner syndrome.
- Apert syndrome.

Abnormalities in tooth size

Microdontia
See ➔ Microdontia.

Macrodontia

Definition
- Refers to teeth that are larger in size.

Aetiology
- Multifactorial. Environmental and genetic factors have been suggested.

Prevalence
- Rare.
- Permanent dentition: 1%.
- Upper central incisors most commonly affected followed by lower second premolars and third molars.

Management
- Dependent upon the effects of the macrodont, that is, the presence and severity of crowding and the dental aesthetics.
- May require multidisciplinary approach with orthodontics.
- Could involve:
  - acceptance and no treatment
  - reshaping the crown (macrodont may require elective root canal treatment which can be complicated by abnormal root canal morphology and therefore has a low success rate)

- aesthetic coronal restoration
- extraction and prosthetic replacement as part of an orthodontic treatment plan.

Associated dental anomalies

Generalized macrodontia has been described with other anomalies including invaginations and evaginations affecting premolars (➔ Invaginations).

Commonly associated conditions

- Unilateral facial hyperplasia (localized macrodontia).
- Pituitary gigantism (generalized macrodontia).

Abnormalities of dental morphology

Double teeth

Definition

- Double teeth is the preferred term to describe when two teeth appear joined together. Varied presentation from a small notch in the incisal edge of a wider than normal tooth to the appearance of two almost separate crowns with a common root.
- Replaces the previous terms of germination and fusion.

Aetiology

- Multifactorial with genetic factors implicated.

Prevalence

- Primary dentition: 0.5–1.6%.
- Permanent dentition: 0.1–0.2%.
- Males = females.
- Upper and lower incisors most commonly affected.

Management

- Usually multidisciplinary where crowding is present.
- Could involve:
  - acceptance and no treatment
  - reshaping the crown
  - aesthetic restoration
  - extraction.

Associated dental anomalies

Anomalies in the permanent dentition occur in 30–50% of cases where there are double teeth in the primary dentition.

Accessory cusps

Most commonly affect the molar teeth and occur in the primary and permanent dentition.

- Cusp of Carabelli:
  - Located on the palatal surface of the mesiolingual cusp of maxillary molars.
  - If there is a deep groove present, this should be sealed with a fissure sealant.
- Talon cusp:
  - Located on the palatal surface of anterior teeth and extends at least halfway from the cementoenamel junction (CEJ) to the incisal edge.
  - Permanent > primary dentition.

- May require intervention for both aesthetic and functional reasons if it causes occlusal interference. Prior to intervention, the pulp size and morphology should be determined by radiographic examination. Management options include selective reduction of the cusp over time or sectioning the cusp from the tooth often combined with an elective partial pulpotomy (➲ Pulp therapy).

Invaginations

Definition

- Refers to a defect characterized by a palatal pit which may extend beyond the CEJ.
- Also referred to as 'dens in dente'.

Classification

- Oehlers classification (1957):
  - Type 1: invagination is lined by enamel and confined within the crown.
  - Type II: enamel-lined invagination extends apically beyond the CEJ. It may/may not communicate with pulpal tissue but never reaches the periapical tissue.
  - Type III A: invagination extends through the root and communicates laterally with the PDL space. There is usually no communication with the pulp tissue.
  - Type III B: invagination extends through the root and communicates with the PDL at the apical foramen. Usually no communication with the pulp.

Aetiology

Early invagination of the enamel epithelium into the dental papilla with local and genetic factors implicated.

Prevalence

- Primary dentition: rare.
- Permanent dentition: 0.3–10%.[1]
- Most frequently affects the maxillary permanent lateral incisor.
- Occur bilaterally in ~40% of cases.

Management

- Where palatal pits are seen clinically, these should be fissure sealed. Palatal invaginations may also be visible on radiographs.
- There is a risk of pulp necrosis where the invagination communicates with the pulp tissue. Where pulp necrosis has occurred, root canal treatment can be complicated by abnormal root canal morphology and a specialist referral may therefore be indicated.

Dilaceration

Definition

- Refers to a deviation in the long axis of a tooth.
- Most frequently affects the maxillary permanent central incisor.

---

1 International Endodontic Journal, 41, 1123–1136, 2008

Aetiology
Can be developmental or result from trauma to the primary predecessor:
- Developmental:
  - Crown deviated upwards and labially.
  - Enamel and dentine formation normal.
  - Females > males.
- Traumatic:
  - Palatal deviation of crown.
  - Enamel and/or dentine defects may be seen.
  - No sex predilection.
  - Often caused by intrusion of the primary predecessor during the developmental stages of the permanent tooth.
  - Usually causes failure of eruption.

Management
- Dependent on severity. May involve:
  - composite restoration
  - orthodontic repositioning
  - surgical exposure and orthodontic alignment
  - extraction and replacement.

Turner teeth
- Refers to enamel ± dentinal defects of permanent teeth (often premolars) resulting from chronic infection associated with the overlying primary teeth.
- Management depends upon severity and may involve the placement of restorations or extraction of the affected tooth/teeth.

Taurodontism
Radiographic appearance of a molar tooth in which the pulp chamber is enlarged, there is apical displacement of the pulpal floor, and reduced/no constriction at the level of the CEJ.

Enamel defects

Classification of enamel defects
Enamel defects arise when there is a disturbance during one of the stages of amelogenesis (secretory, mineralization, maturation). There are two main categories of enamel defects:
- Hypoplasia:
  - Defect during secretory stage of amelogenesis resulting in hypoplastic enamel which is fully mineralized but of abnormal morphology due to disrupted matrix formation.
  - Quantitative defect.
- Hypomineralization:
  - Hypocalcified: defect during the mineralization stage of amelogenesis resulting in poorly mineralized teeth which are of normal morphology.
  - Hypomature: defective protein withdrawal during the maturational stage of amelogenesis.
  - Qualitative defects.

Diagnosis of enamel defects

History

- Positive family history of enamel defects.*
- Obstetric history:**
  - Maternal illness during pregnancy (e.g. cytomegalovirus).
  - Birth trauma.
  - Preterm.
  - Low birth weight.
  - History of neonatal intubation (can result in localized enamel defects in the anterior region).
- Medical history:**
  - Nutritional deficiencies.
  - Renal and liver disease.
  - Endocrine disorders (e.g. hypocalcaemia, hypoglycaemia).
  - Coeliac disease.
  - Cardiac defects.
  - Cleft lip and palate.
  - Bacterial/viral infections during amelogenesis.
  - Chemotherapy/radiotherapy.
- Dental history:
  - Trauma to primary dentition.***
  - Chronic infection of primary teeth.***
  - Generalized defects affecting primary and permanent dentition.*
  - History of excessive fluoride intake.

(* Consistent with a diagnosis of AI; ** may lead to chronological defects; *** associated with localized defects).

Examination

- Ensure teeth are clean.
- Examine the teeth for:
  - white/brown/yellow opacities
  - abnormal morphology which could represent enamel hypoplasia or PEB (Box 3.6)
  - atypical restorations
  - previous extraction of FPMs which could have been due to molar–incisor hypomineralization.

Box 3.6 Differences between hypoplasia and PEB associated with hypomineralization

- Hypoplasia:
  - Enamel usually of normal colour.
  - Enamel feels hard to gentle probing.
  - Margins of defective enamel often smooth.
- PEB:
  - Enamel often discoloured (e.g. white/yellow/brown defects).
  - Enamel feels soft to gentle probing.
  - Margins where PEB has occurred are irregular.

- Teeth with enamel defects can be *hypersensitive* and therefore *careful use of the air from the triple syringe is required*. Where a history of sensitivity is given, consider using cotton wool rolls to dry the teeth instead of air from the triple syringe.
- Determine whether the defects are localized (i.e. affecting a small number of teeth), generalized (i.e. affecting all the teeth), or chronological (i.e. affecting the teeth that form during the same time frame) to assist your diagnosis.
- Where enamel defects are identified, clinical examination should be supported by radiographic examination for caries diagnosis.

Amelogenesis imperfecta
See ➋ Amelogenesis imperfecta.

Molar incisor hypomineralization

Definition
- Hypomineralization of one or more FPM teeth often associated with hypomineralized permanent incisors.

Presentation
- Affected teeth show well-demarcated yellow/brown/white defects which tend to be asymmetrically distributed.
- In severe cases, PEB may be seen.

Aetiology
- Environmental insult during the calcification or maturation stages of amelogenesis (usually between 18th week of gestation and 3 years of age).

Prevalence
- Ranges from 2.8% to 40.2% depending upon the population studied.[2]

Management
- Referral for a specialist opinion is often indicated as management can be complicated by the young age at presentation, presence of behaviour management problems and difficulties achieving LA in some cases.[3]
- Early diagnosis is essential.
- Intensive prevention:
  - Including oral hygiene instruction, diet analysis, and regular fluoride varnish applications.
  - Care with placement of resin-based fissure sealants due to hypersensitivity. GIC sealants are preferable in these cases after using cotton wool (not air from 3-in-1) to dry the teeth.
  - Daily home-application of casein phosphopeptide-amorphous calcium phosphate (e.g. GC Tooth Mousse®) may be beneficial for those experiencing hypersensitivity—creates a supersaturated solution of calcium and phosphate that deposits at the enamel surface. Contraindicated in patients with milk allergies.
- Definitive operative management for posterior teeth may involve composite restorations, PMCs, or extractions.

2 Jälevik B (2010). *Eur Arch Paediatr Dent* 11, 59.
3 Lygidakis N (2010). *Eur Arch Paediatr Dent* 11, 75.

- Operative management for affected incisors is guided by any aesthetic concerns reported by the child and may involve micro-abrasion, resin infiltration, bleaching, and anterior composite restorations.

Associated conditions
- Hypersensitivity of affected teeth.
- Post eruptive breakdown.
- Increased susceptibility to dental caries.
- Rapid caries progression.
- Behaviour management problems and dental anxiety in children with severe defects[4]:
  - By 10 years of age, children with severe defects were shown to have undergone treatment on their FPMs nearly 10× more frequently than control children.

Hypomineralized second primary molars
Also referred to as deciduous molar hypomineralization.

Definition
- Hypomineralization affecting the enamel of one or all of the second primary molars.

Presentation
- As for MIH but involving second primary molars.

Aetiology
- Same risk factors as for MIH as there is some overlap in the developmental stages of the FPMs, permanent incisors, and second primary molars.
- Enamel of the second primary molars starts to form around the 13th week of gestation to around 3 years of age when they erupt.

Prevalence
- 9%.[5]

Management
- Dependent upon severity, presence of symptoms, and cooperative ability of the child.
- Intensive prevention (➔ Prevention).
- Can also involve:
  - placement of GIC sealants
  - PMCs via the Hall technique
  - conventional PMCs under LA if the child is deemed to have sufficient cooperative ability
  - extraction.

Associated conditions
- Increased risk of caries of the affected primary molars.
- Hypersensitivity.
- MIH.[2]

4 Jälevik B (2002). *Int J Paediatr Dent* 12, 24.
5 Elfrink M (2012) *J Dent Res* 91, 551.

Fluorosis

Definition
- Developmental disturbance of dental enamel caused by excessive exposure to high concentrations of fluoride during tooth development.
- Qualitative defect of enamel.

Presentation
- Types: demarcated, diffuse, hypoplastic, combinations.

Classification
Dean's fluorosis index (1942):
- Normal (0): smooth, glossy, white translucent surface.
- Questionable (1): a few white spots.
- Very mild (2): small white areas scattered over 10–25% of the surface of the tooth.
- Mild (3): white opaque areas involving 25–50% of the tooth.
- Moderate (4): all enamel surfaces affected. Brown discolouration is often present.
- Severe (5): all enamel surfaces affected. Hypoplasia present and brown discolouration.

There are other specific indices for fluorosis such as the Total Tooth Surface Index (TSIF) and the Fluorosis Risk Index (FRI).
   The modified Developmental Defects of Enamel (DDE) index could also be used.

Dentine defects
See ➲ Dental defects.

Periodontal diseases in children

Gingival diseases

Plaque-induced gingivitis

- Primary aetiological agent = plaque.
- Local and systemic factors can modify the host's response:
  - *Local risk factors*: high fraenal attachments, fixed appliances, plaque retention factors, incompetent lips, mouth breathing.
  - *Systemic risk factors*: poorly controlled diabetes mellitus, medication.
- Can occur at any age, often with a peak prevalence around puberty.
- Important to diagnose and manage as teeth with consistently inflamed gingiva showed greater clinical attachment loss (CAL) and tooth loss.[1]
- Management: oral hygiene instruction and regular review.

Necrotizing ulcerative gingivitis

- Presentation:
  - Pain.
  - Necrosis of interdental papillae ('punched out' appearance).
  - Secondary foetor oris (halitosis).
  - Pseudo-membrane may be present.
- Fusiform-spirochaetal microbial aetiology.
- Risk factors: smoking, immunosuppression, stress, malnutrition.
- May be associated with human immunodeficiency virus (HIV).
- May progress to necrotizing ulcerative periodontitis.
- Management:
  - Consider referral to paediatrics to exclude undiagnosed immunosuppression.

Non-plaque-induced gingival lesions

- Bacterial infections: rare in children.
- Viral infections:
  - Human herpesviruses (HHVs; e.g. primary herpetic gingivostomatitis).
  - Varicella zoster virus (VZV; chicken pox).
  - Coxsackie virus (herpangina).
- Fungal infections: candidosis, linear gingival erythema (HIV-associated candidosis).
- Genetic: hereditary gingival fibromatosis.
- Manifestations of systemic disease:
  - Haematological: neutropenia, acute lymphoblastic leukaemia.
  - Granulomatous inflammation: Crohn's disease, sarcoidosis, tuberculosis.
  - Immunological: lichen planus, hypersensitivity reactions.
- Trauma: chemical/physical/thermal.
- Foreign body reactions (e.g. amalgam tattoo).
- Drug induced:
  - Immune complex reactions (erythema multiforme, lichenoid drug reactions).
  - Cytotoxic drugs (e.g. methotrexate).
  - Antiretroviral drugs.

1 ॐ www.bsperio.org.uk

The classification of periodontal diseases has been updated (2017)[1] (➲ Classification of periodontal diseases). The guidelines for periodontal screening and management in children have been updated to include this latest information (latest guidelines 2021).[2]

Generalized periodontitis (grade A, B), previously chronic periodontitis

- Presentation:
  - CAL.
  - Apical migration of junctional epithelium.
  - Alveolar bone loss.
- Prevalence of CAL of >1 mm on at least one of the molar, premolar, or incisor teeth increased from 3% to 77% in a 5-year longitudinal study of 14 to 19-year-olds.[2]
- Local and systemic risk factors.
- Slow/moderate progression.
- Periodontal pathogens: *Porphyromonas gingivalis*, *Prevotella intermedia*, *Aggregatibacter actinomycetemcomitans*.
- Management:
  - Early diagnosis and referral to specialist in periodontology or paediatric dentistry.
  - Intensive periodontal therapy.
- Oral hygiene instruction should be provided and reinforced in primary care.

Periodontitis (grade C), previously aggressive periodontitis

- Common features:
  - Patients healthy except for periodontitis.
  - Rapid attachment loss and bone destruction.
  - Familial aggregation.
- Secondary features:
  - Amounts of deposits are consistent with severity of periodontal of periodontal disease.
  - Increased proportions of *A. actinomycetemcomitans*.
  - Host defence defects.
  - Hyper-responsive macrophage phenotype.
  - Progression of attachment loss and bone loss may be self-arresting.
- Localized and generalized forms (Table 3.7):
  - Localized AP may affect around 0.1% of white Caucasians and 2.6% of black Africans.
  - Management:
  - Early diagnosis and referral to specialist in periodontology or paediatric dentistry.
  - Intensive periodontal therapy required with adjunctive microbial therapy.
  - Oral hygiene instruction should be provided and reinforced in primary care.

2 Clerehugh V (2021). Guidelines for periodontal screening and management of children and adolescents under 18 years of age. ℑ www.bspd.co.uk

Table 3.7 Localized and generalized forms of aggressive periodontitis

Localized aggressive periodontitis	Generalized aggressive periodontitis
Onset around puberty	Usually affects patients <30 years old
Robust serum antibody response	Poor serum antibody response
Localized interproximal CAL on at least two permanent teeth, one of which is a first molar, and involving no more than two teeth other than first molars/incisors	Generalized interproximal CAL affecting at least three permanent teeth other than first molars and incisors
	Pronounced episodic nature

Periodontitis as a manifestation of systemic disease

- Haematological disorders:
  - Neutropenia.
  - Leukaemia.
- Genetic disorders:
  - Down syndrome.
  - Papillon–Lefèvre syndrome.
  - Chediak–Higashi syndrome.
  - Ehlers–Danlos syndrome (types IV and VIII).
  - Hypophosphatasia.

Necrotizing periodontal disease

- Rare in developed countries.
- Necrosis of gingival tissues, PDL, and bone.
- May be an extension of necrotizing ulcerative gingivitis.

Abscesses of the periodontium

- *Periodontal abscess*: localized purulent infection in the tissues adjacent to a periodontal pocket. Destruction of PDL and alveolar bone. Requires debridement under LA.
- *Gingival abscess*: localized purulent infection involving marginal tissues or interdental papilla. Fluctuant in 24–48 hours, points, and discharges. Often resolves spontaneously.
- *Periocoronal abscess*: localized purulent infection in the tissues adjacent to a partially erupted tooth. Commonly involves erupting third molars. Management approach varies and is dependent upon the severity of symptoms.

Periodontitis associated with endodontic lesions

- Inflammatory lesions of pulpal or PDL origin with the potential to involve both tissues.
- Management is dependent upon the origin of the primary lesion and may involve root canal treatment, periodontal therapy, or extraction.

Developmental or acquired deformities and conditions

- Recession—apical migration of the gingival tissues:
  - When the sulci are normal, recession is often associated with abnormal anatomy, tooth position, orthodontic tooth movement, trauma (e.g. toothbrushing trauma), or plaque retention factors.
- Where pockets are present, recession relates to periodontal disease.

Oral pathology in children

This section covers the most common conditions that affect the mouth in children. For additional conditions, please refer to ➲ Further reading.

Infection

Bacterial infections

- Odontogenic infections:
  - Most common cause of facial swelling in children = dentoalveolar abscess/cellulitis associated with a primary molar.
  - Immediate management dependent on severity of swelling.
  - Where there are no signs of systemic infection and swelling is localized: place antibiotic dressing in the tooth and make arrangements for the extraction of the non-vital tooth.
  - Where there are signs of systemic infection (malaise, pyrexia) or swelling is large: systemic antibiotic therapy and arrangements for the extraction of the non-vital tooth.
  - For severe infections such as if airway is at risk (bilateral involvement of submandibular/sublingual spaces, raised floor of mouth, trismus) or there is reduced eye opening due to periorbital swelling: an urgent referral to A&E should be made. Child may require admission for IV antibiotics, extraction of the infected tooth/teeth, and drainage of the infection.
- Impetigo:
  - Highly infectious skin infection usually caused by *Staphylococcus aureus* or *Streptococcus pyogenes*.
  - Children > adults.
  - Clinical presentation: vesiculobullous lesions, often involving the perioral region, that rupture resulting in crusted lesions.
  - Management: avoid dental treatment in the acute stages and advise the family to see their GMP. Management often involves the use of topical or oral antibiotics.
  - Complications: scarring, cellulitis, scarlet fever, septicaemia.

Viral infections

- Primary herpetic gingivostomatitis:
  - Most common cause of severe oral ulceration in young children and infants.
  - Majority of cases caused by herpes simplex virus 1 (HSV-1).
  - Peak incidence occurs between 2 and 4 years of age.
  - Incubation time 3–5 days with a prodromal phase of 48 hours.
  - Clinical presentation: stomatitis and intra-epithelial vesicles that may appear on any part of the oral mucosa, including around the lips, and breakdown to form painful ulcers. Child is often pyrexic, has a sore throat, drools, and has difficulty eating and drinking.
  - Management: analgesia, encourage fluids to avoid dehydration, soft diet. Topical agents such as benzydamine/lidocaine gel may be of use during the acute phase. If the child is immunocompromised, contact their medical specialist urgently as they are likely to require antiviral medication.
  - Self-limiting condition. Ulcers heal within 2 weeks.

- Mumps:
  - Acute viral infection that mainly involves the parotid glands, but submandibular and sublingual glands can also be affected.
  - Caused by a paramyxovirus.
  - Clinical presentation: low-grade fever and malaise. One or both of the parotid glands become tender and swollen for ~7 days. There may be pain on chewing.
  - NB: subclinical infection in 30–40% of cases.
  - Complications include ascending bacterial sialadenitis, orchitis, and epididymitis.
  - Management: analgesia and adequate hydration.
- Measles:
  - Highly infectious notifiable disease.
  - Caused by a paramyxovirus.
  - Clinical presentation: fever, runny nose, conjunctivitis, cough. Koplik's spots (irregular patches of erythema with central minute white specks similar to the appearance of grains of salt) on buccal and labial mucosa are pathognomonic of measles.
  - Complications: risk of opportunistic infections due to transient immunosuppression.
- Other viral infections with oral manifestations:
  - Chicken pox (varicella zoster virus) (➋ Zoster (shingles)).
  - Herpangina (coxsackie virus).
  - Hand, foot, and mouth disease (coxsackie virus).
  - Papillomas (human papillomavirus).

Fungal infections

The two most common types of candidiasis seen in children (➋ Patches affecting the oral mucosa) are as follows:

- Acute pseudomembranous:
  - Seen in newborn babies, immunocompromised children, or those on broad-spectrum antibiotics or steroids.
  - Often widespread creamy yellow patches that can be wiped off to expose erythematous mucosa.
  - Management is dependent on underlying cause but often involves the prescription of miconazole gel.
- Chronic erythematous:
  - Associated with removable appliances and dentures.
  - Management involves appliance/denture hygiene advice alongside oral hygiene advice and the prescription of miconazole gel.

Cystic lesions

Epstein's pearls

- Common: 75–80% of newborns.
- Hard raised nodules in the midline of the palate (often posterior palate) that result from trapped epithelial remnants.
- Tend to disappear within a few weeks and therefore management simply involves reassurance.

Dental lamina cysts

- Remnants of dental lamina found on crests of the dental ridges.
- Often occur bilaterally in the first primary molar region.
- No treatment required as often disappear by 3 months of age.

Bohn's nodules
- Remnants of salivary gland epithelium.
- Nodules/papules that usually occur on the labial/buccal aspect of the maxillary alveolar ridge in the newborn.
- No treatment required as often disappear by 3 months of age.

Eruption cyst
- Fluctuant soft tissue cyst associated with an erupting tooth.
- Caused by separation of the dental follicle from around the crown of the erupting tooth.
- Colour ranges from normal to blue-black depending on the amount of blood within the cyst.
- Treatment is usually not required as the cyst often ruptures spontaneously. However, if the cyst is still present after 4 weeks or if it becomes infected, consideration should be given to cutting a small window in the cyst.

Dentigerous cyst
- Fluctuant soft tissue cyst associated with an erupting tooth.
- Caused by separation of the dental follicle from around the crown of the erupting tooth.
- Most common jaw cyst in children.
- Encloses part or all of the crown of an unerupted tooth.
- Usually involve teeth that are commonly impacted (e.g. mandibular third molars and maxillary canines).
- Prevents eruption of the affected tooth.
- Management dependent upon its size and location and may involve marsupialization or enucleation of the cyst ± extraction of the tooth.

Mucoceles
- Common in children and most frequently involve the lower labial mucosa.
- See ➔ Mucoceles.

Conditions associated with trauma
Ulceration
- See ➔ Traumatic ulceration.
- Riga–Fede ulceration (➔ Mucosal disease).

Linea alba
- See ➔ Linea alba.

Idiopathic conditions
Recurrent aphthous ulceration
- See ➔ Recurrent aphthous ulceration.

Geographic tongue (erythema migrans)
- See ➔ Erythema migrans.

Further reading
Academy of Medical Royal Colleges (2013). Safe sedation practice for healthcare procedures. ℅ https://www.aomrc.org.uk/wp-content/uploads/2016/05/Safe_Sedation_Practice_1213.pdf
Academy of Medical Royal Colleges (2021). Safe sedation practice for healthcare procedures: an update. ℅ https://www.aomrc.org.uk/wp-content/uploads/2021/02/Safe_sedation_practice_for_healthcare_procedures_update_0521.pdf

American Academy of Paediatric Dentistry (2013). Guideline on dental management of heritable dental developmental anomalies. ℗ https://www.aapd.org/assets/1/7/G_OHCHeritable2.PDF

American Academy of Paediatric Dentistry (2014). Guideline on paediatric oral surgery. ℗ https://www.aapd.org/assets/1/7/g_oralsurgery.pdf

American Academy of Pediatric Dentistry (2020). Management considerations for pediatric oral surgery and oral pathology. In *The Reference Manual of Pediatric Dentistry* (pp. 433–442). American Academy of Pediatric Dentistry. ℗ www.aapd.org

Drummund PK, Kilpatrick N (Eds) (2015). *Planning and Care for Children and Adolescents with Dental Enamel Defects: Etiology, Research and Contemporary Management*. Springer.

Duggal MS, Curzon MEJ, et al. (2002). *Restorative Techniques in Paediatric Dentistry: An Illustrated Guide to the Restoration of Carious Primary Teeth* (2nd ed). Informa UK Ltd.

National Institute for Health and Care Excellence (NICE) (2004). Dental recall: recall intervals between routine dental examinations. NICE Clinical Guideline CG19. ℗ www.nice.org.uk/guidance/cg19

National Institute for Health and Care Excellence (NICE) (2010). Sedation in children and young people. NICE Clinical Guideline CG112. ℗ www.nice.org.uk/guidance/cg112

Public Health England (2014). *Delivering Better Oral Health: An Evidence-Based Toolkit for Prevention* (3rd ed). Public Health England.

Scottish Dental Clinical Effectiveness Programme (2012). Oral health assessment and review. ℗ https://www.sdcep.org.uk/published-guidance/oral-health-assessment/

Scottish Dental Clinical Effectiveness Programme (2018). Prevention and management of dental caries in children (2nd ed). ℗ https://www.sdcep.org.uk/media/2zbkrdkg/sdcep-prevention-and-management-of-dental-caries-in-children-2nd-edition.pdf

Vaidyanathan M (2010). Clinical guidelines in paediatric dentistry. Update of management and root canal treatment of non-vital immature permanent incisor teeth. Microsoft Word Immature incisor Clinical Guideline final (bspd.co.uk)

Welbury R, Duggal MS, Hosey MT (Eds) (2018). *Paediatric Dentistry* (5th ed). Oxford University Press.

Wright JT (2021). Developmental defects of the teeth. UpToDate. ℗ https://www.uptodate.com/contents/developmental-defects-of-the-teeth

Chapter 4

Orthodontics

Introduction to orthodontics

- Orthodontics is the branch of dentistry concerned with growth of the face, development of the dentition, and prevention and correction of occlusal anomalies.[1]
- The purpose of this chapter is to provide the DFT/DCT with relevant information regarding orthodontic management and diagnosis of the developing dentition and referral where appropriate, when there is an appreciable deviation from normal development. It is the ability to diagnose deviation from normal that is key to orthodontic management and appropriate referral, and all dentists need to develop this skill.
- The dental practitioner should develop their skills in orthodontic assessment to adequately monitor the developing occlusion and to possibly prevent the need for complex interventions when ideally timed referrals may intercept developing anomalies.
- The aim of this chapter is to provide the young practitioner with sufficient orthodontic knowledge to enable safe practice consistent with the curriculum in DCT. It does not provide a comprehensive guide to orthodontics as the majority of orthodontic treatment is now at postgraduate level training.
- There are often few opportunities as trainees in DCT for orthodontics to be provided as part of your training, and so orthodontic mechanics and treatment is beyond the scope of this text. For trainees in DCT who have exposure to orthodontics, the authors would recommend further texts in orthodontics (◑ Further reading).
- Orthodontics is becoming more of a postgraduate specialty, but there are many opportunities for the DFT/DCT to get involved in orthodontic audit, case presentations and publications. These are essential if the DCT wishes to go on to undertake specialty training.

Chronology of dental development

There will always be a variation between individual patients as to when their teeth erupt. Table 4.1 gives average values for dental development. Abnormalities in dental eruption outside of these figures may need further investigation in the permanent dentition (Table 4.1).

---

1 Houston (1986). *A Textbook of Orthodontics*. Wright.

Table 4.1 Tooth eruption dates

Tooth		Tooth germ fully developed	Dentine formation begins	Calcification begins	Crown formation complete	Eruption into the oral cavity	Root complete
Deciduous	Incisors	3–4 mths i.u.	4–6 mths i.u.		2–3 mths	6–9 mths	1–1.5 yrs after eruption
	Canines				9 mths	16–18 mths	
	1st molars				6 mths	12–14 mths	
Permanent	Upper 1s	30th wk i.u.	3–4 mths	3–4 mths	4–5 yrs	7–9 yrs	2–3 yrs after eruption
	Lower 1s		10–12 mths	10–12 mths	9 mths	6–8 yrs	
	Upper 2s		3–4 mths	3–4 mths	6 mths	7–9 yrs	
	Upper 3s	30th wk i.u.	4–5 mths	4–5 mths	6–7 yrs	11–12 yrs	2–3 yrs after eruption
	Lower 3s					9–10 yrs	
	Upper 4s	30th wk i.u.	1.5–2.5 yrs	1.5–1.75 yrs	5–6 yrs	10–11 yrs	2–3 yrs after eruption
	Lower 4s			1.75–2 yrs	5–6 yrs	10–12 yrs	
	Upper 5s			2–2.25 yrs	6–7 yrs	10–12 yrs	
	1st molar	24th wk i.u.	Before birth	Birth	2.5–3 yrs	6–7 yrs	2–3 yrs after eruption
	2nd molar	6th mth	2.5–3 yrs	2.5–3 yrs	7–8 yrs	11–13 yrs	
	3rd molar	6th yr	7–10 yrs	7–9 yrs	12–16 yrs	17–21 yrs	

i.u., *in utero*, mth(s), month(s); wk, week; yr(s), year(s).

Scott JH, Symons NBB (1990). *Introduction to Dental Anatomy* (9th ed). Churchill Livingstone.

Classification of occlusion

- Malocclusion has been defined as an appreciable deviation from normal occlusion.[2]
- It is classified in several ways, but the most normally accepted description is based on the incisor classification along with the skeletal component of the malocclusion.

British Standards Institute classification of incisor relationship

- Class 1:
  - The lower incisor edges occlude or lies immediately below the cingulum plateau of the upper incisors.
- Class II/1:
  - The lower incisor edges lie posterior to the cingulum plateau of the upper incisors. The upper incisors are of average inclination or are proclined.
- Class II/2:
  - The lower incisor edges lie posterior to the cingulum plateau of the upper incisors. The upper central incisors are retroclined.
- Class III:
  - > The lower incisor edges lie anterior to the cingulum plateau of the upper incisors. The overjet will be reduced or reversed (Fig. 4.1).[3]

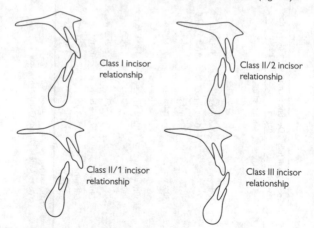

Class I incisor relationship

Class II/2 incisor relationship

Class II/1 incisor relationship

Class III incisor relationship

Fig. 4.1 Diagram of incisal relationship. Reproduced with permission from Rushworth B, Kanatas A (2020). *Oxford Handbook of Clinical Dentistry* (7th ed). Oxford University Press.

2 Houston W (1992). *A Textbook of Orthodontics*. Wright.

3 British Standards Institute (2020). Dentistry. Vocabulary. BS EN ISO 1942:2020. BSI.

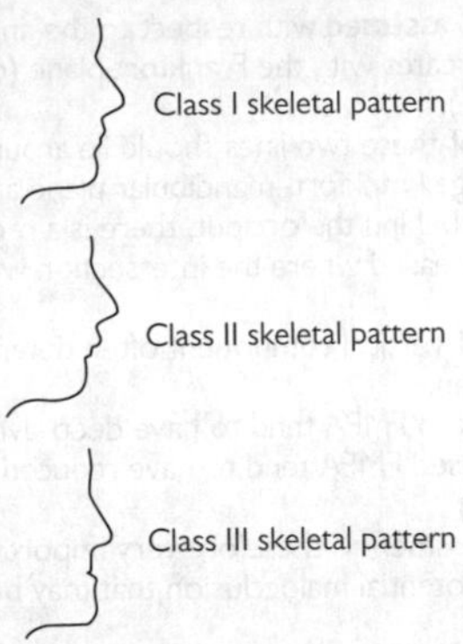

Class I skeletal pattern

Class II skeletal pattern

Class III skeletal pattern

Fig. 4.2 Diagram of AP relationship. Reproduced with permission from Rushworth B, Kanatas A (2020). *Oxford Handbook of Clinical Dentistry* (7th ed). Oxford University Press.

Skeletal relationship
Anteroposterior (AP)

- AP classification (Fig. 4.2):
  - Class I.
  - Class II.
  - Class III.
- Class I skeletal pattern: the maxilla should lie around 2–4 mm in front of the mandible.
- Class I skeletal pattern: the maxilla lies >4 mm ahead of the mandible.
- Class III skeletal pattern: the maxilla lies <2 mm ahead of the mandible.
- Class II and class III are further subdivided into mild, moderate, and severe (based on subjective and cephalometric analysis).
- This is based on the soft tissue assessment of the dental bases of the maxilla and mandible with palpation of the concavities of the anterior maxilla (soft tissue A point) and the concavity of the anterior mandible in the labiomental fold (soft tissue B point).
- This allows the relationship between the maxilla and mandible to be estimated without radiological assessment (lateral cephalogram).

Vertical component

- The lateral face can be divided into thirds and the relationship between the thirds gives a clinical estimation of the relative lower anterior face height.
- This is important in determining the vertical skeletal component to the malocclusion.
- Vertical assessment can be in the AP and frontal planes.
- The lower third is further subdivided into the upper 1/3 and the lower 2/3, with the upper 1/3 being the upper lip length (subnasale to stomion).

- The vertical is also assessed with respect to the angle the lower border of the mandible creates with the Frankfort plane (clinical estimation is the alar–tragal line).
- The intersection of these two lines should lie around the occiput in a normal or average Frankfort–mandibular plane angle (FMPA). If the intersection is behind the occiput, there is a reduced FMPA, and vice versa with increased where the intersection would be before the occiput.
- The importance of vertical component often determines the type of overbite that is seen.
- Patients with reduced FMPA tend to have deep overbites, whereas a patient with increased FMPA tend to have reduced overbites or anterior open bites (AOBs).
- The extraoral assessment is therefore very important as it gives an indication of the potential malocclusion that may be seen intraorally.

Transverse component

- The frontal face can be divided into vertical fifths, with the alar base width representing the middle fifth, the eyes (medial to lateral canthus) medial to this, and the external fifths from lateral canthus to the ear.
- Each fifth is around the size of the eye.
- A difference in the size of these fifths indicates some asymmetry.
- The intercanthal distance is around equal to the alar base width in Caucasians (32 ± 3 mm). Interpupillary distance is equal to the width of the mouth.
- If the interpupillary line is horizontal (no orbital dystopia), then the transverse occlusal plane should be parallel to this line. Non-parallelism indicates a transverse occlusal cant.

Further reading

Atack N. Postgraduate Notes in Orthodontics. University of Bristol.
British Orthodontic Society: ☞ www.bos.org.uk
Cobourne MT, DiBiase AT (2015). Handbook of Orthodontics (2nd ed). Mosby Elsevier.
Littlewood S, Mitchell L (2019). An Introduction to Orthodontics (5th ed). Oxford University Press.
Naini F (2008). Facial aesthetics: 2. Clinical assessment. Dent Update 35, 159–162.
Your Jaw Surgery. Information resource for patients: ☞ www.yourjawsurgery.com

Assessing the orthodontic patient

- Normal dental examination of children and young adults should include an orthodontic assessment of the malocclusion and this should be recorded in the dental notes.
- Good knowledge of the normal eruption of the dentition is integral to a good orthodontic examination.
- Important transitions from the deciduous dentition to the permanent dentition should be noted and we would always suggest asking the patient's age to remind you of where they are in their dental development. You will be aware that chronological age and dental age do not always correlate but deviations from normal eruption should be noted and investigated, especially if there has been >6 months between the eruption of the contralateral tooth. Asymmetry of dental development must be noted and investigated appropriately.

Key average transitions to the permanent dentition

- Age 6: first molars and lower incisors.
- Age 7: upper incisors and lower lateral incisors.
- Age 9: upper lateral incisors.
- Age 10: lower canines, palpate upper canines.
- Age 10–12: premolar eruption.
- Age 12: upper canines and second molars.
- Age 18+: third molars.

Key orthodontic assessment

- Dental development stage (mixed dentition/permanent dentition).
- Degree of crowding/unerupted teeth.
- Incisor classification.
- Overjet.
- Overbite.
- Crossbites and any displacements from retruded contact position (RCP) to intercuspal position (ICP).
- Index of Orthodontic Treatment Need (IOTN).

This will then alert you to any deviation from normal and further investigations may be appropriate such as radiological assessment of unerupted teeth.

Basic orthodontic assessment

- An orthodontic assessment should be performed as part of a routine dental examination to ensure that the developing dentition and occlusion is within normal parameters or whether it requires further investigation, orthodontic assessment, or treatment. The more confident you become at performing this, the quicker it will become.
- A basic assessment should include:
  - developmental stage (primary, mixed, secondary)
  - oral hygiene
  - incisor relationship
  - overjet and overbite
  - palpation of unerupted teeth
  - crossbites.

- The basic assessment should alert the practitioner to any abnormalities in tooth number, position, eruption, or the underlying developing malocclusion.

Full orthodontic assessment

It is useful to determine the patient's concerns regarding their malocclusion as this can alert the practitioner to any potential problems, such as bullying or trauma.

- A full medical, dental, and social history, including ability to attend regular appointments, digit habits, and previous trauma or treatment.
- Assessment of the malocclusion starts on the outside and works in (extraoral to intraoral).

Extraoral assessment
- AP: class I, II, III.
- Vertical: average, increased, or decreased.
- Transverse: any asymmetry?
- Lip position (nasolabial angle) and competence.
- Temporomandibular joint (TMJ) assessment.

Intraoral assessment
- Oral hygiene and periodontal assessment.
- Teeth present: dentition phase, missing teeth, unerupted teeth?
- Caries, decalcification, and MIH.
- Degree of crowding of the upper and lower arches.
- Incisor relationship: class I, II/1, II/2, III.
- Overjet and overbite.
- Centrelines.
- Molar and canine relationship: class I, II, III, and subdivisions ¼, ½, ¾.
- Crossbites and displacements.
- IOTN (➔ Index of Orthodontic Treatment Need).

Following this assessment, a determination is made to any further special investigations such as vitality testing, radiographs, and so on. Generally, an OPT is taken prior to orthodontic treatment to assess the dentition, bone levels, root length, morphology of the condyles, and assessment of any pathology.

The assessment will highlight any 'problem' areas, indicating whether further investigation is warranted or referral as appropriate.

Useful orthodontic definitions

- IOTN: Index of Orthodontic Treatment Need.
- Overjet: the distance between the upper and lower incisors in the horizontal plane.
- Overbite: overlap of the upper and lower incisors.
- Anterior open bite (AOB): the upper incisor fails to overlap the lower incisors in the horizontal plane.
- Crossbite: deviation from the normal buccolingual relationship. All crossbites should be examined to determine if it is a true crossbite in RCP and ICP or whether there is some deviation into ICP. It is always worth measuring the differences between RCP and ICP for displacements due to crossbite. To achieve this, determine which

direction the displacement is observed. An AP slide should be measured by the overjet in RCP and ICP. Any lateral movements are best measured by determination of centreline discrepancies between RCP and ICP. This is important for determining IOTN (→ Index of Orthodontic Treatment Need) of crossbites with associated displacements.

- This can be further subdivided into:
  - buccal crossbites: where the lower buccal cusps lie buccal to the upper buccal cusps
  - lingual crossbite: where the lower buccal cusps lie lingual to the upper palatal cusps
  - anterior crossbite: crossbite involving the incisors and canines
  - posterior crossbite: crossbite involving the premolars and molars.
- Recording which teeth are in crossbite: standard convention is the position of the lower teeth relative to the upper teeth. Do not count the number of both maxillary and mandibular teeth in the same crossbite (e.g. UR2 and UL2 in lingual crossbite is two teeth in crossbite, not four teeth UR2, UL2, LL2, LR2).
- Mandibular displacement: on full closure into ICP, the mandible deviates to avoid premature contact.
- Displacement of contact points: measurement of contact point displacement from the normal arch form.
- Crowding: discrepancy between the size of the dental arch and the size of the teeth present/unerupted:
  - Divided into mild (0–4 mm), moderate (5–8 mm), and severe (>8 mm).[1]

1 Proffit W (2012). *Contemporary Orthodontics* (5th ed). Elsevier.

Medical considerations for orthodontic treatment

Orthodontic treatment generally has fewer medical contraindications than other aspects of dental treatment owing to the non-invasive nature of treatment, but there are certain conditions that need to be considered when planning treatment.[1]

Allergies

Nickel:
- Type IV hypersensitivity.
- Less reported hypersensitivity noted intraorally.
- Alternatives to nickel-titanium archwires can be used.

Latex:
- Type I and type IV hypersensitivity.
- Use of non-latex orthodontic elastomerics.

Cardiovascular system (CVS)

Infective endocarditis:
- Liaison with physician regarding the risk of infective endocarditis.
- Avoid use of orthodontic bands and fixed acrylic appliances to reduce the risk of infective endocarditis.

Coagulopathies:
- Orthodontic treatment is not contraindicated but extractions need further consideration and possible liaison with the haematologist.
- Orthognathic surgery needs liaison with haematologist, but may be contraindicated.
- Temporary anchorage devices are not contraindicated.

Sickle cell anaemia:
- Orthodontic treatment is not contraindicated provided there are no complications.
- Non-extraction approach is preferred.

Leukaemia:
- Avoid treatment during chemotherapy/radiotherapy.
- Delay orthodontic treatment until 2 years following bone marrow transplants.
- Immunosuppression will delay growth.
- Patients may be prescribed bisphosphonates so at risk of medication-related osteonecrosis of the jaw (MRONJ) with extraction-based plans.

Endocrine

Diabetes mellitus:
- Higher risk of periodontal disease. Good oral hygiene and regular maintenance therapy programme.
- Avoid orthodontics in poorly controlled IDDM due to increased susceptibility to periodontal disease.

1 Patel A (2009). *J Orthod* 36, 1.

Genetic

Down syndrome:
- 1:700 live births; 50% may have cardiac defects which may impact treatment; particular consideration is needed for any planned GA.
- Orthodontic treatment tailored to patient's compliance and understanding (learning difficulties).

Medication

Corticosteroids:
- Supplementary corticosteroids may be indicated for dentoalveolar surgery under GA.

Bisphosphonates:
- Patients have a risk of MRONJ, less with oral.
- Consider non-extraction treatment to reduce the risk of MRONJ with extractions.
- Consent for slower tooth movement.
- Avoid temporary anchorage devices or orthognathic surgery.

Musculoskeletal

Rheumatoid arthritis:
- Characterized by symmetrical stiffness of the joints; 15% may develop Sjögren syndrome—xerostomia, higher risk of caries, and discomfort with fixed appliances.
- TMJs can be affected with erosive changes leading to AOB.

Juvenile idiopathic arthritis:
- Severe disease in late childhood which may have an effect on growth, condylar hypoplasia, and mandibular retrognathia.
- Higher risk of caries and periodontal disease.
- Bite splints may be advised during acute periods. Functional appliances may be considered. Orthognathic surgery may be required to fully correct.

Neurological

Epilepsy:
- Orthodontic treatment is not contraindicated in well controlled epilepsy.
- Consideration to fixed appliances over removable (potential airway obstruction). Functional appliances can be used with good retention.

Respiratory system

Cystic fibrosis:
- Avoid GA for extractions if feasible.
- No orthodontic contraindication.

Interceptive orthodontics

- The late mixed dentition is probably the most advantageous time for considering any interceptive orthodontic treatment. The aim is to reduce the necessity for orthodontic treatment in the future by early correction of the occlusal trait.
- Interceptive orthodontics includes any treatment which eliminates or reduces the severity of a developing malocclusion. It should eliminate or simplify the need for future treatment.
- The aims of interceptive orthodontics are to:
  - maintain centrelines
  - maintain class I incisor relationship
  - maintain good vertical and transverse relationship
  - eliminate crossbites associated with displacement/pathology
  - prevent trauma
  - minimize crowding
  - minimize psychological factors/teasing.
- Possible interceptive orthodontic traits are:
  - failure of or delayed eruption
  - extraction of poor prognosis first molars
  - extraction of primary canines (➔ Impacted maxillary canines)
  - correction of crossbites with displacements
  - early correction of skeletal class II or III discrepancies.

Further reading

British Orthodontic Society (2016). Orthodontic management of patients with relevant medical histories. https://www.bos.org.uk/

Fleming P, Johal A, DiBiase AT (2008). Managing malocclusion in the mixed dentition: six keys to success. Part 1. *Dent Update* 35 607, 612–613.

Fleming P, Johal A, DiBiase AT (2008). Managing malocclusion in the mixed dentition: six keys to success part 2. *Dent Update* 35, 673–676.

Dental eruption anomalies

Ectopic eruption of first permanent molars

Infraeruption of primary molars

Dental eruption anomalies

Ectopic eruption of first permanent molars

- This occurs when the FPM is blocked from eruption by the second primary molar (E).
- This most commonly occurs in the maxilla and more frequently in males.
- Although this impaction may present with significant resorption of the primary molar, it is rarely symptomatic.
- Two types have been described: reversible (66%) and irreversible (34%) types.

Potential problems

- Caries of second deciduous molar tooth and FPM tooth.
- Root resorption of second primary molar tooth.
- Space loss if the second primary molar tooth is lost.

Treatment

- Observe as the majority of cases will self-correct.
- Disimpact by placing separator/brass wire.
- Distalize 6 with orthodontic appliance.
- If non-viable, extract E and distalize 6 once erupted.

Infraocclusion of primary teeth

Infraocclusion or submerging primary teeth is more commonly seen in the primary molars. The infraocclusion occurs due to ankylosis of the tooth to the alveolar bone, caused by a loss in periodontal ligament in any part of the root. This may just be a 'spot' ankylosis, but the result is the whole tooth appears to submerge. The reality of this phenomenon is that the tooth is not submerging, but more the child is growing around the ankylosed tooth with an increase in vertical height of the alveolar bone. The ankylosis may be transient.

Potential causes

- Genetic.
- Developmental absence of the permanent successor.
- Failure of the normal resorptive process.
- Deflection of the permanent successor/ectopic position of the permanent tooth.
- Caries causing pulpal infection.
- Trauma.

Treatment options with a permanent successor

- Observe, particularly if there is a successor, as in the majority of cases the permanent successor will erupt, and the primary tooth will exfoliate.
- Extract if there is significant infraocclusion (below the contact point of the adjacent teeth) and evidence of the permanent successor being deflected off course.

Treatment options without a permanent successor

- Observe. If there is significant infraocclusion, a decision is needed regarding the long-term prognosis and maintenance of this tooth.

- Occlusal onlay to increase the occlusal height, normalizing the occlusal plane and preventing overeruption of the opposing dentition.
- Extraction. An orthodontic decision is then needed as to whether the space can be utilized for correction of the malocclusion and closure of space or whether the space needs to be maintained for prosthetic replacement in the future.

Primary failure of eruption

Primary failure of eruption is a condition in which non-ankylosed teeth fail to erupt fully or only partially erupt because of cessation of the eruption mechanism without any obvious cause.[1,2]

Clinical features
- Primarily posterior teeth and most frequently first molars.
- Any number of quadrants involved.
- Teeth distal to the most mesially involved tooth are also affected.
- Lateral open bites develop.
- Ankylosis can occur if orthodontic forces are applied.

Mechanical failure of eruption has a similar presentation to primary failure of eruption, but is characterized by only a single tooth ankylosis, with teeth distal apparently normal. This may also affect more than one quadrant.

Indeterminate failure of eruption is a diagnosis of exclusion where it is too early to determine the distinction between primary failure of eruption and mechanical failure of eruption as the teeth posterior to those ankylosed have not erupted yet.

Unerupted maxillary central incisors

The maxillary central incisor erupts around 7–8 years of age. Failure of eruption of maxillary central incisors should be investigated if the contralateral tooth erupted >6 months previously. If both maxillary central incisors have failed to erupt and the lower central incisors erupted >12 months previously, this warrants investigation.[3]

Incidence
- 0.13%.

Aetiology

Developmental
- Presence of a $.

Genetic
- Hereditary gingival fibromatosis.
- CLP.
- Cleidocranial dysplasia.
- Down syndrome.

1 Ahmad S (2006). *Eur J Orthod* 28, 535.
2 Mistry V (2017). *J Paediatr Dent* 27, 428.
3 ⅋ https://www.rcseng.ac.uk/-/media/files/rcs/fds/guidelines/management-of-unerupted-maxillary-incisors-2022-update.pdf

Local/environmental factors
- Crowding or space loss.
- Trauma leading to dilacerations.
- Retained primary incisor.

Management
- Create space (orthodontically).
- Remove the cause:
  - Extract retained primary tooth or surgical removal of $/odontomes.
  - If there is to be removal of $ teeth or odontomes, it is often preferable to undertake exposure of the unerupted central incisor to prevent further surgery if the tooth still fails to erupt, although the limited evidence would show that creating space will allow these teeth to erupt naturally.
  - This is all case dependent and should be assessed by an orthodontist. Repeated GAs are not advisable and so many operators choose to expose the unerupted tooth at the same time as $ removal.
  - In more severe cases, it may not be possible to align a severely ectopic incisor and may require surgical removal and prosthetic replacement.
- Surgical exposure:
  - Closed exposure with gold chain and orthodontic alignment.
  - Open exposure for a more superficial incisor using an apically repositioned flap followed by orthodontic alignment.
- Severe dilacerations with unfavourable root formation may preclude orthodontic alignment or may risk the pulp vitality following alignment. In these cases, endodontic treatment may be necessary and potential apical surgery.

Impacted maxillary canines

Maxillary canines can become impacted and prevented from eruption by bone, tooth, or soft tissue. Normal eruption occurs at the age of around 12 years and should be palpated in the buccal sulcus from around 10 years of age.

Incidence
- 2% of the population with 61% of these being palatal, 34% in the line of the arch and 4.5% are buccal.[4]
- Females > males; 70%:30%.

Aetiology
- Multifactorial.
- Theories:
  - Guidance theory. This theory is based on the lateral incisor as a guide for the canine to erupt. Patients with diminutive or developmentally absent lateral incisors have a higher incidence of impacted canines, also class II/2 malocclusions.[5]
  - Genetic theory.[6]

4 Stivaros N (2000). *Br J Orthod* 27, 169.
5 Becker A (1995). *Angle Orthodontist* 65, 95.
6 Peck S (1994). *Angle Orthodontist* 64, 249.

Clinical examination

- Palpate in the buccal sulcus at the age of 10 years adjacent to the lateral incisor.
- Assess the presence of palatal or buccal bulges and their location.
- Assess the mobility of the primary canine.
- Colour and inclination of the adjacent lateral incisor.

Radiographic examination

- To establish: presence, position, and any pathology.
- Parallax: use of two radiographs with an X-ray tube shift either vertical or horizontal:
  - Two periapicals.
  - OPT and anterior occlusal.
- CBCT may be ultimately used by orthodontists to further investigate the position of the unerupted canine in three dimensions and evaluate any possible resorption of adjacent teeth.

Potential consequences of impacted canines

- Resorption of roots of adjacent teeth.
- Loss of vitality of resorbed adjacent teeth necessitating complex endodontics or extraction.
- Extended complex orthodontic treatment times.
- Aesthetic impairment if unerupted and primary tooth lost.

Risk factors for root resorption

- There is a greater risk in females <14 years.
- Horizontal palatal canines.
- Medial position of the canine.
- Evidence of resorption of other teeth or shorter/blunted roots.

Interceptive treatment for ectopic canines

- Historically, extraction of the primary canine has been advocated to normalize the eruption of a maxillary canine that appeared to be deviating in its eruptive path.[7,8]
- A Cochrane review[9] found that no high-level evidence was currently available to support these conclusions although studies that have aimed to increase the space available with headgear or arch expansion have shown there to be increased success with the extraction of the primary canine. More recent higher-level evidence from randomized controlled trials[10,11] shows that extraction of the primary canine was effective in normalizing palatally displaced canines.
- If an impacted canine is suspected and your investigations confirm this (palpation and radiograph), refer to an orthodontist for an opinion so that each case can be assessed.

7 Ericson S (1988). *Eur J Orthod* 10, 283.

8 Power S (1993). *Br J Orthod* 20, 215.

9 Parkin N (2012). *Cochrane Database Syst Rev* 12, 12.

10 Naoumova J (2015). *Eur J Orthod* 37 209, 219.

11 Bazargarni F (2014). *Angle Orthodontist* 84, 3.

Surgical exposure

- Depending on the position of the unerupted ectopic canine, these can be exposed using a closed or open technique; the preferred method of exposure is very operator dependent.
- Open technique requires a good wide exposure to prevent re-covering and good postoperative oral hygiene.
- In some cases, surgical exposure and alignment may be inadvisable due to:
  - position
  - patient compliance
  - good 2–4 contact
  - acceptable primary canine and the patient being aware of the long-term restorative consequences.
- Advice to patients having undergone open surgical exposure:
  - Early light brushing of the area with a small-headed toothbrush.
  - Regular saltwater mouthwashes in the first week.
  - Ensure a parent/carer can regularly visualize the exposed tooth.
  - Orthodontic review around 2 weeks after the procedure.
- Advice for patients having undergone closed surgical exposure:
  - Keep the area clean with gentle brushing around the area.
  - Regular saltwater mouthwashes in the first week.
  - The gold chain may be sutured to the gingivae and care needs to be taken around this to prevent dislodging.
- When performing closed surgical exposures, good suturing of the end of the gold chain to tissue that is not hypermobile is needed. An alternative to suturing is to bond the end of the gold chain to an adjacent tooth with composite.

First molars of poor prognosis

- Timing of extractions is usually around age 8–10 years for interceptive extraction aiming for spontaneous space closure.
- A two-surface restoration in the first molars of a young child can be considered a tooth of poor long-term prognosis (➔ Molar incisor hypomineralization for poor prognosis first molars).
- First molars are not necessarily the orthodontist's first choice of extraction as part of an orthodontic plan, but in some cases, the first molar may be of choice especially when:
  - they are of poor prognosis/apical pathology or large restorations when the premolars are sound
  - high maxillary mandibular planes angle/AOB cases and space closure can gain overbite.
- Extractions as part of an orthodontic plan (for the creation of space) are most likely to occur in the permanent dentition, when full orthodontic treatment is planned, not to be confused with interceptive loss for spontaneous space closure.
- Delaying extraction of first molars of poor prognosis needs to be carefully managed as the tooth will need to be restored to enable survival until the planned time of extraction.
- Timing the extraction of the lower first molar is critical for spontaneous space closure:
  - Calcification of the bifurcation of the lower first molar.

- Ideally long axis of the crypt of lower second molar and the lower first molar is <30°.
- Ideally minimal/mild crowding at this stage.
- Ideally third molars present. Often the first molars are of such poor prognosis that maintenance of these teeth just because the third molars are not present is usually problematic and unwise. Accepting a shortened dental arch is much more pragmatic.
- Lack of evidence of third molars at this stage is common, and does not mean that they are not present, they have just not developed sufficiently to be seen radiographically.
- Timing the extraction of the upper first molar is less critical as spontaneous mesial drift occurs more readily.

Balancing extractions

- Extraction of the same tooth on the contralateral side to maintain the centreline.
- Rarely advised for first molars. Although it may have an effect on the midline, this may be better dealt with by alternative extractions especially if the contralateral tooth is of good prognosis.

Compensating extractions

- Extraction of the same opposing tooth in the opposite arch.
- Extraction of the upper first molar when the lower is extracted is advised to preserve the molar relationship and prevent overeruption.
- Extraction of the lower first molar when the upper is extracted is not necessary.

Treatment planning for extraction of first molars

- First molars that have a hopeless long-term prognosis and are unrestorable do not require an orthodontic opinion as there would be very little to add to the assessment as the teeth need to be lost.
- An orthodontic opinion may be required for more complex decisions, but this needs to be arranged in a timely manner as to not leave children in pain.
- An orthodontic opinion is required if the malocclusion is to be treated utilizing the first molars for space creation. This is quite a difficult concept to determine for the referrer but consider: is temporization of the molar a possibility if a plan was to keep the tooth for extraction at a later date; can the patient cope with treatment to temporize the tooth? By keeping the tooth, is the patient at risk of developing problems later if the tooth were to flare up? Is the patient appropriate for orthodontic treatment (oral hygiene/cooperation)? Answering these questions to yourself will give you an idea of what is potentially possible and the potential treatment plan.
- Appropriate timely referral for orthodontic assessment, dependent on the:
  - malocclusion (class I/II/III)
  - stage of development
  - restorability of the first molars if to be temporized until the second molars have erupted.
- It is of great use to provide as much information about your thoughts on the long-term prognosis of each tooth when requesting an

orthodontic opinion. This will assist the orthodontist in planning the potential extraction pattern.
- In general, if there is enforced loss of a lower first molar (at the ideal time), which is the occlusal stop for the upper first molar, consider compensating the extraction to prevent overeruption of the upper molar, which may prevent the mesialization of the lower second molar into the first molar space, thus closing the extraction space spontaneously.
- Consider the method of extraction. Is the patient going to need a GA? If so, a more radical extraction pattern may be indicated.
- Early enforced loss of first molars can create significant spacing, especially in the lower arch between premolars and molars. Ideally, if possible, wait for a better time to extract teeth. This is not always feasible, and the dental/medical health of the patient takes priority over timing extractions. It is clear that the risks of facial swellings and the need for hospitalization far outweigh the potential for leaving a spaced arch.
- If there is enforced loss of first molars, not at the ideal time, then correction of the malocclusion can still be possible, but may require further extractions of premolars at a later stage. Ideally, there will be evidence of third molars if further extractions are planned. Remember, it is not always possible to gain a perfect occlusal result just by the loss of timed first molars.
- In a high proportion of cases, oral hygiene will not be adequate for consideration of orthodontics at the time of assessment, so reinforce the need for good oral hygiene.

Treatment planning for specific malocclusions
It can be difficult to provide 'rules' to aid treatment planning cases for the loss of the first molars. The following can provide some suggestions, but each case will be different and may require further advice. It is also useful to take into consideration some of the suggestions in the previous sections regarding the feasibility of delaying extractions due to cooperation or pain/infection.

Class I
- Minimal incisor crowding or moderate premolar crowding: aim for extraction at the optimal time.
- Moderate–severe crowding: may require space for the correction of the malocclusion and may be more appropriate to delay extractions (if this is possible) until after the eruption of the second molars. If extractions are enforced, consent for the possibility that further extractions may be necessary for orthodontic purposes at a later stage.
- Spaced dentitions: significant spacing requiring the loss of first molars is likely to result in residual spacing, but if there is enforced loss, aim for the optimal time.

Class II/1
- The extraction of the first molars can be important as space may be required in the maxillary arch to reduce an overjet, but similarly, space may not be required in the lower arch as any retroclination of the lower incisors will only worsen the overjet, so timing can be very important.

- Extraction of first molars at the optimal time to enable spontaneous space closure, and then the use of a functional appliance (around the pubertal growth spurt).
- If space is going to be used to retract the upper incisors, the 6 extraction will need to be timed after the 7 has erupted and may require anchorage reinforcement for utilization of this space.

Class II/2

- These malocclusions may have similar requirement considerations as to class II/1. Some class II/2 are treated by converting to a class II/1 then the use of a functional appliance to correct or by extraction in the upper arch.
- The treatment planning of these cases is dependent on the space requirements.
- Class II/2 tend to have deeper overbites and on a reduced vertical skeletal base, so often extractions can be contraindicated due to the potential for worsening of the overbite and the difficulty in correcting this orthodontically.

Class III

- These malocclusions can be challenging to plan, particularly due to the age at which these decisions are being made. It may not be clear as to whether orthodontic camouflage is possible or whether the patient may require orthognathic correction in the future.
- Often there is a space requirement in the upper arch due to the reduced maxillary length, so space may be created by loss of the 6, timed after the eruption of the 7.
- Space may be required in the lower arch to retract the lower incisors to improve the overjet, so timing would be following the eruption of the lower second molar.
- Specialist advice is recommended for these more challenging decisions.

Early loss of primary teeth

- Early loss of primary teeth can have an impact on the developing dentition and occlusion.
- The primary dentition is considered the normal space maintainers for the permanent dentition.
- The mesial–distal size of the C, D, and E is larger than that of the permanent successors, 3, 4, and 5. This additional space is known as the Leeway space.
- The earlier the loss of the primary teeth, the greater the potential for loss of space and development of crowding (➜ Chronology of dental development), particularly if there is the existing potential for crowding.
- Early loss of primary teeth can lead to detrimental effects on the occlusion such as centreline shifts and loss of space and therefore planning needs to consider limiting these detrimental effects such as balancing and compensating extractions (➜ Balancing/compensating extractions).
- The requirement for balancing/compensating is dependent on each specific tooth.
- Common sense also needs to be applied when considering balancing and compensating extractions. It may not be feasible to provide multiple

extractions due to cooperation requiring sedation or GA, especially if this is of sound teeth and the extraction of a single tooth is possible under LA/sedation alone. The risks of GA need to be considered and likely outweigh the benefits of interceptively extracting teeth to prevent centreline shifts.

Incisors (A, B)
- There is no need to balance or compensate in either arch.
- Minimal effect on the centreline.

Canine (C)
- Balancing extractions are recommended to prevent a centreline shift.
- Compensating is not required.

First primary molar (D)
- Unilateral loss can have an effect on the centreline and balancing should be considered, particularly in the presence of crowding.
- Consider compensating extraction to prevent alteration of the buccal segment relationship.

Second primary molar (E)
- Unilateral loss is unlikely to have an effect on the centreline and balancing is not necessary.
- Early loss of the E is likely to lead to mesialization of the 6 and crowding of the 5.
- Consider compensating extraction to prevent development of a class II buccal segment relationship.

Space maintenance
- Early loss of primary molars can lead to rapid space loss.
- Consideration should be made to whether space maintenance would be required or is appropriate.
- Early loss due to caries indicates that the patient may not be suitable for space maintenance.
- Consider the length of time the space maintainer would be required and whether this is appropriate for the individual.
- Ideally space maintenance where a single tooth has been lost early, in a well-cared for dentition and a low caries risk to prevent localized crowding.
- If there is the potential for crowding in all quadrants requiring extractions, it may not be worth space maintaining.
- Space maintenance in the posterior dentition is likely to be using a band and loop.

Early treatment of crossbites
Anterior crossbites
- Correction in the mixed dentition is indicated if there is significant hard (attrition/abrasion) or soft tissue (periodontal attachment loss) damage caused by an anterior crossbite with displacement.
- Correction can be achieved by:
  - removable appliances
  - sectional fixed appliances.
- Usually, any periodontal attachment loss improves following correction of the crossbite.

Posterior crossbites

- The idea of early correction in the mixed dentition is to prevent the crossbite being perpetuated into the permanent dentition.[12]
- Correction can be achieved by removable or fixed orthodontic expanding appliances (midline screws, quad helix appliance, expansion arches, or rapid maxillary expansion).
- The majority of UK orthodontic correction of posterior crossbites occurs in the permanent dentition during definitive orthodontic correction, potentially due to waiting lists, funding, and cooperation of patients.

Early treatment of skeletal discrepancies

Class II skeletal

- Ideally, timing of functional appliances coincides with the pubertal growth spurt (10–12 years in girls, 11–13 years in boys).[12]
- Early treatment would be considered before the age of 10 years.[13]
- Prevention of trauma to the upper incisors (due to increased overjet) is one of the reasons authors have advocated early treatment.
- Research has shown that early treatment has:
  - reduced outcomes
  - increased length of treatment
  - more attendances
  - no less trauma experienced.
- Recommendations are that treatment is delayed until the appropriate developmental stage to enable a smooth, timely transition into fixed appliances in the permanent dentition.[14,15]
- Severe bullying may be considered a reason to provide early treatment.

Class III skeletal

- Use of protraction facemasks to correct a class III skeletal and incisal relationship.
- Early treatment is defined as between 8 and 10 years.
- Early treatment may reduce the need for orthognathic correction in the future.[16]

Dummy or digit habits

Dentists are often asked by parents for advice on dummy (pacifier) use or digit sucking in their children. There are many opinions and thoughts on the use of dummies for children and you may have limited experience in this area to provide advice. The evidence in this area is also limited.

Dummy habit

- Often used from an early age to provide comfort to the baby/child.
- A natural suckling urge is present which is not always satisfied by feeding and use of a dummy can satisfy the baby/child.

12 Agostino P (2014). *Cochrane Database Syst Rev* 8, 8.
13 O'Brien K (2003). *Am J Orthod Dentofacial Orthop* 124, 234.
14 Batista K (2018). *Cochrane Database Syst Rev* 13, 3.
15 Thiruvenkatachari B (2015). *Am J Orthod Dentofacial Orthop*. 148, 47.
16 Mandall N (2016). *J Orthod* 43, 164.

- Recommend orthodontic dummies (flatter in shape) to minimize the effect on the dentition.
- It is rare that a dummy habit will continue beyond the primary dentition.
- A dummy can affect the occlusion with a reduction in overbite and reduction in maxillary arch width, tending to crossbite formation.
- Effects into the permanent dentition are rare due to cessation earlier.

Digit habit

- Often used from an early age to provide comfort to the baby/child but is more likely to persist into an older age group and therefore have an effect on the permanent dentition.
- Can be much more difficult to stop the habit as the 'digit' is freely available.
- The overall effect on the occlusion is dependent on the frequency and intensity of the habit.
- Can have significant effects on the occlusion with:
  - proclination of the upper incisors and an increase in the overjet
  - retroclination of the lower incisors
  - constriction of the maxillary arch width and crossbite development plus displacement
  - AOB which may be asymmetric, depending on the pattern of the habit
  - asymmetric development of the occlusion
  - potential for modification of the underlying facial growth, tending to a more class II, open bite tendency.

Management options

- Encouragement to stop the habit with positive reinforcement.
- Plasters, bitter nail varnish, cotton gloves, sock, or thumb guards.
- False nails also appear to have a good success (if appropriate).
- Habit breaker orthodontic appliances if the habit persists such as:
  - removable appliances
  - fixed palatal arch.

Further reading

RCS England (2014). First molars extractions in children. 🔗 https://www.rcseng.ac.uk/-/media/files/rcs/fds/publications/a-guideline-for-the-extraction-of-first-permanent-molars-in-children-rev-sept-2014.pdf

RCS England (2016). Management of the palatally ectopic maxillary canine. 🔗 https://www.rcseng.ac.uk/-/media/files/rcs/fds/publications/canine-guideline-2016.pdf

Orthodontic treatment

Treatment mechanics are beyond the scope of this text as most trainees in DCT will not be providing orthodontic treatment.

The purpose of this section is to advise the reader on the range of appliances that may be used and what they will come across in their practising careers.

Types of appliances

Removable appliances

- Conventional removable appliances are now used much less in the UK as fixed appliance therapy is the mainstay of treatment.
- Removable appliances still have their benefits for certain aspects of treatment:
  - Anterior crossbite correction.
  - Reduction of deep overbites using a flat anterior biteplane.
  - Biteplanes in the lower arch for correction of class III incisor relationships in combination with fixed appliances.
- Aligner style appliances can be considered in this category:
  - Use three-dimensional (3D) digital technology.
  - Series of aligners are created to correct a malocclusion.

Functional appliances

- Fixed or removable.
- Generally, to correct class II malocclusions although available for class III malocclusions.
- Use postured bites to encourage dentoalveolar tipping/minor skeletal enhancement to correct to class I.
- Mainly used during pubertal growth spurts (10–12 in girls, 11–13 in boys), aiming to utilize the growth potential but also compliance is better in this age group.

Fixed appliances

- Majority of orthodontic treatment is carried out using fixed appliances due to their ease of use and sophisticated mechanics to allow 3D correction of tooth position.
- Types include:
  - metal (stainless steel, cobalt chrome, gold)
  - ceramic
  - composite (less hard wearing and prone to fracture).
- Lingual fixed appliances:
  - Customized or direct placement.
  - Difficulty in access and may be more traumatic to the soft tissues.
  - Benefits are that lingual appliances are not visible.

Orthodontic referrals

Most NHS orthodontic patients are referred by their GDPs to commissioned providers of orthodontics.

- Provision of orthodontics is different across the regions within the UK, with some areas having provision from a variety of sources such as dentists with enhanced skills in orthodontics, specialists within primary care, specialists within community dental services, and consultant orthodontists within secondary care hospital services.
- These roles are defined in the NHS commissioning guide for England based on the different levels of care complexity:
  - Level 1: GDP.
  - Level 2: GDP with enhanced skills.
  - Level 3a: specialist.
  - Level 3b: consultant.
- This enables the referrer to determine the level of care a patient may require.
- Currently the referral process is dependent on the referrer to choose a provider in their local area. This may be via a regional electronic referral management system (eRMS) or may be individual practice referrals. Identify the correct method of referral in your area by contacting your local area team/commissioner or health board.
- This relies on the referrer choosing the most appropriate provider for the type of malocclusion and the potential treatment needed. This has been simplified with the introduction of the eRMS, as the algorithm will determine the most appropriate location to refer. It also enables appropriate triage of more time-sensitive cases and urgent cases requiring review.
- Urgent referrals will require radiographs to be attached, to demonstrate the urgent nature (e.g. periapicals/OPT of impacted/unerupted teeth).
- All areas are slightly different depending on the provision in that region.
- All referrals need to include an assessment of the appropriateness of the patient for orthodontic treatment, confirming caries status and good oral hygiene. Attach recent bitewing radiographs to demonstrate this.

The hospital orthodontic service provides the following:
- Advice and second opinions.
- Treatment plans for primary care providers of orthodontics.
- Treatment of complex malocclusions usually involving interdisciplinary management with other dental/medical specialties, such as restorative dentistry, paediatric dentistry, oral surgery, cleft/craniofacial/OMFS, and sleep medicine.
- Complex cases for training.
- Medical complications or behavioural management.

Hospital level referrals include the following[1]:
- Patients with clefts of the lip and/or palate or craniofacial syndromes.
- Patients with significant skeletal discrepancies requiring combined orthodontics and orthognathic surgery.

1 ⌁ https://www.england.nhs.uk/commissioning/wp-content/uploads/sites/12/2015/09/guid-comms-orthodontics.pdf

- Patients who require orthodontics and complex oral surgery input (e.g. multiple impacted teeth requiring complex orthodontic alignment).
- Patient with complex restorative problems (i.e. severe hypodontia) requiring secondary care input in a multidisciplinary environment.
- Patients with complex medical issues, including psychological concerns, which require close liaison with medical personnel locally.
- Patients with medical, developmental, or social problems who would not be considered suitable for treatment in specialist practice.
- Complex orthodontic cases not considered suitable for management in specialist practice.
- Referrals where advice or a second opinion is required from a secondary care consultant (i.e. to those providing level 1, 2, 3a care).

The majority of orthodontics is provided within primary care with practitioners providing treatment for a wide range of malocclusions but usually will have less need for input from other specialties.

Timings of referrals

Most orthodontic malocclusions are treated in the permanent dentition when patients are around 12 years and older. There are certain time-dependent referrals that need to be noted (there will be some individual variation in timings):
- Unerupted central incisors: 7–9 years.
- Anterior crossbite correction: 8–10 years.
- Molars of poor prognosis: 8–10 years.
- Early class III skeletal correction: 8–10 years.
- Impacted canines: 10–12 years.
- Functional appliance treatment for class II: 11–13 years.
- Most malocclusions: 12 years+.
- Orthognathic correction: 17 years+.

NHS orthodontics in the UK is limited to patients with specific malocclusion traits as defined by the IOTN. The referrer needs to be able to have a working knowledge of the IOTN and be able to assess a patient appropriately to determine the occlusal traits requiring assessment or intervention. This assessment provides the basis for appropriate referral and identification of time-sensitive cases, which they feel is the reason for the referral. We acknowledge that all practitioners are not calibrated in the IOTN and therefore there will be errors made, but the IOTN should provide a guide as to what malocclusion traits are eligible for treatment on the NHS.

Index of Orthodontic Treatment Need

- IOTN was developed as a method in which to determine whether a patient would benefit from orthodontics, based on the benefits outweighing the risks of treatment.
- IOTN has two components; the dental health component (DHC) and the aesthetic component (AC).[2]
- The DHC was based on an index used by the Swedish Dental Health Board to determine whether a patient required an orthodontic assessment and potentially treatment.

- The DHC is divided into five grades with a grade of 1 being no treatment needed to grade 5 being very great need for treatment.
- The five grades are then subdivided dependent on the malocclusion trait and assigned a letter. It is the most severe trait that determines the DHC score.
- There is a hierarchy within the DHC that determines the most severe trait and follows the acronym 'MOCDO':
  - Missing teeth/impacted teeth.
  - Overjet.
  - Crossbites.
  - Displacement of contact points.
  - Overbite.
- Once the DHC score has been attributed, the AC is a subjective score using the ten photographs.
- The need for the AC is only really for those patients scoring DHC 3 as this will determine eligibility for orthodontics care on the NHS which is limited to IOTN DHC 3, AC 6 and above.

IOTN DHC

Grade 5 (very great need for treatment)

5i Impeded eruption of teeth (except third molars) due to crowding, displacement, the presence of $, retained primary teeth and any pathological cause.

5h Extensive hypodontia with restorative implications (>1 tooth missing in any quadrant) requiring pre-restorative orthodontics.

5a Increased overjet >9 mm.

5m Reverse overjet >3.5 mm with reported masticatory and speech difficulties.

5p Defects of cleft lip and palate and any other craniofacial anomalies.

Grade 4 (great need for treatment)

4h Less extensive hypodontia requiring pre-restorative orthodontics or orthodontic space closure to obviate the need for prosthesis.

4a Increased overjet >6 mm but ≤9 mm.

4b Reverse overjet >3.5 mm with no masticatory or speech difficulties.

4m Reverse overjet >1 mm but <3.5 mm with recorded masticatory and speech difficulties.

4c Anterior or posterior crossbites with >2 mm discrepancy between RCP and ICP.

4l Posterior lingual crossbite with no functional occlusal contact in one or both buccal segments.

4d Severe contact point displacements >4 mm.

4e Extreme lateral or AOB >4 mm.

4f Increased and complete overbite with gingival or palatal trauma.

4t Partially erupted teeth, tipped and impacted against adjacent teeth.

4x Presence of $.

Grade 3 (borderline need for treatment)

3a Increased overjet >3.5 mm ≤6 mm with incompetent lips.

3b Reverse overjet >1 mm ≤3.5 mm.

3c Anterior or posterior crossbites with ≤2 mm discrepancy between RCP and ICP.

3d Contact point displacements >2 mm ≤4 mm.
3e Lateral or AOB >2 mm ≤4 mm.
3f Deep overbite complete on gingival or palatal tissues but no trauma.

Grade 2 (little need for treatment)

2a Increased overjet >3.5 mm but ≤6 mm with competent lips.
2b Reverse overjet >0 mm but ≤1 mm.
2c Anterior or posterior crossbites with ≤1 mm discrepancy between RCP and ICP.
2d Contact point displacements >1 mm but ≤2 mm.
2e Lateral or AOB >1 mm but ≤2 mm.
2f Increased overbite ≥3.5 mm without gingival contact.
2g Pre-normal or post-normal occlusions with no other anomalies (includes up to ½ unit discrepancy).

Grade 1 (no need for treatment)

1 Extremely minor malocclusions.
(IOTN reproduced from Brook P, et al. (1989). The development of an index of orthodontic treatment priority, *Eur J Orthod* 11, 309–320, by permission of Oxford University Press on behalf of the European Orthodontic Society.)

IOTN AC

- The AC is a series of ten photographs arranged in two rows of five, with 1 being the most attractive and 10 being the least attractive.
- Images available by searching for IOTN AC or at ℘ www.dental-referr als.org
- The AC is only really used to grade IOTN DHC 3 as the NHS only funds treatment of IOTN 3 (DHC), 6 and above (AC).
- The photographs do not represent all malocclusions and the dentist/orthodontist has to make a judgement as to the severity of the dental appearance.
- Some conventions used:
  - Class II malocclusions overjet in mm = AC (e.g. 6 mm overjet = AC 6).
  - Class III malocclusions:
    - Edge-to-edge aligned = 5.
    - Edge-to-edge malaligned = 6.
    - Increasing reverse overjet = AC 7+.
  - Class II/2 classic appearance = AC 6.
  - Missing teeth/crossbites:
    - one gap/anterior crossbite = 7.
    - two gaps/anterior crossbite = 8.
  - AOB:
    - 2 mm and aligned =5.
    - >2 mm = 6+.
  - Deep overbite = 6+.

Orthognathic surgery

As a trainee in DFT/DCT, you will assess patients who may benefit from orthognathic surgery to correct their dentofacial discrepancy, or you may be working in a unit that provides this treatment. A basic knowledge of the process is beneficial to assist explanation of treatment and referral or assisting in the surgery itself.

- Orthognathic treatment is usually provided through a multidisciplinary team (MDT) within a hospital setting involving orthodontics and OMFS/oral surgery with potential input from restorative dentistry and psychology.
- Orthognathic surgery is maxillofacial surgery to correct dentofacial disharmony and/or severe malocclusions and is usually performed on non-growing patients.

Patient journey

- Assessment in orthodontics, diagnostic records, and treatment planning.
- Orthognathic MDT clinic to discuss the treatment plan, risks, and benefits of treatment or any alternative options. There may be a psychological assessment as part of the MDT, to ensure that patients are prepared for potential surgery and to ensure that patients are considering treatment appropriately (assessing for body dysmorphic disorder).
- Usually, orthodontic treatment is commenced prior to surgery, with the aim to:
  - decompensate the arches (removing the existing dentoalveolar compensation for the underlying skeletal pattern, with either extractions or expansion)
  - coordinate the dental arches for the postsurgical result to enable a stable, functional occlusion.
- Presurgical planning: photographs, facebow mounted models, cephalometric analysis, and model surgery or 3D virtual planning.
- Presurgical orthognathic MDT clinic to reassess the patient and finalize the surgical plan, rediscussing surgery and its risks:
  - Discussion on discontinuing drugs, such as oral contraceptives, due to increased risk of DVTs.
- Construction of surgical acrylic wafers to guide the surgical movement of the maxilla and mandible:
  - Ensure that any laboratory work (wafers) is ready prior to surgery and have been tried in the mouth (ortho/OMFS) and surgical hooks have been placed on the appliances.
- Orthognathic surgery:
  - Usually, an inpatient stay of 1–2 days.
  - Surgery can be a combination of maxilla (Le Fort I, most common) and mandible (bilateral sagittal split osteotomy) ± genioplasty.
- Postsurgical recovery:
  - On average around 4–6 weeks off work.
  - Immediately post surgery, this author prefers no intermaxillary elastics. Any elastics placed should be directed by a member of the team with good knowledge of the force, direction, and frequency

required. Elastic traction can move the jaws, so any intermaxillary elastics need to be used with care.
- Soft/liquid diet for 2 weeks, increasing to normal soft diet around 6–8 weeks.
- OMFS review 1 week.
- Orthodontic review 10–14 days to assess the need to guide the jaws into position.
- Postsurgical orthodontics:
  - Guiding the jaws and dentition into maximum intercuspation and finalizing tooth position.
- Retention.
- Orthognathic clinic:
  - Review at 1 year post surgery, 2 years post debond.

Risks of orthognathic surgery

The main risks associated with surgery are pain and discomfort, swelling (especially up to 4 weeks after surgery, but persisting for around 3–6 months), infection of fixation plates (5–10% of cases, increased in smokers or poor oral hygiene), surgical relapse of the corrected jaw position, change in facial appearance with widening of the nasal base, paraesthesia of the inferior dental nerve (10–20% cases), and paraesthesia of the lingual nerve (5%).

Further reading

Your Jaw Surgery. Information resource for patients. ♒ www.yourjawsurgery.com

Cleft lip and palate

As a trainee in DFT and DCT, you will see, treat, and be involved with the care of patients with orofacial clefts, and it is useful to have an under-standing of the treatment that is required or has already been performed. It is the most common craniofacial anomaly. Cleft lip/palate (CL/P) is a feature of >400 recognized syndromes. Cleft care in the UK was centralized to regional units to improve surgical outcomes by increasing the numbers seen in each unit. Many regional centres operate a 'hub and spoke' model of care across a number of hospitals. Cleft teams involve input from cleft surgeons, orthodontists, ear, nose, and throat (ENT) specialists, speech and language therapists (SALTs), dietitians, psychologists, audiologists, paedia-tricians, paediatric dentists, restorative dentists, and nursing. The care for patients with CL/P is complex and long term. The overall aim of treatment is to provide a good facial appearance and improve function for speaking, hearing, eating, and swallowing.

Incidence
- 1:700 live births (all clefts), 1:2000 (CP).
- 14% CL/P associated with a syndrome; 55% CP associated with a syndrome.
- Unilateral CLP left:right, 2:1.
- Unilateral CLP 40% > CP 30% > bilateral CLP 10% = CL 10% = submucous 10%.
- Japanese > Caucasian > Afro-Caribbean.

Aetiology
- Largely unknown; epigenetic/polygenic multifactorial.
- Syndromes: single gene mutations.
- Environmental: smoking, alcohol, methotrexate, retinoids, ani-folate, diet vitamin B_{12} deficiency, social class.

Embryology
The 5th–9th weeks *in utero* is the most important period in the developing face:
- 6 weeks:
  - CL: failure of fusion of medial and lateral nasal processes and maxillary prominence.
- 8–10 weeks:
  - Palatal shelves elevate at 8 weeks and fuse at 8–10 weeks. Breakdown of mesial edge epithelium allows fusion.
  - CP: failure of shelves to elevate; failure of contact between shelves; failure of breakdown of mesial edge epithelium; rupture following fusion.

Dentofacial features in clefts
There is a normal growth potential, but surgery to the palate will cause scarring and restriction of growth:
- Retrusive maxilla and mandible.
- Increased vertical proportions.
- Delayed dental development/eruption.

- Hypodontia; $\underline{2}$ on cleft side absent ~30%, non-cleft side ~15%; increased hypodontia other than cleft site (⮕ Hypodontia).
- Supernumeraries (⮕ Supernumerary teeth).
- Hypoplasia/microdontia (⮕ Microdontia and ⮕ Enamel defects).
- Caries (⮕ Prevention).
- Impacted teeth: $\underline{3}$ in the cleft site (⮕ Impacted maxillary canines); $\underline{6}$ due to reduced maxillary arch length (⮕ Ectopic eruption of first permanent molars).

Management

Treatment and advice will be from diagnosis (possibly *in utero*) until adulthood across multiple specialties. There are also specific time points that audit records are taken: birth, 5 years, 10 years, 15 years, and 20 years. These are used as assessments of the overall care outcome.[1]

- Birth:
  - Advice and support. Feeding advice and hearing assessments.
  - Presurgical orthopaedics—occasionally used such as lip strapping or orthodontic feeding plates.
- 3–6 months (this may vary across different units with some favouring earlier repair):
  - Lip repair ± alveolar repair.
  - Z-plasty (Millard, Tennison), Delaire or Veau repairs. Surgeon dependent.
- 9–12 months (this may vary across different units):
  - Palate repair.
  - Von Lagenbeck, Veau, or Delaire repairs.
- 2–10 years:
  - Speech assessments and therapy.
  - ENT assessments. Grommet surgery.
  - Paediatric dentistry assessments, prevention, advice, and treatment.
- 7–10 years (this may vary across different units):
  - Orthodontic preparation for alveolar bone grafting.
  - Secondary alveolar bone grafting to provide bone into the cleft site, to enable eruption of the permanent teeth (e.g. $\underline{3}$).
- 11–15 years:
  - Orthodontic treatment.
  - Restorative replacement of missing teeth.
- 18 years+:
  - Orthognathic assessment and treatment as required.

Further reading

Cleft Lip & Palate Association: ℘ www.clapa.com

1 Akram A (2015). *Br Dent J* 218, 129.

Syndromes of the head and neck

There are several hundred syndromes that may be relevant to the trainee in DFT and DCT, but it is beyond the scope of this handbook to provide detail on this. There are >400 syndromes conditions associated with orofacial clefting. Some of the details of more relevant syndromes are included here, but again, it is not possible to provide all details for each syndrome. Details of syndromes can be found at ℜ www.omim.org, if you come across a patient with a syndrome you have not heard of before. The website is also very useful for images of some of the terminology used. It is useful to know some of the clinical presentations, particularly with respect to cardiac anomalies.

Velocardiofacial (DiGeorge, 22q11 deletion, CATCH 22)
* 1:2000.
* Microcephaly; long face; retrognathia; low-set ears/small/hearing defects; narrow palpebral fissures; hypertelorism; square nasal root; CP (CL); velopharyngeal insufficiency.
* *CVS*: abnormality in 85%; tetralogy of Fallot; ventriculoseptal defect (VSD).
* *Neurological*: learning difficulties; autistic features.

Pierre Robin sequence
* 1:8500–30,000.
* Defect of first arch structures.
* Mandibular micrognathia; glossoptosis; isolated wide CP.
* *Birth*: requires tracheostomy—medical emergency.
* May require distraction osteogenesis.

CHARGE syndrome
* 1:10,000.
* CHARGE:
  * C: Coloboma of iris/retina.
  * H: Heart defects (tetralogy of Fallot atrial septal defect/VSD, etc.).
  * A: Atresia of choanae (blockage between nose and pharynx).
  * R: Retardation of growth/development.
  * G: Genital anomalies.
  * E: Ear anomalies.
* CL/P.

Van der Woude syndrome
* 1:28,000.
* Lower lip pits or mucous cysts.
* CLP/CP; cleft/bifid uvula; narrow high-arched palate.
* Ankyloglossia; hypernasal; hypodontia.

Oral–facial–digital syndromes
* 1:50,000–250,000.
* *Oral*: CL (midline); CP; cleft tongue/bifid; hypodontia; $.
* *Facial*: frontal bossing; midface hypoplasia; broad nasal root; hypertelorism; telecanthus; epicanthal folds; down slanting palpebral fissures.
* *Digital*: brachydactyly; syndactyly; clinodactyly.
* *CVS*: cardiac anomalies.
* *Neurological*: learning difficulties (variable).

Treacher Collins syndrome
- 1:50,000.
- First and second arch abnormality.
- Malar hypoplasia; zygomatic hypoplasia; malformation of auricle; conductive hearing loss; ear tags; blindness; choanal stenosis/atresia; downward slanting palpebral fissures.
- CP; mandibular hypoplasia; macrostomia.
- Normal intelligence.

Hemifacial microsomia
- 1:3000–5000.
- *Aetiology*: unknown. Failure of neural crest cell migration/haemorrhage of stapedial artery/disturbance in blood supply to first/second arches *in utero*.
- *Facial*: asymmetry; small half of face; hypoplasia of facial muscles/mala/maxilla/mandible.
- *Dental*: crowding on affected side; hypodontia; delayed dental development.
- *Ears*: unilateral external ear deformity; pre-auricular tags; external auditory canal atresia; microtia/anotia; hearing loss.
- *Eyes*: epibulbar dermoid; upper eyelid coloboma; microphthalmia/anophthalmia; strabismus.
- *Mouth*: macrostomia; CL/P; parotid agenesis; soft palate malformation.
- *CVS*: VSD; tetralogy of Fallot; aortic coarctation.
- *Genitourinary*: ectopic kidney; renal agenesis.
- *CNS*: variable learning difficulties.
- *Classification*: OMENS+:
  - O: Orbital distortion.
  - M: Mandibular hypoplasia.
  - E: Ear anomaly.
  - N: Nerve involvement.
  - S: Soft tissue deficiency.
  - +: Extracranial features.

Goldenhar syndrome (oculo-auriculo-vertebral syndrome)
- 1:3500–26,000.
- Spectrum of hemifacial microsomia.
- Unilateral right > left; 30% bilateral.
- Small ear; pre-auricular tags; epibulbar dermoids (benign tumours inside opening of the eye).
- Internal organ disruption; scoliosis.

Ectodermal dysplasia
- 1:17,000; >150 syndromes associated.
- Affects the ectodermal structures: teeth; hair; nails; sweat glands.
- Severe hypodontia/microdontia.
- Sparse, lightly pigmented hair.
- May be associated with CLP.

Holoprosencephaly
- 1:15,000 (live), 1:250 miscarriages.
- Developmental defect with failure of cerebral hemispheres to split.

- Cyclopia (most severe—not compatible with life).
- Midline CLP; midline solitary maxillary incisor (mild form).

Fetal alcohol syndrome
- 1:100.
- *Aetiology*: alcohol during pregnancy. Severity proportional to amount/time.
- Characteristic facies. Short/flat nose; midface hypoplasia; thin vermilion border upper lip; indistinct philtrum.
- Learning difficulties.
- Cerebral palsy.

Marfan syndrome
- 1:5000, connective tissue disorder.
- *Growth*: disproportional tall stature.
- *Head*: dolichocephalic; long, narrow face; malar hypoplasia; micrognathia; retrognathia.
- *Eyes*: enophthalmos; myopia; down-slanting palpebral fissures.
- *Mouth*: high-arched narrow palate.
- *CVS*: aortic/mitral regurgitation; valve prolapse; aortic dilation/dissection; ascending aneurism.
- *Skin*: pectus excavatum; scoliosis; arachnodactyly.

Down syndrome
- 1:700, trisomy chromosome 21.
- *Aetiology*: increased maternal age.
- *Growth*: short stature.
- *Head*: brachycephaly; flat profile; mid-face hypoplasia.
- *Ears*: small ears; conductive hearing loss.
- *Eyes*: upslanting palpebral fissures; epicanthal folds.
- *Mouth*: macroglossia; macrostomia; hypodontia; microdontia; supernumeraries; delayed eruption; class III malocclusion; aggressive periodontal disease.
- *CVS*: congenital heart defects; atrial septal defect/VSD 40%.
- *Skin*: atlanto-axial instability.
- *CNS*: learning difficulties (variable); increased risk of epilepsy.

Gorlin–Goltz syndrome (multiple basal cell naevi syndrome)
- 1:50,000–150,000.
- *Head*: broad facies; frontal and biparietal bossing; mandibular prognathism; odontogenic keratocysts of the jaws.
- *Eyes*: hypertelorism; strabismus; iris coloboma.
- *Mouth*: CL/P; $/hypodontia; ectopic teeth; dental malformations.
- *Skin*: basal cell naevi; basal cell carcinoma.
- *CNS*: learning difficulties; calcification of falx cerebri.

Achondroplasia
- 1:15,000–40,000.
- Short-limb dwarfism.
- *Head*: frontal bossing; megalocephaly; mid-face hypoplasia.
- *Mouth*: high-arched palate; macroglossia.
- *Skin*: foramen magnum stenosis; lumbar lordosis; spinal stenosis; bowing of legs; brachydactyly; trident hand.

Ehlers–Danlos syndrome
- Group of disorders that affect connective tissue.
- Affect joints and skin: hypermobility; weak muscle tone; arthritis.
- *Head and neck*: narrow maxillary; hypermobile ears; myopia; epicanthal folds; microdontia.
- *Mouth*: TMJ hypermobile; fragile mucosa; dilacerated roots; pulp obliteration; tooth mobility; early-onset periodontal disease.
- *CVS*: mitral valve prolapse.

Cleidocranial dysplasia
- 1:200,000.
- *Head*: frontal bossing; midface hypoplasia; micrognathia; brachycephalic.
- *Eyes*: hypertelorism.
- *Mouth*: CP; narrow high-arched palate; Skeletal class III; delayed eruption of primary teeth, delayed eruption of secondary teeth; supernumeraries; retention cysts; enamel hypoplasia.
- *Body*: narrow thorax; aplastic/hypoplastic clavicles; Wormian bones; scoliosis; brachydactyly.

Acromegaly
- 80:1,000,000.
- *Aetiology*: anterior pituitary tumour (adenoma); produces excess growth hormone after epiphysial plate closure.
- *Features*: renewed growth of jaws, hands, feet, and soft tissues; prognathism; frontal bossing; coarse features/skin; enlarged lips/nose/macroglossia.
- *Systemic*: cardiovascular hypertension; congestive heart failure; impaired glucose metabolism; sleep apnoea.

Craniosynostoses
Premature fusion of the sutures of the skull. Non-syndromic 75–80% single suture. Syndromic 20–25%. Associated with increased paternal age

Apert syndrome
- 1:65,000.
- Coronal suture synostosis (early); multisuture fusion.
- *Head*: acrobrachycephaly; turribrachycephaly; megalocephaly; large fontanelle (late closing).
- *Face*: high forehead; midface hypoplasia; mandibular prognathism.
- *Ears*: hearing loss.
- *Eyes*: shallow orbits; proptosis; hypertelorism; down-slanting palpebral fissures.
- *Nose*: depressed nasal bridge.
- *Mouth*: CP 30%; narrow, high palate; delayed eruption.
- *CVS*: VSD; overriding aorta.
- *Skin*: symmetric syndactyly of hands/feet.

Crouzon syndrome
- 1:25,000.
- Multi-suture craniosynostosis.
- *Head*: brachycephaly; frontal bossing; maxillary hypoplasia; mandibular prognathism.
- *Ears*: conductive hearing loss.

- *Eyes*: optic atrophy; shallow orbits; proptosis; hypertelorism; poor vision.
- *Nose*: parrot-like.
- *Mouth*: crowding; high-arched palate; CP 3%; sleep apnoea.
- Limbs unaffected.

Further reading

Akram A, McKnight MM, Bellardie H, et al. (2015). Craniofacial malformations and the orthodontist. *Br Dent J* 218, 129–141.

Hennekam RCM, Krantz ID, Allanson J (2010). *Gorlin's Syndromes of the Head and Neck* (5th ed). Oxford University Press.

OMIM®. An Online Catalog of Human Genes and Genetic Disorders: ℘ www.omim.org

Risks of orthodontic treatment

Risks of orthodontic treatment

The young practitioner should be aware of the risks of orthodontic treatment to enable them to advise their patients more effectively on the benefits of treatment weighed against the risks. In some cases, the risks of treatment outweigh the benefits and this needs to be assessed and conferred to the patient. One of the frequently occurring risks is decalcification due to poor oral hygiene or diet. Patients who clearly cannot maintain good oral hygiene should not be considered for orthodontic treatment and should be counselled to improve prior to referral for active orthodontic treatment. Although these are not all the risks of treatment, they are the more common areas to discuss.

- Discomfort and pain: usually for several days after initial appliance fitting or adjustment. Easily controlled by pain relief.
- Tooth demineralization: early caries more likely on the buccal surface caused by poor diet and oral hygiene regimen.
- Tooth damage: enamel surface damage with removal or brackets—not common.
- Loss of tooth vitality: more likely to occur to previously traumatized teeth or teeth with large restorations.
- Root resorption: orthodontically induced inflammatory root resorption occurs in most cases but on average this is about 1–2 mm of the overall root length. Around 2–4% will experience more severe resorption, which is most likely a genetic predisposition to root resorption.
- Gingival recession: minor periodontal attachment loss is common. Adult orthodontics is more likely to lead to 'black triangles'.
- Periodontal bone loss: minor bone loss may occur. In the presence of active periodontal disease, orthodontic treatment may accelerate further bone loss.
- TMJDS: there is currently no evidence that links orthodontics to increased or decreased symptoms, although this is possible.
- Facial profile: this can be affected by treatment; in particular, excessive retraction of the upper incisors may lead to reduced lip support.
- Relapse of tooth position: long-term retention is required to maintain tooth position.

Retention

- Following a course of orthodontic treatment, most malocclusions will need to be retained using some form of retention regimen if tooth position is to be maintained.
- Orthodontic retention is paramount for the success of the active treatment.
- Most orthodontic cases will show some form of relapse if retainers are not worn.
- General advice on retainer regimens differs, but tends to follow a similar pattern:
  - Initial full-time or part-time wear except for eating/drinking for 3 months.
  - Night-time wear for 12 months.
  - Titrate wear depending on tooth movement, usually advising reduction in the number of nights worn on a gradual basis.
  - Patients will need to continue to wear their retainers life-long if they wish to maintain the corrected occlusion.
- Most orthodontists will monitor retention for at least 12 months following appliance removal.
- Following this period, patients will be referred back to their GDP for continued monitoring of retention.
- NHS patients will be provided with retainers, in most cases, with a guarantee for 12 months. Following this period, replacement removable retainers will be chargeable and can be replaced by either the GDP or the orthodontist on a private basis.
- Types of retainers:
  - Vacuum-formed retainers.
  - Hawley retainers (removable appliances with no active components).
  - Bonded retainer wires.
- Within the 12-month period following appliance removal, patients should seek advice for their orthodontist. After this period, any replacements or repairs may be chargeable.

Further reading

Fleming PS, Littlewood SJ (Eds). (2021). Orthodontic retention special issue. *Br Dent J* 230(11). ᐧ
  https://www.nature.com/bdj/volumes/230/issues/11

Orthodontic emergencies

- As a trainee in DFT/DCT, you may only come into contact with orthodontic emergencies out of hours, or if the patient cannot see their orthodontist.
- There are very few true emergencies within orthodontics.
- The only true emergency would be eye penetration with headgear, and this must be immediately referred to the eye department within your local hospital.
- Common orthodontic 'emergencies':
  - Long archwire causing discomfort/trauma.
  - Loss of orthodontic brackets.
  - Loss of modules (elastomerics holding the wire *in situ*).
- The aim would be to make the appliance safe. This can be achieved by:
  - cutting long wires short with distal-end cutters. Do not try to do this with any other wire cutters as you are more likely to cause more problems
  - do not attempt to replace lost brackets as they are unlikely to adhere, unless you have new brackets and are comfortable doing this. Cutting the archwires short to prevent irritation may be the best solution
  - if you have no way to improve the situation, remove the archwire by disengaging each elastomeric module off each bracket using a short probe. This will then enable removal of the archwire until the patient can see their orthodontist.
- Orthodontic advice on irritation caused by appliances is to use orthodontic wax or an equivalent vegetable-based wax (e.g. the wax around a well-known small cheese). Warm a small piece of wax in your fingers. Dry the area with a tissue and apply the wax to the area of the appliance causing irritation against the mucosa. This can alleviate the trauma caused by appliances.
- It is very common for appliances to cause ulceration and discomfort, especially within the first week after placement. Advice is often the best remedy in that this is very normal and that over the next several weeks, the lips/cheeks will become accustomed to the appliances and discomfort will improve.

Bonded retainer repair

- Breakages of bonded retainers:
  - You may feel confident that you can repair a broken bonded retainer (most will fail at the bond/enamel interface at some point).
  - Remove any residual composite from the tooth using a tungsten carbide debonding bur (this will not cut enamel).
  - Remove existing composite from the wire by gentle pressure with a Weingart orthodontic plier (or similar), this will debond the excess composite remaining on the wire. Try to not distort the wire as placing any activity within the wire could potentially become an active component and move the tooth it is bonded to.
  - Etch/bond or use self-etch primer on the area and apply composite resin and light cure. There are specific bonded retainer composites, but any composite is an option. Bonded retainer composite has less

filler content and so is easier to apply than composite for dental restorations.
- If you do not feel confident in providing the above treatment, refer the patient back to their orthodontist or to a local orthodontist for private repair (if outside of the 12 months).
• If in doubt, get advice.

Bonded retainer replacement

- Replacement of bonded retainers are within a GDP's remit, but, as with all treatment, you should be comfortable in providing this treatment. If there are any concerns, refer to an orthodontist.
- Bonded retainers can be of several varieties, sizes, and materials and it is operator preference as to which one you use.[1]
- Bonded retainers can be direct placement or laboratory construction. Some will provide a jig to enable accurate placement, others rely on operator positioning.
- The key to successful placement is good moisture control and placement not in the occlusion or subject to excusive movements.
- Placement tips and advice:
  - Ensure that any residual composite has been removed with a tungsten carbide debonding bur.
  - Good isolation with OptraGate™ or Dry Dam®.
  - Good moisture control with a saliva ejector.
  - Airway protection using gauze or Dry Dam®.
  - Etch/prime or self-etch primer.
  - Place flowable composite onto the lingual surface where you intend to place the wire.
  - Seat the laboratory-made wire into the flowable composite and cure into position.
  - Cover the wire on the tooth with a bonded retainer composite and shape using a microbrush with primer.
  - Check the occlusion and adjust as necessary.

1 Kirschen R (2021). *Br Dent J* 230, 709.

Chapter 5

Restorative dentistry

Introduction to restorative dentistry

- Restorative dentistry is a specialty defined by the GDC as 'The restoration of diseased, injured or abnormal teeth to normal function. Includes all aspects of endodontics, periodontics, and prosthodontics'.[1]
- The majority of restorative dentistry in the UK is carried out in general practice; however, there are a large number of hospital units that are commissioned to offer specific specialist services.
- The specific services offered can vary considerably depending on capacity and the type of clinicians working there. For example, in a district general hospital with one consultant and one postgraduate trainee, the service may be limited to an advisory capacity with treatment for priority groups only, whereas a teaching hospital linked with an undergraduate dental school and multiple postgraduate trainees may have wider acceptance criteria to facilitate training as well as priority groups.
- Priority groups of patients are those that may require restorative dental treatment as part of multidisciplinary care including maxillofacial defects such as head and neck cancer, cleft and craniofacial abnormalities, hypodontia, and trauma.
- Patients may also be referred by the GDP to the unit for advice on treatment planning or second opinions and in some cases provision of treatment, particularly if the GDP feels it is out of their remit.
- As a trainee in DCT in these units, part of the role may be to contribute to new patient assessment consultations for diagnosis and treatment planning for referred or priority group patients.
- A larger role of the trainee in DCT would be in the delivery of the consultant-led treatment plan, which may include more complex and advanced procedures then would normally be carried out in general practice.
- Once the agreed treatment plan has been completed, the patient is often discharged back to the continuing care of the GDP. Some treatment plans may require some or all care to be provided in general practice, or the long-term maintenance to be carried out in general practice even if the treatment was provided in hospital.
- The purpose of the hospital unit is not to take over the role of the GDP in providing regular routine, emergency, and preventative care. This can be done more cost-effectively in general practice.
- As an exception to this, many units may provide emergency treatment or a walk-in clinic for the provision of urgent dental treatment to patients who are currently undergoing a course of treatment at the hospital or those who are not under the care of a dentist but require urgent care.

Introduction to maxillofacial defects

Head and neck cancer

TNM staging

Introduction to maxillofacial defects

Restorative dentistry forms part of several multidisciplinary teams for the management of patients with head and neck cancer and developmental anomalies such as cleft lip and palate. Defects in orofacial anatomy as a result of development, disease or treatment may require complex dental management.

Head and neck cancer

Consultants in restorative dentistry have a key role in the head and neck oncology multidisciplinary clinic and are responsible for the dental health of head and neck oncology patients prior to, during, and after treatment.[1] As a DCT trainee in restorative dentistry, you are likely to be involved in the management of these patients under the guidance of the team. Due to the severity of the disease and the need to initiate treatment quickly following referral and diagnosis, it is imperative that the restorative team are involved from an early point to assess the dental needs of these patients prior to commencing treatment for the cancer.

TNM classification

The main aim for management of head and neck cancer would either be curative or palliative. Options for treatment vary depending on the type of cancer, size, and its location and also any metastases (TNM classification):

T	*Primary tumour*	**N**	*Cervical nodes*
T1	<2 cm diameter	N0	No nodes
T2	2–4 cm diameter	N1	Single nodes <3 cm
T3	>4 cm diameter	N2	Single node 3–6 cm (N2a)
T4	Massive, invading beyond mouth		Multiple nodes (N2b)
			Contralateral nodes (N2c)
		N3	Node >6 cm
M	*Distant metastasis*		
M0	Absent		
M1	Present		

Treatment of cancer patients

The main modalities for treatment, which may include a combination of treatment, are:

- Surgery
- Radiotherapy
- Chemotherapy.

The effects of each of these treatment modalities can have a significant impact on the dental health in the short and long term, so decisions are needed regarding the potential effects and minimizing the side effects of treatment. The restorative assessment will be discussed at the head and neck oncology MDT with a plan for pre- and post-treatment (NICE 2004).[2]

1 Colloc T (2020). *Br Dent J* 229, 655.

2 NICE (2004). *Improving Outcomes in Head and Neck Cancers*. NICE Guidance CSG6. ℘ https://www.nice.org.uk/guidance/csg6

The surgical treatment will create changes in the anatomy, function, and appearance. Radio- and chemotherapy will create changes in the oral and facial region, all of which may have an adverse effect on speech, mastication, taste, swallowing, salivary gland function, and mouth opening.

Pre-treatment restorative management
- Assessment of the oral health, preventative advice, and support:
  - Instigating the necessary oral hygiene and diet measures that will be required to maintain oral health throughout treatment and throughout the side effects of any treatment planned.
  - Radiotherapy treatment may lead to an increased risk of caries due to radiation-induced xerostomia.
  - Bear in mind that these patients have recently been given a cancer diagnosis so may not be in a position to process oral hygiene advice at the first visit. Be prepared to go over all information again at a later stage.
- Treatment of dental disease and loss of poor prognosis teeth:
  - If the field of radiotherapy involves the oral cavity, then this can put the patient at risk of osteoradionecrosis of the jaw (ORNJ) should subsequent extractions be required. For that reason, teeth with a poor long term prognosis may be electively extracted prior to radiotherapy.[3]
  - The field of radiotherapy often aims to spare the anterior teeth; however, scatter may occur and these too may be at risk should extraction be necessary.
  - Prior to surgery, extractions may also be required as they may fall within the proposed resection site.
  - Prediction of the ability to maintain oral health with trismus and the removal of teeth that may be difficult to access.
- Plan any adjuncts to minimize the unwanted effects of radiotherapy on the oral cavity:
  - Lead shielding oral appliances.
- Plan for the future restorative rehabilitation:
  - No flap reconstruction: patients may require the construction of a temporary obturator or cover plate to seal the defect.
  - Input into the oncology reconstruction plan to facilitate restorative rehabilitation with dentures, bridges, or implants.
  - Consideration of primary implant placement.

Preventative management
- Oral hygiene instruction, toothbrush advice, and interdental cleaning.
- Dietary advice in conjunction with dietitians to manage potential cariogenic diets/supplements.
- Topical fluoride, such as Duraphat 5000 ppm.
- Sodium fluoride mouthrinse (0.05%).
- Daily GC Tooth Mousse™.
- Saliva replacement therapy.
- Jaw exercises.

3 Bruines H (1998). *Oral Surg Oral Med Oral Pathol* 86, 256.

Management during treatment
- Oral mucositis:
  - 1–2 weeks after radio-chemotherapy treatment lasting ~6 weeks.
  - Oral mouth wash (e.g. benzydamine m/w (Difflam™)).
  - Reinforce oral care.
- Candidal infections:
  - Antifungals.
- Xerostomia:
  - Salivary stimulants (e.g. pilocarpine).
  - Saliva substitutes (e.g. Glandosane®, Biotene Oralbalance® gel).
- Trismus:
  - Exercises.

Post-treatment considerations
- Patients following head and neck radiotherapy may have the following complications: xerostomia, poor saliva quality, radiation caries, ORNJ, trismus, worsening periodontitis, mucositis, taste disturbance, and/or opportunistic infections.[4]
- Following surgery there may be reconstructions using different flaps which would vary in size, shape, anatomical region, bone support, and soft tissue support.
- Some patients may not have any kind of reconstruction and have an open defect, and this is more so for the maxilla. Both the width and depth of the defect need to be considered in these cases.
- There are some patients who have had both surgery and radiotherapy and they will have to be considered accordingly.
- There may be a small number of patients who may also have chemotherapy and they may require blood investigations to check for healing.

Post radiotherapy restorative management
- Asymptomatic radiation caries can occur in areas that are less typically affected by caries, in particular on root and labial surfaces of the incisors, which can occur quickly after radiotherapy. Intuition would advise caries removal and restoration; however, in doing so this may initiate pulpal symptoms. These are often best managed with topical fluoride to slow the caries progression. Eventually the caries may become so extensive that they can no longer support the crown which may fracture off leaving a root stump.[5]
- By intervening in such cases, a pulpal response may occur, triggering further intervention such as root canal treatment. However, this may cause further problems with failure and possible risk of ORNJ should it require extraction. In asymptomatic radiation caries, preventing the rate of progression of caries should be considered as the main treatment.
- Emphasis on prevention is important to slow the rate of caries progression and advancing periodontal disease. Use of high-fluoride

4 Restorative Dentistry (RD-UK). Predicting and managing oral and dental complications of surgical and non-surgical treatment for H&N cancer. ℜ www.restdent.org.uk
5 Ray-Chaudhuri A (2013). *Br Dent J* 214, 387.

toothpastes (e.g. 5000 ppmF) and emphasis on good mechanical plaque control is important.
- Trismus is another major problem for these patients:
  - Asking them to maintain wide opening for good oral access can be demanding.
  - Use of mouth props can be helpful, applying paraffin wax to the lips can aid comfort.
  - Use of a rubber dam can be particularly helpful for restorative work to gain clearer access.
  - Taking impressions can also cause difficulty—when using alginate, it may be worth quickly applying material around all the surfaces of the teeth prior to seating the tray. Turning the tray by 90° on approach and gently pulling the labial commissure from the opposite side, then swiftly turning and seating the tray can facilitate this.
  - When using silicone, applying a light-bodied material to all fissures and gingival margins prior to seating the tray could be done instead.

Post-surgery restorative management

Following resection of the tumour, the patient may have reconstruction with a flap (which may be composed of skin, muscle, bone, or various combinations) or no reconstruction with an open defect.

Oral rehabilitation options:
- Osseointegrated implants:
  - *Primary implants*: placed at the time of surgery. May have increased integration rates if radiotherapy is planned post surgery.
  - *Secondary implants*: placed postoperatively. Higher risk of failure if bone irradiated post surgery. Better planning available.
  - *Zygomatic implants*: used to retain obturators.
- Conventional prostheses:
  - Dentures/obturators.

Management techniques are described below, in particular with impression taking and removable prosthetics:
- Great care needs to be taken when dealing with open defects. The size and depth are important as they present different challenges. While small defects may seem negligible, there is a high risk of impression material separating within the defect on removing the tray which may not be retrievable. The use of gauze with paraffin wax applied that completely covers the defect with a generous margin will capture material the passes into the small defect.
- Larger defects may consume more of the normal anatomy. Assessment of the depth of the cavity and if there are any walls that could retain the prosthesis. Due to the size of the defect, there is a lower likelihood of the bulk material separating into the defect.
- Flaps can present several challenges depending on the location and properties of the reconstruction.
- The presence of a flap would create a loss of basic anatomy and this must be kept in mind—there may be an absence of a buccal sulcus and alveolar ridge.
- Primary impressions should aim to be overextended and cover the entire denture-bearing area.

- Stock trays should be modified by trimming sections that may impede on the reconstruction. However, the reconstruction should be included in its entirety as far as the denture-bearing area is concerned.
- Once the stock tray is trimmed, the use of beauty wax or impression compound can be used to modify the tray to extend around the aberrant anatomy.
- Flaps can vary in properties. A particularly bulky flap may cause problems as it may not provide any support. Using it as a secondary area or support may reduce the retention. Consider using a perforated region on the special tray, or even having a spaced region and using a low-viscosity material such as a light-bodied silicone to reduce the displacement of this region while impression making.
- It may be worth creating a set of heat-cured bases for the patient to try as training plates.
- Due to the loss of anatomy, it may also be difficult to establish the position of the denture teeth. To overcome this, it may be worth taking a neutral zone impression. This can be done once the base plate is constructed; wire fins can be applied to the occlusal surface by the laboratory. In clinic, apply two stubs of impression composition to the most posterior part of the denture and get the patient to close to correct the vertical dimension while the material is setting. Once this is done, mix cold cure denture acrylic conditioning material to 'snow-like' consistency and apply to the fins. Insert the baseplate and ask the patient to make the full range of tongue and lip movements to displace the conditioning material into the neutral zone. This can be given to the laboratory to position the denture teeth.

Restorative management of cleft lip and palate

Restorative management of CLP patients following surgical and ortho-dontic care is usually aimed at replacement of developmentally absent teeth and to improve dental aesthetics and function with conventional restorative techniques, such as composites, bridges, and implant-retained prostheses (➔ Cleft lip and palate and ➔ Hypodontia).

Older patients who have had repaired or unrepaired CLP surgery can present with different challenges:

- The maxillary arch form tends to deviate from the normal pattern with a wide distance between the posterior teeth, narrowing at the premolar region, and potentially multiple absent anterior teeth.
- The palate can have an open defect (fistula) or this is most likely closed, but will have scarring and tends to be deep and narrow.
- A standard stock tray may not fit the arch form and may require significant modification.
- Again, trimming the tray in the premolar and molar regions and recreating the borders of the tray with impression compound can help create a tray that is correctly extended.
- While getting an adequately wide impression tray for the posterior part of the arch form may be possible, this can be very difficult to get past a narrow mouth opening and even removing the tray out of the mouth.
- A way of overcoming this may be to get an impression as best as possible then note any deficiencies (i.e. lack of buccal surfaces and sulcus) then trim the cast in these areas and construct a special tray

around this (as this would be more closely fitting then a stock tray and hence smaller). The use of small stub handles in the mid palate region rather than the labial region can help also. This means there can be a greater possible degree of rotation to pass the tray into the mouth.

- It is important to find out what the patient wants from the prosthesis. As mentioned, the patient may simply want replacement of missing teeth, alternatively they may want to disguise a cross bite. This can be achieved by the use of an onlay denture. The fit surface of such a denture would cover part or all of the existing dentition and the denture teeth would be placed in the more ideal position.
- Using a chrome denture there can be meshwork running over the natural dentition, with tissue stops and internal clasps to aid retention.
- When constructing such dentures, it is important that the patient can tolerate a large increase in vertical dimension to account for the chrome, acrylic, and denture teeth over the existing natural dentition. The advantage of using chrome, however, is that if there is only a small amount of interocclusal space on the last standing teeth, then this can be overlayed with chrome only as a bite plane.

Restorative management of dental developmental anomalies

Hypodontia

Definition

- The developmental absence of one or more teeth, excluding the six molar teeth:
  - *Severe hypodontia*: six or more missing teeth.
  - *Anodontia*: absence of all teeth either primary/permanent or both.

Aetiology

- Genetic in origin or associated with an environmental insult during tooth development (e.g. radiation/chemotherapy).
- Isolated and non-syndromic or part of a syndrome.

Prevalence

- Primary teeth: 0.1–0.9%:[1]
  - In cases of primary hypodontia, dental anomalies affecting the permanent dentition can be expected in 30–50% of cases.
- Permanent teeth: 4.6–6.3%[2] (white European populations); 6.1–7.7% (Chinese populations).
- Females > males.[2]
- Tends to affect the end of a dental series (e.g. 2s, 5s, 8s).
- In permanent dentition affects lower 5s > upper 2s > upper 5s > lower 1s.[2]

Associated dental anomalies

- Microdontia (➜ Abnormalities in tooth size).
- Infraocclusion of primary molar teeth (➜ Dental eruption anomalies).
- Ectopic eruption of maxillary permanent canines (➜ Impacted maxillary canines).

Commonly associated conditions

- Ectodermal dysplasia.
- Down syndrome (40–60%).
- CL/P.
- The condition is complicated by the following:
  - Size and shape of the remaining permanent teeth.
  - Position, spacing, and alignment of the remaining teeth.
  - Malocclusion.
  - Retained primary teeth and their prognosis/infraocclusion.
  - Any previous interventions taken.

Assessment

- Elicit the patient's main concerns, which may be related to the missing teeth but is often due to the appearance of the dentition/spacing. The patient may also report symptomatic teeth or mobile primary teeth in addition to other dental problems.

1 Brook A (1974). *J Int Assoc Dent Child* 5, 37.
2 Polder B (2004). *Community Dent Oral Epidemiol* 32, 217.

- Medical history should investigate any possible ectodermal conditions that may be present or other developmental/congenital conditions affecting the head and neck.
- Age: this has a major impact on planning treatment and prosthetic options.
- Social and family history: this should include any previous family history including siblings who have hypodontia. Assess parental involvement if appropriate and current education or work situation.
- Dental history: attitudes to dental care and long, complex treatment with the need for modifications.
- Clinical examination[3]:
  - *Skeletal pattern and facial profile*: a higher proportion of patients exhibiting reduced lower vertical proportions due to lack of alveolar development.
  - *Periodontal health*: oral hygiene and periodontal assessment. Provision of complex treatment involving multiple specialties requires an excellent level of periodontal health and maintenance for treatment and stability of the final result/restorations.
  - *Orthodontic assessment of the malocclusion* (➔ Assessing the orthodontic patient): presence and position of teeth. Assessment of crowding and spacing. Classification of the malocclusion and molar relationship.
  - *Size and shape of remaining teeth*: this may be complicated by microdontia and conical-shaped teeth. Recording the shape and size will help identify normal proportions.
  - *Prognosis of teeth*: assessment of the viability of retained primary teeth and the long-term prognosis of the permanent teeth.
  - *Edentulous spaces*: size and position of spacing. Clinical assessment of the alveolar height and width, either for consideration of the viability of orthodontic tooth movement through edentulous areas or for prosthetic replacement of teeth
  - *Gingival aesthetics*: the amount of gingival display can influence decisions regarding restoration outcome.
- Radiographic examination: any radiographic exposure needs to be justified, so careful consideration is needed as to the type or radiographs required to assess each case:
  - *Periapical*: a periapical parallel to a single tooth space can be useful in assessing the intra radicular space and the convergence of the adjacent teeth. Ideally, a minimum of 7 mm space is required between the roots, with parallel roots of the adjacent teeth for implant placement.
  - *OPT*: this is a useful diagnostic aid for treatment planning of these complex cases as it provides significant information on the whole dentition and supporting structures for consideration of orthodontic treatment and for restorative replacement of teeth. Although it has been described as the 'distortogram' due to multiple artefacts, it provides a useful assessment of the prognosis of the dentition, such as root length of primary teeth; useful in locating any ectopic teeth; proximity to other structures such as the maxillary sinus, inferior

3 Gill D (2015). *Br Dent J* 218, 143.

dental canal; as well as the root formation. Further intraoral views may also be necessary for greater detail.
* *CBCT*: 3D scans can be invaluable for identifying the 3D nature of the dentition and associated structures, which are not demonstrated accurately on 2D imaging. It provides accurate information on the position of ectopic teeth and their association with adjacent structures. Identification of structures such as the maxillary sinus or inferior dental bundle for consideration of implant placement. It shows the volume of bone and in conjunction with a rigid radiographic stent with radiographic marker can indicate the volume of bone at a proposed implant site. CBCT data can now be combined with 3D scans of the dentition for fully digital assessment.
* Diagnosis[4]:
  * Mild: one or two missing teeth.
  * Moderate: three to five missing teeth.
  * Severe: six or more missing teeth.
  * Anodontia: no teeth present.

Management
* Multidisciplinary specialist management involving orthodontics, restorative dentistry, and paediatric dentistry as part of a MDT with support from primary care is often required, particularly for more severe hypodontia.
* The joint team will require models/scans, radiographs, and photographs to enable treatment planning.
* Aimed at improving aesthetics and function.
* Generalized management options:
  * Accept the current position of the teeth and any retained primary teeth ± restorative improvement of the dental appearance.
  * Open space for prosthetic replacement of missing teeth.
  * Close spaces to obviate the need for prosthetic replacement or reduce the number of spaces present.
  * Redistribute space to facilitate improved restorative restoration.
* Factors which affect these options:
  * The underlying malocclusion is likely to determine the treatment options available.
  * Extent of hypodontia.
  * Patient motivation.
* The team should provide a treatment plan for each specialty, with specific aims and objectives, space description, and location, along with any additional objectives such as gingival emergence or root positioning.

Paediatric management
The paediatric dentistry team will be involved in early assessment and restorative treatment in the mixed and permanent dentition as required. Final restorative replacement of absent teeth may also be provided by this team. The paediatric team will be instrumental in instituting a prevention regimen and maintenance of primary teeth as required. Some teams also provide autologous tooth transplants, with movement of developing third molars into developmentally absent premolar regions.

4 Gahan M (2010). *Dent Update* 37, 74.

Orthodontic management

The orthodontic assessment[5] will determine decisions regarding space opening or closing, which are:

- Incisor relationship:
  - Class II may require space for incisor retraction and overjet reduction, which may favour space closure.
  - Class III may favour space opening as retraction would potentially create a reverse overjet.
- Molar relationship:
  - Class I requires equal numbers of mandibular and maxillary teeth.
  - Class II would require two fewer teeth in the maxillary arch.
  - Class III would require two fewer teeth in the mandibular arch or sometimes just a lower incisor.
  - Molar relation can be corrected by the use of functional appliances, headgear, or temporary anchorage devices, which may influence the overall decisions, but some of these will be age dependent.
- Space requirement in the arch:
  - Assessment of crowding or spacing.
  - It may not be possible to close large spaces orthodontically due to atrophic ridges. Occasionally, orthodontic tooth movement will be required to develop the alveolar ridge as tooth movement can create bone deposition behind the direction of tooth movement.
- Size, shape, colour, and gingival contour of teeth to be masked as missing teeth:
  - Masking canines as lateral incisors needs consideration of these factors as to whether camouflage is viable.
- Facial profile and smile aesthetics:
  - Determining whether a space-opening procedure would provide optimal facial and dental aesthetics or whether a camouflage option is appropriate.
  - Often there is a compromise that needs to be reached with respect to treatment in these cases as there are multiple factors involved in the decision-making, but ultimately the underlying skeletal pattern, and size and shape of the dentition will affect the overall aesthetic outcome. Often, aiming for symmetry is the preferable option as lay people rarely can distinguish camouflaged teeth if symmetrical, but asymmetry is discernible, and this may affect the treatment planning process.

Restorative management

- Following a joint assessment to formulate a treatment plan, the restorative team may require further impressions for facebow articulated study casts or 3D articulated digital models either for diagnosis and assessment of aesthetics or for treatment planning of the final restorative phase.[6,7]

5 Gill D (2015). Br Dent J 218, 143.
6 Gahan M (2010). Dent Update 37, 74.
7 Lewis B (2010). Dent Update 37, 138.

- *Diagnostic set-up*: used to determine the feasibility of a proposed plan or to determine the most appropriate of several plans. The set-up may be:
  - diagnostic wax up of models/Kesling set-up
  - chairside build up
  - 3D virtual planning/2D image manipulation.
- An index of the waxed-up/3D model can be taken using silicone putty and then using a temporary crown and bridge material such as bis-acryl composite; the waxed-up result can be shown in the patient's mouth.
- This enables the patient to be able to make judgements about the proposed treatment.

Missing lateral incisors

- *Space closing*: it may be necessary to disguise canine teeth as lateral incisors. This may require reduction in the width and reduction of the cusp tip. Composite addition may be required to alter the morphology to that of the lateral incisor ± external bleaching. Often it may also be required to increase the size of adjacent teeth to enable ideal proportions. Orthodontics may aim to extrude the canine to improve the gingival height or gingival crown lengthening may be required to adjacent teeth to improve proportions and levels.
- *Premolar as a canine*: the orthodontic treatment will aim to rotate the premolar to disguise the palatal cusp. Intrusion of the premolar will also improve the gingival height but requires composite addition to the cusp to bring the tooth into occlusion or gingival crown lengthening. Grinding of the palatal cusp may be required if interfering in the occlusion.
- *Space opening*: the plan to open space for prosthetic replacement will have been a decision between the patient and clinicians. Opening space will require prosthetic replacement and long-term maintenance so the patient should be fully consented and appraised of the potential future costs. Options for tooth replacement include:
  - resin-retained bridges
  - conventional bridges
  - partial dentures
  - implant-retained prosthesis.
- Each case is unique and the options available will be dependent on several factors such as space created, medical history, patient preference, gingival display, age of the patient, and further growth potential.

Missing second premolars

- Options:
  - Accept the space.
  - Retain the primary tooth for as long as possible with potential for onlays to improve the height.
  - Extraction of the primary tooth and prosthetic replacement.
  - Reduction in the mesial–distal width of the retained primary tooth and orthodontic space closure.
  - Full orthodontic space closure.
  - This may not be feasible due to the malocclusion but may be achievable with the use of temporary anchorage devices.
- Options for replacement, as above.

Missing lower incisors

- *Space closing*: depending on the malocclusion, orthodontic space closure may be an option, either accepting three lower incisors or if bilateral developmental absence, masking the lower canines as lateral incisors. This will require some alteration of the morphology ± composite addition.
- *Space opening*: replacement of one lower incisor can be easily achieved with resin-retained bridges. Where there is bilateral absence of the central incisors, it may not be ideal to restore the space due to atrophic bone preventing implant placement or poorer bonding to small lateral incisors for bridge placement. Orthodontic redistribution of space may be required to either provide a double abutted resin-retained bridge or bridges supported off the canines.[8] If implants are planned, it may be desirable for one central implant with a restoration of the two incisors. Bone grafting may still be required.

Severe hypodontia

These cases are more difficult to plan, usually due to limited bone availability and significant space around the arch or if abutment teeth are retained primary teeth. Where spaces are distributed between multiple teeth, the above mentioned options may be appropriate. Where there are large spans, occasionally the most appropriate restoration is a partial denture or implant-retained prostheses, depending on bone availability/grafting potential.

General restorative considerations in hypodontia

- Restorative treatment for hypodontia cases will most likely involve several types of restorations such as composites, veneers (composite or ceramic), onlays, bridges (resin-retained or conventional), and implants.
- Where conical teeth exist, particularly in older patients, consideration for conventional bridges by simply preparing the finishing line on the tooth and using this as a bridge abutment. This may not be ideal in many circumstances such as a tooth with a large pulp.[9]
- Restorations should be split into small units, rather than a few large span restorations. Having a shortened dental arch is also an option.

Microdontia

Definition

- Teeth that are smaller than normal, usually with a conical or peg-shaped crown.

Aetiology

- Isolated microdontia may have an autosomal dominant pattern of inheritance.
- Generalized microdontia is rare and may be associated with congenital hypopituitarism.

8 King P (2015). *Br Dent J* 218, 423.
9 Drury K (2014). *Br Dent J* 216, 25.

Prevalence
- Primary dentition: <1%.
- Permanent dentition: 2.5%.
- Generalized microdontia: 0.2%.
- Females > males.
- Most commonly affected tooth is the permanent upper lateral incisors.

Management
- May require a multidisciplinary approach with orthodontics depending on the amount of space available to restore the crown to ideal dimensions.
- Aesthetic restoration with composite is usually the treatment of choice in paediatric patients.

Associated dental anomalies
- Hypodontia. Developmentally absent permanent upper lateral incisors are associated with microdontia of the contralateral lateral incisor.

Commonly associated conditions
- Ectodermal dysplasia.
- Downs syndrome.
- Cleft lip and palate.

Fixed management of missing teeth

Introduction to the fixed management of missing teeth
- Hypodontia can present with both missing teeth and teeth of abnormal shape and not in the ideal position.
- This presents with particular difficulty as the surface area and alignment of teeth adjacent to missing spaces may not be ideal to support the prosthesis.
- Management options for missing teeth include dentures, bridges, or implants.
- Patients should be dentally fit with good oral hygiene.
- The treatment plan may be part of a joint orthodontic–restorative dental team.
- The patient's expectations should be discussed, in particular the time for both the initial treatment and the level of maintenance they are prepared to undergo.
- NHS funding for dental implants is usually restricted to the following groups, this may vary according to local commissioning arrangements[10]:
  - Patients with congenital, inherited conditions leading to absent teeth such as hypodontia, CLP, and dental abnormalities such as dentinogenesis imperfecta.
  - Tooth loss due to trauma.
  - Surgical intervention leading to tooth loss such as resection of malignant tumours.
  - Developmental conditions with extraoral defects.
  - Edentulous patients where repeated conventional dentures have been unsuccessful.

10 Restorative Dentistry-UK (RD-UK), Faculty of Dental Surgery, Royal College of Surgeons (2019). Guidance on the standards of care for NHS funded dental implant treatment. ♫ https://www.rcseng.ac.uk/-/media/files/rcs/fds/publications/implant-guidelines.pdf

- Where conventional treatment would be detrimental to mucosal disorders.
- Patients whose existing teeth cannot be used for anchorage for orthodontic therapy.
- Patient selection[10]:
  - *Age*: while there is no upper age limit provided the patient is medically well enough and able to undergo treatment, young adults whose dentofacial growth is yet to be completed should not undergo implant therapy.
  - *Medical history*: contraindications include poorly controlled diabetes, bisphosphonates treatment, and psychiatric conditions which could impact a patient's ability to comprehend and comply with extensive treatment. General surgical contraindications such as haematological conditions, immune deficiency, bone conditions, and neurological conditions such as epilepsy.
  - *Social history*: smoking and poor dental health is a contraindication.
- Following NHS-funded implants, the patient must be aware that the long-term maintenance may not be NHS funded and the patient may have to bear the cost of this.[10]

Implant assessment

The trainee in DCT may have some input into implant planning and placement, but this is a rough guide and direction under supervision should occur.[11]

History taking in implant assessment

Understanding the patient's main concerns, and full medical, social, and dental history should take place ensuring that there are no contraindications and the patient is medically and dentally healthy.

Examination in implant assessment

- Extraoral examination: in addition to examination of soft tissue abnormalities and pathology, examination should occur of:
  - TMJ to ensure no pain or pathology,
  - degree of mouth opening, particularly for molar replacement where there needs to be enough space to use screwdrivers and handpieces
  - identification of the lip line at rest and on smile particularly for aesthetic zone cases, where recession around an implant could cause an aesthetic problem.
- Intraoral examination:
  - Full intraoral soft tissue examination for soft tissue abnormalities and pathology, examination of the teeth for caries and restoration defects, and basic periodontal examination to check if dentally fit.
  - Examine the gingivae for the band of keratinized tissue: ideally a thick band of keratinized tissue would be required to support peri-implant health.
  - Check for gingival biotype—thin biotypes are more prone to recession. A simple way of assessing this would be to see if the roots shape is visible or palpable, or use a periodontal probe into

11 Barker D (2012). *Dent Update* 39, 128.

the gingival sulcus to see if it shines through: both of these would indicate thin gingival biotype.
- Check for scalloping or flat gingival biotype—flat is more favourable.
- Examine the tooth shape: ideally, rectangular teeth with small embrasures and long contacts are more favourable, whereas triangular teeth can make management of the papillae more difficult.
- Check for the mesiodistal space of the propose implant site: minimum 7 mm space is needed as the minimum implant diameter would usually be 3.5 mm and a minimum of 1.5 mm between implant and tooth root would be needed. Between implants, 3 mm of space would be needed.
- Check the vitality of adjacent teeth, particularly if they have been restored.
- Occlusion, static and dynamic occlusion including intercuspal position, slide from the retruded contact point to the intercuspal position, and lateral excursions and protrusion. Non-working side interferences should be assessed and to identify if there would be any occlusal overload particularly due to parafunction such as bruxism.

Assess the ridge: Cawood and Howell's classification[12] of the ridge is as follows:
   1: dentate.
   2: post extraction.
   3: good height and width and well rounded.
   4: good height and narrow width.
   5: poor height and width.
   6: some basal bone loss, depressed ridge.
- The bone loss tends to occur more labially and then the ridge height may be lost.
- In the anterior maxilla this can be more of a problem as aesthetically the loss of the labial bone can require the use of bone augmentation. Typically, loss of horizontal bone loss can possibly be managed with guided bone regeneration; however, loss of bone height would often need a block graft.
- In the posterior maxilla, there is less of an aesthetic demand; however, as a patient ages, there is pneumatization of the maxillary sinus which results in reduced available bone height over time.
- In the anterior mandible, there tends to be sharp labial bone at the crest of the ridge. Any loss in the ridge height usually results in widened flatter ridge. As a result, any minor loss in ridge height may not be of significance.
- In the posterior mandible, as bone loss occurs there may be less bone available to the inferior alveolar canal.

Diagnostic wax-up of implant planning
- A wax-up of the aesthetic preview should be constructed.
- Ideally this should then be mocked up in the patient's mouth to check the aesthetic preview with temporary crown and bridge material.

---

12 Sethi A (2012) *Practical Implant Dentistry*. Quintessence.

- Should this be satisfactory in terms of aesthetics and occlusion then the wax-up should be used to create a radiographic stent. This stent should ideally be made of a colourless material that is reasonably rigid such as an Essex retainer material and the waxed-up tooth should be filled with a radiopaque (non-metallic) material. This should fit comfortably in the patient's mouth to show the proposed tooth position. A small hole should be placed through the radiopaque material to indicate the direction of axial loading on the restoration.
- This can then be placed in the patient's mouth and used as a radiographic stent while taking a CBCT scan.

Radiographs in implant planning
- Plain film radiographic examination:
  - BWs should be taken to ensure no caries and sound restoration of posterior teeth.
  - Periapical radiograph should be taken of root-treated teeth to ensure no presence of apical pathology. A further periapical radiograph should be taken parallel to the space in question to ensure minimum 7 mm of space between roots and the root alignment. Using a calibrated radiopaque object such as a 5 mm ball bearing can help with more precise measurements. Check the distance between the crestal position and the proposed contact of the final restoration. Ideally, there should be 5 mm or less between the contact point and the crestal bone to ensure papillae infill.
  - Using the periapical assess the vertical bone position, it is often difficult to augment >1 mm vertically using guided bone regeneration and therefore a block graft may be needed.
  - Ideally, aim for parallel roots of the adjacent teeth. Convergent roots may mean that there is sufficient bone at the crestal position, but insufficient subcrestally.
  - Divergent roots may mean sufficient bone subcrestally as the roots will be further away from the tip of the implant but may mean deep undercuts on the proximal surfaces meaning a very coronal contact point. This would mean a greater likelihood of 'black triangles' due to lack of papillae.
  - This should be a prerequisite to a CBCT scan.
- CBCT scan:
  - Where there is clinical doubt on the shape of the alveolar ridge then a CBCT scan is often justified.[13]
  - Where a single implant is being placed, often a small volume CBCT scan is all that is required; where the edentulous arch is being planned, a full volume may be needed.[13]
  - Use the radiographic stent fabricated so that the position of the proposed restoration is visible on the scan with respect to the bone.
  - CBCT imaging data can be integrated with a 3D scan of the dentition/arch, and a purely digital workflow may be used.

---

13 FGDP (UK) (2018). Selection criteria for dental radiography. ℘ https://cgdent.uk/selection-criteria-for-dental-radiography/

Planning the implant placement

Key anatomy when planning implant placement

Any vital structures that could be injured should be noted, in particular:

- Anterior maxilla:
  - Nasopalatine canal: at the incisive papillae, contains the nasopalatine nerve. If >6 mm diameter, possible cyst.
  - Canalis sinuosis: a branch of the anterior superior alveolar nerve which branches from the infraorbital nerve which runs through the anterior wall of the maxilla and the lateral wall of the nasal cavity—can be injured during upper lateral incisor implant placement.
- Posterior maxilla:
  - The maxillary sinus: the floor of the sinus can reduce the vertical bone height present to place implants. Thickening of the Schneiderian membrane may be pathological and require ENT input.
- Anterior mandible:
  - Mandibular incisive canal: runs anteriorly from the mental foramen and carries a neurovascular bundle that supplies the anterior teeth which usually exits the mandible at the lingual foramen; however, it can reach the midline and be present in the mid third of the mandible.
  - Mental foramen: typically, at the region of the second premolar, but if there is significant bone loss then it may be present on the ridge. The mental nerve exits here.
  - Anterior loop of the mental foramen: prior to the inferior alveolar nerve leaving the mental foramen to the branch off as the mental nerve it may pass anteriorly in a short loop which can be several millimetres in length before moving posterior and laterally out of the mental foramen. Care needs to be taken to identify this if placing implants in the lower canine or premolar region.
- Posterior mandible:
  - The position of the inferior alveolar canal should be identified as well as any branches of the neurovascular bundle.
  - Submandibular fossa: a depression inferior and lingual to the crest of the posterior mandible.

Virtual implant planning

- Using the implant planning software, any key anatomy should be marked.
- Aim to have a restoratively driven implant placement, rather than simply placing the implant where there is bone.
- This would involve placing the implant along the path of axial loading based on the position of the hole placed in the radiopaque marker.
- The implant platform should ideally be placed 4 mm from the horizontal plane of the gingival zenith if using subcrestal implant or 3 mm if using crestal implants.
- When planning the diameter of the implant, it should be at least 1.5 mm from adjacent tooth roots and 3 mm from adjacent implants and 1 mm of labial bone.
- A minimum length of 7 mm is usually needed for standard implant length.
- When considering the dimensions of the implant greater than this, take into account the expected occlusal load. Greater bone to implant contact may be needed in these cases and therefore increasing the

dimensions of the implant may be needed. If there is a chance in the future that the implant will fall into lateral excursion or if the implant will have some cantilever (particularly in molar replacement where there is likely to be either a mesial or distal cantilever if a single implant is used), then greater bone to implant contact may be needed.

- Increasing the implant dimensions should not violate vital anatomical structures, teeth, or other implants.
- It may not be desirable to use the entire available bone volume to place the largest implant possible. Should failure of the implant occur late on, having more bone volume gives the option of another implant.
- Once the ideal implant position is planned virtually it can be identified on the CBCT scan whether further bone augmentation procedures would be needed to facilitate the ideal implant placement.
- Where the implant placement is within the natural bone then no further augmentation procedures would be necessary.
- Where the direction of the implant placement follows the natural bone, but there is insufficient buccolingual thickness than it may be amenable to ridge expansion to increase the volume of bone.
- If the proposed implant site is not in the direction of the bone in the ridge, then guided bone regeneration may be needed.
- Where the implant position is grossly out of the natural bone, more complex augmentation procedures such as block grafts may be needed or placement in a less than ideal position using angulated abutments.

Implant placement

Placing an implant at DCT level should be done under close supervision and the guidance on this book alone should not be used as the sole means of planning and placing implants.

- Full aseptic field should be set up for implant placement.
- Local anaesthesia should be given as required for other types of minor oral surgical procedures.
- A three-sided flap should ideally be used extending one tooth either side when considering the relieving incisions. This is to accommodate guided bone regeneration should it be needed.
- From the crevicular incisions, rather than make a crestal incision the flap should ideally be extended palatally. This would be a palatal rotation flap—the benefit of this would be that the entire implant platform can be covered and if augmentation techniques are used they too are unlikely to come out of the incisions which may occur if a crestal incision is used.
- For the lower arch, be aware of the mental foramen and lingual aspect. A three-sided flap would still be necessary but avoid extending too lingually.
- Using the Essex retainer-made or a laboratory made surgical drill guide using the CBCT scan, the osteotomy should be made in accordance with the protocol set by the implant manufacturer.
- Place the cover screw to prevent soft tissue entering the implant platform.
- When suturing ideally use a fine (6-0) monofilament suture.

Implant exposure

- About 3–6 months after implant surgery it would be necessary to expose the implant head to get adequate soft tissue healing.
- This would involve making a small incision over the implant platform. A typical exposure would be an 'H incision'. This involves making a full

thickness incision crestally over the implant platform and two incisions just on either side of the implant platform.

- The cover screw is removed, and a healing abutment is screwed into the implant. The healing abutment is exposed to the oral environment. The purpose of the healing abutment is to form healthy epithelium from the implant opening to the oral environment.
- Usually this takes about 2 weeks.
- Following this, the soft tissue is evaluated to ensure that it has healed.

Impression taking for implants

- The next stage involves the manufacture of the restoration. Once the soft tissues have healed, an abutment is needed.
- An abutment is a connecting component that is fitted into the implant at one end and the restoration is fitted to it at the other end.
- The abutment can either be a standard design, available in various angles, or customized by taking an impression.
- Open impression:
  - This involves using an impression post that fits into the implant opening and screws into position.
  - An impression tray with a hole in it to accommodate the protruding impression post is used.
  - The impression material is placed into the impression tray and seated.
  - The impression post should be visible out of the tray in the hole and any impression material is cleared from the impression post.
  - Once the impression material is set, the impression post is unscrewed from the implant and the whole of the impression is removed with the impression post bound within it.
  - The healing abutment is replaced.
  - The impression is sent to the laboratory for either a customized abutment or the restoration and abutment.
- Closed impression:
  - Once the healing abutment is removed, a standard abutment is fitted and a coping is placed on the abutment. Alternatively, the final customized abutment (constructed previously from the open impression) is placed and the final coping is fitted on the abutment.
  - Impression material is placed on the impression tray and seated.
  - On removal of the impression tray, it would pick up the coping and this is sent to the laboratory for construction of the restoration.

Fitting the implant restoration

Cement retained

- The final restoration is fitted on the abutment using cement.
- Typically, this is zinc oxide eugenol cement.
- Excess cement must be removed as it is implicated in peri-implant disease.

Screw retained

- There is easier maintenance with screw-retained style.
- The restoration has a screw through and access hole usually along the path of axial loading.
- This is then screwed into the abutment or alternatively the abutment and crown come as a single unit and the crown restoration is screwed directly into the implant.

- A medium is used to cover the screw such as a cotton pellet or PTFE tape.
- Composite restoration material is then used to seal this.

Resin-bonded bridges

Implants may not be the desirable option and should not necessarily be considered as the best option for replacement of missing teeth in all cases, as resin-bonded bridges have several advantages.

Advantages of resin-bonded bridges over implants
- Take a shorter length of time to deliver.
- No invasive surgical procedure.
- Cheaper and easier to maintain.
- Easier placement where the ideal space is not possible (e.g. <6 mm).

Factors to gain optimal outcome
There are several factors that can be used to gain success in bridges[14]:
- Aesthetics can be good; however, the patient should be warned about alteration of the shade of the abutment tooth as a result of the metal wing and cement as well as the need for improved oral hygiene around the pontic and adjacent teeth including interdental cleaning.
- The tooth needs to be ideally positioned with a good surface area of enamel for bonding and should not be periodontally compromised.
- Ensure only light contact in intercuspal position and no contact in lateral excursion on the pontic. Parafunction will increase the rate of debond.
- Ideally cantilever design. Can be used as fixed orthodontic retention with multiple retainers (e.g. double abutting central incisors).
- Maximize the surface area that the retainer covers. Use of electrosurgery to expose greater anatomical crown height.
- The retainer connector is at least 0.7 mm thick to ensure rigidity.
- Use opaque resin cement to try to disguise the dark colour of the metal through the translucent tooth.
- Ovate pontics have good aesthetics and facilitate oral hygiene.
- Preparation should be restricted to enamel only and should not expose dentine unless preparation is into restorations.
- Sandblast the wing prior to cementation.
- Ensure adequate moisture control with either cotton rolls or rubber dam split dam technique.
- Consider some ridge alteration by using a bur to make a minor alteration into the ridge to allow greater emergence of the pontic. Explain clearly to the laboratory where this is required so they can adjust the cast accordingly and then carry out ridge preparation at the fit stage.

Management of suboptimal shape, size, and space
- Check just prior to debond of the orthodontic appliance that the space, position, and alignment is optimal for restorative management—if not, discuss with orthodontist.
- If the shape of adjacent teeth or the proportions are less than ideal, again discuss with the orthodontist to consider redistributing the space and use composite to improve the shape, bonding surface, or proportion of the adjacent teeth.

14 Durey K (2011). *Br Dent J* 211, 113.

Introduction to dental defects

Amelogenesis imperfecta (AI)

Definition

- This is a group of several developmental conditions affecting the appearance and structure of enamel. Most or all of the teeth are affected and there may be other systemic conditions involved. There may be a genetic component—this may be autosomal dominant, autosomal recessive, or sex linked.
- Characteristics of the enamel include:
  - discoloration
  - sensitivity
  - hypoplastic
  - hypomineralized
  - susceptible to breakdown.

Classification

- Many classifications exist. Some are based on the clinical appearance whereas others use the appearance and mode of inheritance.
- Four major categories:
  - Type I: hypoplastic.
  - Type II: hypomature.
  - Type III: hypocalcified.
  - Type IV: hypomature/hypoplastic with taurodontism.

Presentation

- Hypoplastic:
  - Crown size may be smaller than usual.
  - Enamel thickness varies: can be thin and smooth/grooved or pitted.
  - Radiographic appearance of normal or thin enamel.
- Hypomature:
  - Enamel may appear white and opaque or can have yellow/brown defects.
  - Enamel usually of normal thickness but can display breakdown and tooth surface loss (TSL).
  - Enamel appears of similar radio-opacity to dentine on radiographs.
- Hypocalcified:
  - Enamel appears creamy or yellow/brown.
  - AOB common.
  - Enamel appears of similar or reduced radio-opacity to dentine on radiographs.
- Hypomature/hypoplastic with taurodontism:
  - White or yellow/brown mottling of enamel which is usually of reduced thickness.
  - Radiographs usually show normal radio-opacity of enamel and taurodontism of molar teeth.

Aetiology

May show autosomal dominant, autosomal recessive, X-linked, or sporadic inheritance patterns.

Prevalence
- 1:12,000–14,000 (Michigan, USA).[1]
- 1:700 (Sweden).[2]

Associated conditions
- Early definitions of AI excluded the involvement of other structures. However, the concept of AI as a feature in some syndromes is now largely accepted.
- Tricho-dento-osseous syndrome: AI, curly hair, and skeletal abnormalities.
- Cone-rod dystrophy.
- Nephrocalcinosis.

Assessment
- Presenting complaint: pain and sensitivity particularly to mildly cool liquids. Other complaints may include the appearance of the teeth and breakdown of teeth.
- Medical history: aware of any particular syndromes and otherwise general health.
- Social and family history: there is a genetic component so other family members may be suffering from this. Pedigree plotting can be done.
- Dental history: attitude to potentially long and complex treatment and acceptance of failure and require maintenance.
- Clinical examination: all the teeth would be affected in general, no particular chronological effect, hypoplastic, hypomineralized, or hypomature enamel. There may be pitted sections, rough and discoloured enamel—important to differentiate from fluorosis. The teeth may have broken down—even teeth that have just erupted may have pre-eruptive resorption and so may be defective.[3]
- Radiographs: in hypoplastic cases, enamel and dentine to appear normal in terms of contrast; in hypomaturation cases, enamel and dentine have similar radiodensity; in hypocalcified cases, the dentine is more radiopaque compared to the enamel.[4]
- Diagnosis: there are many classifications of AI. The diagnosis can be aided with four details[3]:
  - Family history.
  - Are all teeth affected?
  - Absence of chronological distribution.
  - Absence of past metabolic disturbance that may have affected the enamel.

Management
Some treatment may have already been provided by the paediatric dentists, including preformed metal crowns. Composite resin is generally the preferred means of restoration. The patient may still be young and have large healthy pulp with incomplete gingival maturation. As a result, crowns can place the pulp at high risk of necrosis and when further gingival maturation

1 Witkop C (1957). *Acta Genet* 7, 236.
2 Bäckman B (1986). *Community Dent Oral Epidemiol* 14, 43.
3 Crawford P (2007). *Orhanet Journal of Rare Diseases* 2, 17.
4 Gadhia K (2012) *Br Dent J* 212, 377.

occurs, there may be additional exposed tooth affected by AI which may continue to cause sensitivity. Composite requires minimal preparation and as the patient becomes older the composite can be added on to the cervical margins. While the composite will wear and accumulate staining, this could be polished and replaced accordingly.

This does not eliminate other restorations in the future as if the process of repairing and replacing the restorations becomes too frequent, the patient would probably be older and problems with gingival recession and pulp health would be less of an issue provided that the patient maintains the oral hygiene.

Maintaining the oral hygiene can be difficult as the enamel is rough and may accumulate more plaque and cold water can make brushing of the teeth painful. Advise the patient to use warm water and with well-polished restoration it can help to provide smoother tooth surfaces.

Dentinogenesis imperfecta (DI)

Definition
- These are autosomal dominant genetic conditions affecting the dentine of the primary or permanent dentitions or both.
- There are different types of these conditions including those that are also inherited with osteogenesis imperfecta (OI).
- The affected dentine results in loss of the overlying enamel with more rapid tooth wear of the susceptible dentine.

Classification
- Shields' classification[5]:
  - Type I: seen in patients with OI.
  - Type II: hereditary opalescent dentine.
  - Type III: typical findings are of multiple pulp exposures and enlarged pulp spaces leading to the appearance of 'shell teeth'.
- Shields' classification remains the most widely used classification, but it is outdated as a different molecular aetiology for type I has since been identified.

Presentation
- Clinical:
  - Discoloration of teeth ranging from blue-grey to yellow.
  - Teeth appear opalescent due to the thinness of the enamel overlying the defective dentine.
  - Enamel chipping and wear of dentine are common features. Primary dentition usually more severely affected than permanent dentition.
- Radiographic:
  - Bulbous crowns with marked cervical constriction.
  - Pulpal obliteration, Short, blunted roots.

Aetiology
- DI type I: autosomal dominant condition resulting from mutations in one of the two collagen type I genes.
- DI types II and III: autosomal dominant conditions caused by mutations in the dentin sialophosphoprotein 1 gene.

5 Shields E (1973). *Arch Oral Biol* 8, 543.

Incidence
- Type I: 1:20,000.
- Type II: 1:8000.[6]
- Type III: rare.

Other genetic caused of dentinal defects
- Hypophosphataemia rickets (X-linked dominant vitamin-D resistant rickets).
- Ehlers–Danlos syndrome.
- Goldblatt syndrome.
- Schimke immuno-osseous dysplasia.

Assessment
- Presenting complaint: pain from the teeth, broken down teeth, and appearance would be frequent complaints, as well as loss of teeth.
- Medical history: patients may also have OI and therefore bones may be affected. It is important to be aware that patients with OI may have historically been treated with IV bisphosphonates and are at risk of medicine-induced osteonecrosis of the jaw particularly with surgical interventions or extractions. There may be other associated conditions such as Ehlers–Danlos syndrome.
- Social and family history: there are likely to be family members also affected due to the autosomal dominant nature.
- Dental history: as with AI (➔ Amelogenesis imperfecta (AI)).
- Clinical examination: the patient with blue sclera from OI, intraorally the teeth may appear blue, purple, amber translucent discoloration, tooth wear with sclerotic dentine present.
- Radiographic examination: enamel and dentine may appear normal; however, the enamel may already have been lost. Crowns may appear bulbous, roots may be short and sharp or missing. Pulp chambers may have stones or be obliterated with periapical radiolucencies in non-carious teeth. In cases without OI, the appearance of the teeth is similar.
- Diagnosis: based on history, examination, and radiographs.[7]

Management
- Aimed at improving aesthetics and preventing wear of the dentition to preserve function.
- Often requires early specialist intervention.
- Commonly involves placement of preformed metal crowns on posterior teeth and anterior composite restorations (using opaque composites placed via a layered approach).
- As with AI, the paediatric dentists may have already made some intervention.
- Manage pain and infection and protect the teeth from further wear.
- Due to possible pulp stones and narrow canals, root canal treatment is often difficult, therefore teeth are more liable for extraction if they become compromised.

6 Witkop C (1957). *Acta Genet* 7, 236.
7 Barron M (2008). *Orphanet J Rare Dis* 20, 31.

- If the teeth are already badly worn, overdentures may be useful.
- Metal onlays with minimal preparation can also help reduce wear occlusally.
- Bear in mind what was mentioned earlier about a possible history of bisphosphonate use in OI and the need for extractions.
- There may be early tooth loss particularly where there are short or absent roots.
- Dentine is more prone to caries then enamel so the patient is at increased risk of carious tooth loss also.

Dentine dysplasia

Definition
- Heritable defect of dentine.

Classification
- Shields' classification[8]:
  - Type I: radicular dentine dysplasia ('rootless teeth').
  - Type II: coronal dentine dysplasia.

Presentation
- Type I: crowns often appear normal clinically. Radiographically, roots are sharp with conical apical constrictions. Pre-eruptive pulpal obliteration occurs. Multiple periapical radiolucencies may be seen in non-carious teeth.
- Type II: the clinical appearance of the primary teeth is similar to that seen in DI type II, but the permanent dentition is either unaffected or shows mild radiographic abnormalities such as thistle-tube deformities or pulp stones.

Aetiology
- Type I: unknown.
- Type II: autosomal dominant condition caused by mutations in the dentin sialophosphoprotein 1 gene.

Prevalence
- Type I: very rare.
- Type II: ~1:100,000.

Management
- Early diagnosis and referral for specialist management.
- Often similar to management approach for DI.

Regional odontodysplasia

Definition
- Developmental abnormality of the teeth which affects all the dental tissues and often involves multiple teeth in one quadrant.

Presentation
- Clinical: teeth are severely malformed and may remain unerupted. Where teeth do erupt, they are often hypoplastic and/or hypomineralized. Abscesses are frequent findings.

8 Shields E (1973). *Arch Oral Biol* 8, 543.

- Radiographic: reduced radio-opacity of teeth with loss of distinction between enamel and dentine ('ghost teeth').
- Maxilla > mandible.

Aetiology
- Suggested aetiological factors include a vascular disorder, trauma, latent virus in tooth germs, metabolic disturbances, and local infections.

Management
- Close monitoring if asymptomatic and infection free.
- Where intervention is indicated, often extraction and prosthetic replacement is the only available management option.

Introduction to advanced restorative treatment

There will be a large number of patients referred by GDPs for advice and/ or treatment of complex restorative dental treatment. While most units would be able to provide advice and treatment planning, many would be restricted to the type of treatment they can offer based on capacity and the commissioned service. As a result, the patient may be referred back to the GDP with a treatment plan or alternatively they may require onward referral to either a specialist or dentist with enhanced skills to manage the case. Depending on the situation, patients may be accepted for treatment for the purposes of training.

Important aspects to bear in mind with these patients are that only specific items of treatment may be provided and long-term maintenance and follow-up would generally rest with the GDP. There may also be shared care, for example, the hospital unit may carry out the chemo-mechanical instrumentation part of the root canal treatment and obturation, but it may be sent back to the GDP for final restoration.

This section will briefly discuss endodontics, periodontics, and management of TSL. Many of these may be managed in a general practice setting, however the trainee in DFT/DCT will probably be involved in some of these procedures as part of the training.

Endodontology

Reasons why a patient may be referred to the hospital include the following:
- Severe curvature of the root canals.
- Incomplete root development.
- Canal obliteration—canals that radiographically appear not to be negotiable to the entire length.
- Resorption of the root (internal/external) (e.g. due to trauma).
- Apical surgery.
- Iatrogenic damage.
- Non-surgical retreatment.

Operating microscopes

These can be extremely useful for locating canals and generally gaining and improving visualization. There are two aspects that can affect this: firstly, the magnification itself can show much more detail than direct vision; secondly the light from the microscope is usually of a much greater power and provides excellent illumination. Many even consider the light to be the superior feature of operating microscopes.
- Aim to gain access to the pulp chamber prior to the use of the microscope—this is often the task that requires less detail and so magnification may not be necessary.
- Avoid using the highest magnification as the default setting—this may not provide any additional detail and is more prone to losing focus if the patient moves compared to lower magnification.
- Set the microscope up before the patient arrives—and get it to the position that you are used to—this can save time when the patient is in the chair; also make sure that it is working and that it focuses well.
- It can also help with posture as it forces an upright position.

Managing curvature of root canals

Severely curved canals can prove a challenge and they are particularly prone to ledge formation and iatrogenic damage which can be difficult to manage.

- Gain access and prepare the coronal part of the root canal first as usual. In doing so, many of the interferences at the coronal part would have been eliminated.
- Using the preoperative radiograph identify the direction of the curvature. Prepare the canal wall opposite to the direction of the curvature more generously, but with caution not to cause iatrogenic damage. This increases the straight-line access and the degree to which the file must curve.
- Pre-bend the file gently—this can be done with Adams cribs pliers; avoid making kinks in the file and keep to a smooth curvature—pass the file down following the curvature of the canal.
- An apex locator can help you identify if you are still in the canal.
- Lubricants such as EDTA can also be helpful.

Incomplete root formation

This can frequently occur with children who have suffered some degree of trauma to the incisors resulting in loss of vitality in the tooth with an immature root.

- Ensure that the tooth is restorable and has a reasonable prognosis.
- Open the tooth and prepare the coronal aspect as normal.
- A preoperative radiograph is necessary for estimating working lengths; working length radiographs are also useful.
- Apex locators are useful; however, they can become unreliable if there is a particularly large apical foramen.
- When establishing a working length, an apex locator can be useful. When confirming the length using paper points, the paper points can be measured at 0.5 mm increments and carefully placed down the canal at the increasing lengths. As soon as fluid is seen on the tip of the paper point it indicates that endpoint is reached. Using the previous paper point which would have been 0.5 mm shorter, check again—if this comes out clean then the working length can be confirmed using this method.[1]
- Historically, this would have been obturated with a large GP point; however, a more modern way would be to use a MTA or tricalcium-based cement for root end closure. Aim for a minimum of 4 mm thickness. Use a plugger that has been pre-measured to be 4 mm short and use this to pack the material carefully—try not to extrude material through the apex; however, extruded MTA is not as harmful as extruded GP. The aim would be to pack the material rather than push it.
- Check with a radiograph that it is in the correct position—if not, MTA can be washed out as it takes 4 hours to become fully set. Once set, backfill with GP and restore the tooth.

Resorption defects

With internal resorption it is difficult to instrument and therefore the main way of managing this is to rely on the effect of the irrigants. Care must be

1 Rosenburg D (2003). *Dentistry Today* 22, 80.

taken—if the resorption extends through the tooth it may result in a hypochlorite accident; use saline or chlorhexidine where possible. Repair the defect using MTA to carefully pack into the area. When obturating it may not be possible to use cold lateral condensation and so using warm backfill in this region can be helpful along with using the pluggers to ensure the material fills the void created by the resorption.

Apical surgery

This is beyond the remit of this handbook (⊃ Further reading).

Non-surgical retreatment

This may be a very common procedure undertaken by the trainee in DCT. The aim would be to disinfect the root canal system to provide an environment conducive to healing—for that reason it is important to be aware that while it may not seem possible to get a better radiographic appearance of the final obturation, it may be possible to further disinfect the canals which may improve the success.

- Assess the coronal restoration to see if there are any leakages; if so, this may be the reason for initial failure—this should then be removed and replaced.
- When removing the coronal restoration or going through a crown, the base of the restoration may be at the floor of the pulp chamber. Great care needs to be taken to prevent iatrogenic damage to the pulp chamber floor. When the bulk of the coronal restoration has been removed to a sufficient depth, open the rest of the cavity to the same depth. Use a fine spherical burr to carefully remove the remaining material on the pulp chamber floor. Alternatively, use an ultrasonic instrument; however, be aware this may dislodge the entire coronal restoration.
- When the canal orifice is located, it is important to check if there is actually any GP within it. In many cases a tooth may have a buccal and lingual canal and only one may be obturated, which may be superimposed on the unfilled canal.
- When the GP is located, use a Gates Glidden burr size 1 to remove the bulk of the GP. Gently go down the canal with the same burr but ensure the shaft of the burr does not begin to bend. Stop when the burr starts to feel resistance, if it no longer removes any further GP, if it begins to bend, or if you are progressing more than one-third of the estimated working length.
- If no more GP is being cut, then use a file with a cutting tip as large as possible that just engages with the most coronal part of the remaining GP.
- Engage the file just into the coronal part of the GP and try to lift it out—rather like a corkscrew effect.
- Use a smaller file that engages with the remaining GP and lift out.
- There will be some GP remaining—place cotton pellets around the opening of the access cavity and use either chloroform or oil of wintergreen with a few drops into the canal and with a paper point blot out any remaining GP. This irrigant has the potential to dissolve the rubber dam and so the cotton pellets should prevent this. Do not use this irrigant prior to removing the bulk of the GP as it will cause it to

become sticky and difficult to remove. Only a small amount is needed so use it very sparsely.
- As you are going along with removing the GP, prepare the canals as usual.

Use of apex locators
- Apex locators are one of the most commonly used devices to enable you to determine the working length.
- There are various factors that can affect the accuracy of the apex locator including:
  - the contents of the root canal
  - the diameter of the apical constriction
  - the file used with the apex locator
  - the distance of the file from the apical constriction.
- Use a file appropriate to the canal. Using a file that is too narrow may not engage the wall adequately, whereas a file that is too large may cause a perforation.
- The apex locator should have a good steady movement that correlates well with the approximate position of the file. There should be no sudden jumps in the apex locator readings from small movements of the file.
- The apex locator is most accurate as it gets closer to the apex. Once the apex locator indicates the file has passed the apical constriction, move back until it indicates it is at the apex and this is the most accurate reading. The working length should be 1 mm short of this reading.

Iatrogenic damage
Repair of such defects can be done by carefully irrigating the region with saline, drying with sterile paper points and cotton pellets, and trying to get haemostasis with moistened sterile cotton pellets. Place sterile paper points into the root canals and apply MTA over the defect ensuring that it does not occlude any of the canal orifices. A relatively thick layer may be required. Remove the paper points and dress and reassess at the following visit as it requires 4 hours to set and so further irrigation of the root canal system at that visit should not happen.

Periodontology

As with endodontics, different units will vary in what they treat and what is sent back to the GDP with advice and treatment planning. Moreover, there are many units that will employ dental hygienists or therapists and have oral health educators available.

A good starting point would be the *Good Practitioners Guide to Periodontology* as this provides a very detailed guide about what can be expected.[2]

Examination and assessment
A full history should be taken including:
- The patient's presenting concerns
- Medical and social history (including smoking and tobacco use)

2 British Society of Periodontology (2017). 🔗 https://www.bsperio.org.uk/assets/downloads/good_practitioners_guide_2016.pdf

- Dental history (including oral hygiene and attitudes to dental care)
- Full hard and soft tissue examination should also occur.

Periodontal indices and investigations

Basic Periodontal Examination

This should be done with a World Health Organization (WHO) 621 periodontal probe or equivalent in the six sextants as follows[3]:

    0: healthy periodontium.
    1: bleeding on probing with no pocketing >3.5 mm.
    2: plaque retention features such as calculus or overhangs.
    3: pocketing >3.5 mm but <5.5 mm.
    4: pocketing >5.5 mm.
    * furcation involvement in addition to the numerical score.

Sextants are based on:

- Upper right is based on the highest score on UR4, UR5, UR6, UR7
- Upper left is based on the highest score on the UL4, UL5, UL6, UL7
- Lower left is based on the highest score on the LL4, LL5, LL6, LL7
- Lower right is based on the highest score on the LR4, LR5, LR6, LR7
- Lower central is based on highest score of the lower incisors and canines
- Upper central is based in the highest score on the upper incisors and canines
- Where one molar is missing, then the third molar tooth should also be included in posterior sextants.

Full mouth periodontal charting (six-point charting)

- This involves using a University of North Carolina (UNC) 15 probe or 10 mm Williams probe to measure in millimetres, six points (mesial, mid-point and distal of the buccal and palatal/lingual surfaces). The probe should be walked around and the deepest point in the region should be the recorded point.
- It should also be use around any implants (or a four-point pocket chart), rather than a BPE score.
- This should be for probing depths ≥4 mm and recession.
- Furcation involvement and mobility score should also be taken.

Radiographs

Radiographs should be taken to identify the crestal bone levels.

A DPT radiograph will show this; however, where there are probing depths <5.5 mm only on posterior sextants, horizontal BWs can also show this. Alternatives include vertical BWs and PA radiographs. The new guidance will require an assessment of percentage bone loss, so the full length of the root will need to be visualized, which will require a DPT or PA radiograph.

Measuring progress of patients

Not all units will use the same methods of measurement, so it is important to familiarize with your unit.

- *Debris index* measures a sample of six teeth and scores them out of 3 and an average is taken in terms of the amount of plaque covering the tooth surface.

3 British Society of Periodontology (2019). ℬ www.bsperio.org.uk

- *Bleeding index* scores the extent of bleeding on probing out of 3 and an average is taken.
- *Plaque distribution charts* split each of the teeth into surfaces and measure the presence or absence of plaque, which is then presented to the patient as a percentage.

Classification of periodontal diseases

The summary of the 2017 classification of periodontal and peri-implant disease and conditions is given below (Figs. 5.1 and 5.2)[4]:

Periodontal health, gingival disease/conditions
- Periodontal health and gingival health:
  - Clinical gingival health on an intact periodontium.
  - Clinical gingival health on a reduced periodontium:
    - Stable periodontitis patient.
    - Non-periodontitis patient.
- Gingivitis—dental biofilm induced:
  - Associated with dental biofilm alone.
  - Mediated by systemic or local risk factors.
  - Drug-induced gingival enlargement.
- Gingival disease—non-dental biofilm induced:
  - Genetic/developmental disorders.
  - Specific infections.
  - Inflammatory and immune conditions.
  - Reactive processes.
  - Neoplasms.
  - Endocrine, nutritional, and metabolic disease.
  - Traumatic lesions.
  - Gingival pigmentation.

Forms of periodontitis
- Necrotizing periodontal diseases:
  - Necrotizing gingivitis.
  - Necrotizing periodontitis.
  - Necrotizing stomatitis.
- Periodontitis as manifestation of systemic diseases: this is based on the primary systemic disease.
- Periodontitis:
  - Stage of periodontitis based on the worst level of interproximal bone loss:
    - Stage 1: less than either 15% or 2 mm attachment loss from the cementoenamel junction.
    - Stage 2: up to coronal third of the root.
    - Stage 3: up to mid third of the root.
    - Stage 4: up to the apical third of the root.
  - Grade of disease determined by percentage of bone loss divided by the patient's age:
    - Grade A: <0.5.
    - Grade B: between 0.5 and 1.0.
    - Grade C: >1.0.

4 Caton JG (2018). *J Clin Periodontol* 89(Suppl 1), S1–S8.

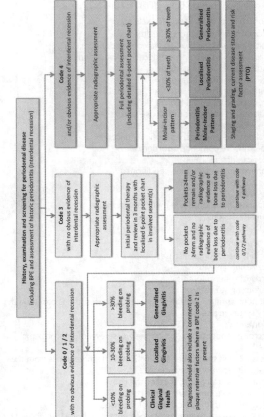

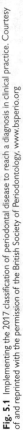

Fig. 5.1 Implementing the 2017 classification of periodontal disease to reach a diagnosis in clinical practice. Courtesy of and reprinted with the permission of the British Society of Periodontology, www.bsperio.org

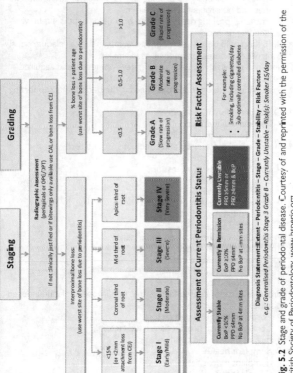
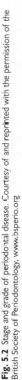

Fig. 5.2 Stage and grade of periodontal disease. Courtesy of and reprinted with the permission of the British Society of Periodontology; www.bsperio.org

- Diagnosis is based on the classification (stage and grade) as well as the extent, current disease stability, and risk factors:
- Extent:
  - Localized: <30% of sites affected.
  - Generalized: >30% of sites affected.
- Stability:
  - Stable: bleeding in probing <10%, no probing depths >4 mm, and no bleeding on probing at 4 mm sites.
  - Remission: bleeding on probing at >10% of sites, but not at 4 mm sites and no probing depths >4 mm.
  - Unstable: probing depths ≥5 mm or probing depths 4 mm with bleeding on probing.
- Risk: this could be any periodontal risk factor such as plaque, poorly controlled diabetes, or smoking as examples.
- Periodontal manifestations of system, developmental, and acquired disease:
  - Systemic disease or conditions affecting the periodontal supporting tissues.
  - Other periodontal conditions:
    - Periodontal abscesses.
    - Endodontic-periodontal lesion.
  - Mucogingival deformities and conditions around teeth:
    - Gingival phenotype.
    - Gingival/soft tissue recession.
    - Lack of gingivae.
    - Decreased vestibular depth.
    - Aberrant frenum/muscle position.
    - Gingival excess.
    - Abnormal colour.
    - Condition of the exposed root surface.
  - Traumatic occlusal forces:
    - Primary occlusal trauma.
    - Secondary occlusal trauma.
    - Orthodontic forces.
  - Prosthesis/tooth-related factors that predispose to plaque-induced disease:
    - Localized tooth-related factors.
    - Localized dental prosthesis-related factors.
- Peri-implant disease and conditions:
  - Peri-implant health.
  - Peri-implant mucositis.
  - Peri-implantitis.
  - Peri-implant soft and hard tissue deficiencies.

Management of periodontal patients

Accepting patients for periodontal treatment will vary according to the referral criteria set by the unit (Fig. 5.3).

- Typically, this would be patients with a classification of the stage 3 or 4 or grade C (individual units will define their own acceptance criteria).
- Modifiable risk factors such as plaque control and smoking would normally need to be controlled prior to acceptance for treatment.

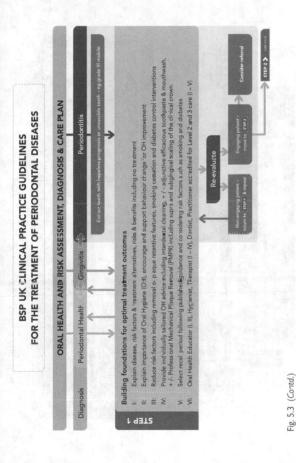

BSP UK CLINICAL PRACTICE GUIDELINES FOR THE TREATMENT OF PERIODONTAL DISEASES

ORAL HEALTH AND RISK ASSESSMENT, DIAGNOSIS & CARE PLAN

Diagnosis	Periodontal Health	Gingivitis	Periodontitis

Extract teeth with hopeless prognosis or unsavable teeth – eg grade III mobile

STEP 1

Building foundations for optimal treatment outcomes

I: Explain disease, risk factors & treatment alternatives, risks & benefits including no treatment

II: Explain importance of Oral Hygiene (OH), encourage and support behaviour change 'or OH improvement

III: Reduce risk factors including removal o– plaque retentive features, smoking cessation and diabetes control interventions

IV: Provide individually tailored OH advice including removal interdental cleaning, + / - adjunctive efficacious toothpaste & mouthwash, + / - Professional Mechanical Plaque Removal (PMPR) including supra and subgingival scaling of the clinical crown

V: Select recall period following published guidance and considering risk factors such as smoking and diabetes

VI: Oral Health Educator (I, II), Hygienist, Therapist (I – IV), Dentist, Practitioner accredited for Level 2 and 3 care (I – V)

Re-evaluate

Non-engaging patient – return to **STEP 1** & repeat

Engaging patient – move to **STEP 2**

Consider referral

STEP 2

Fig. 5.3 (Contd.)

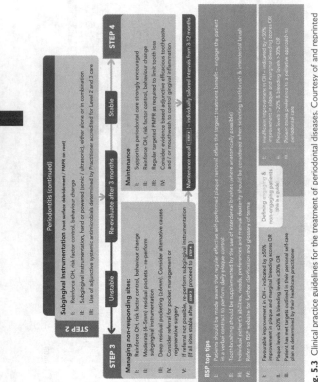

Fig. 5.3 Clinical practice guidelines for the treatment of periodontal diseases. Courtesy of and reprinted with the permission of the British Society of Periodontology, www.bsperio.org

- Where treatment does commence, this would usually start with a course of non-surgical periodontal treatment.
- For periodontitis with a rapid rate of progression such as those with a grade C classification, this may also include the use of antibiotics.
- A typical antibiotic regimen would be either[5]:
  - 500 mg amoxicillin and 400 mg metronidazole three times a day for 7 days or
  - 500 mg azithromycin once a day for 3 days.
- Antibiotic uptake in tissue is usually where the inflammation is greatest; however, penetration of undisturbed biofilm is poor, therefore oral hygiene should be optimal, and the antibiotics should be used as an adjunct to root surface debridement.
- If the patient's oral hygiene at the outset is excellent it may be ideal to provide antibiotics as an adjunct to non-surgical periodontal treatment as part of the first course of treatment. If it is suboptimal, antibiotics may be better as an adjunct on a subsequent course of treatment once plaque control is optimized.
- Subsequent to this, further treatment may include surgical approaches, which would be outside of the remit of this handbook or in stable or remission cases the patient may then be required to have supportive periodontal therapy from the GDP.

Treatment planning of general restorative cases

This should be done as a part of an integrated restorative treatment plan and follow a common strategy:

- *Urgent treatment*: manage pain and any acute infections.
- *Prevention*: eliminate the aetiology of the disease where possible whether this is through diet or oral hygiene changes. This needs to be optimized for the long-term success of any further treatment.
- *Disease control*: remove any active carious lesions which would not otherwise be reversible through prevention and provide appropriate restorations. Removal of plaque to facilitate management of dental health through preventative measures. Removal of teeth as appropriate.
- Assess responses to management so far.
- Elective treatment including any surgery and root canal therapy.
- Provision of final restorations.
- Reassess and maintain.

Provision of treatment

- Any urgent treatment would normally be carried out by the referring practitioner.
- Depending on the unit, preventative management may be undertaken by oral health educators and non-surgical phases of treatment by oral health practitioners such as hygienists or therapists.
- The trainee in DCT may be involved with any of those aspects and surgical phases of treatment or prescribing antimicrobial therapy if needed as part of the treatment plan.

5 Palmer NO (Ed) (2020). *Antimicrobial Prescribing in Dentistry* (3rd ed). FGDP (UK), Faculty of Dental Surgery.

Tooth wear

Background
- Tooth wear is defined as non-carious TSL.
- Tooth wear is a normal physiological process, but excessive tooth wear is classed as pathological, and it is defined as tooth wear exceeding that expected in a patient of a particular age.
- Prevalence:
  - For 15-year-olds: 31% occlusal surface of first molars, 44% palatal surfaces of the upper incisors.
  - For adults: 76%. Severe in 3% of 20-year-olds, 17% of 70-year-olds.

Definitions
- TSL is multifactorial and may be a combination of processes.[6]
- Divided into the following:
  - *Attrition*: loss of tooth substance due to mastication or contact of occlusal surfaces.
  - *Erosion*: chemical process of TSL, not bacterial.
  - *Abrasion*: physical wear of the teeth caused by materials other than tooth contact.
  - *Abfraction*: cervical tooth wear caused by flexural forces in function/parafunction.

Aetiology
- Multifactorial aetiology with possible combination aetiologies in most cases, although difficult to define.
  - *Attrition*: bruxism. Parafunctional activity due to stress of premature contacts.
  - *Erosion*:
    - *Extrinsic*: acidic diet, medications, environmental.
    - *Intrinsic*: gastric acids in the oral environment.
  - Voluntary: bulimia/anorexia, rumination.
  - Involuntary: gastro-oesophageal reflux disease, pregnancy, hiatus hernia.
  - *Abrasion*: toothbrushing, habits (e.g. pen chewing), oral piercings, dental materials.
  - *Abfraction*: possible combination with toothbrush abrasion.
- Prior to any intervention, the aetiology must be identified and modified if possible. The multifactorial nature of TSL will make diagnosis difficult. Where there are clear aetiologies, for example, with attrition, any parafunction caused by stress needs to be addressed. If erosion is the main aetiology, investigation into the source and possible liaison with the GMP should be performed. Symptoms such as sensitivity suggest that the tooth wear is active.
- Operative management is not always indicated. Aesthetics may be the driving force for seeking intervention.
- Preventative measures should be employed.

6 Hemmings K (2018). *Dent Update* 45, 3.

Initial assessment

- *Presenting complaint*: appearance of worn teeth is common—if patients are not concerned about the appearance there may be no need to restore the teeth. Sensitivity is another complaint and usually a sign that tooth wear is active—in these cases the aetiological factor needs to be controlled to prevent further tooth wear. Stress, clenching or bruxism may also feature—again, this needs to be controlled prior to intervention.
- *Medical history*: medication; diagnosed reflux. Any examples of intrinsic erosion such as gastrointestinal reflux must be identified and managed through the GMP; mental health concerns such as anxiety, OCD, eating disorders. Be aware of psychiatric illness with the possibility that it may not be diagnosed, you may be the first person to identify this.
- *Dental history*: patient's readiness for long treatment plans.
- *Social history*: this is very important—identify any occupation causes of stress, and dietary habits such as frequent intake of acidic food and drinks.
- *Clinical examination*: tooth wear is multifactorial, but it is important to identify all the factors that may be involved as well as the predominant one:
  - *Attrition*: flat incisor edges where the teeth have been meeting—common to see in children.
  - *Erosion*: presenting as cupping defects with greater dentine loss and rings of thin enamel with proud restorations. Intrinsic causes tend to affect the palatal surfaces of the upper anterior teeth and the occlusal surfaces of the posterior teeth. Extrinsic causes tend to affect the labial surfaces of the anterior teeth.
  - *Abrasion*: there are usually external causes of physical wear and this is seen where the teeth are in contact with the abrasive medium.
  - *Abfraction*: defects occurring at the cervical margins where the enamel is at its weakest!
    ○ Assess the amount of clinical crown height there is to restore.
    ○ Assess the periodontal status of teeth.
  - *Occlusion*: the incisal relationship (overjet and overbite) may have an influence on the restorability of the teeth and the expected longevity of the restorations.
  - *Condition of the opposing dentition*: if the opposing dentition is restored with ceramic, then this causes a higher failure rate to anterior composite build ups.
  - *Inter occlusal height/space for restorations*.
- *Special investigations*: diet history, duplicated articulated study models, 3D intraoral scans, photographs, and PA radiographs of teeth where retention for restorations may be compromised and elective root treatment with post-core crowns may be required. PA radiographs should also be taken where crown lengthening is being considered and for assessing the root condition and length, and sensibility testing.
- *Diagnosis*: this should include the type of tooth wear, the vitality of teeth, condition of the roots, and restorability.
- *Management options*: identify and manage the aetiological factors if appropriate. If there are no patient concerns regarding appearance,

then no treatment may be necessary. If there is sufficient tooth tissue remaining, then fixed restorative options may be appropriate. Patients with more severe tooth wear or loss of teeth may benefit from the use of removable options such as overdentures or a combination of the above. One of the major aims is to maintain as much tooth tissue as possible and to prevent further loss.

Measuring and monitoring TSL

- There are several indices used for measuring TSL[7]:
  - Tooth Wear Index (TWI).
  - Basic Erosive Wear Examination (BEWE).
  - Anterior Clinical Erosive classification (ACE).
- Study models (sequential) are useful to monitor change.
- 3D intraoral imaging:
  - Digital overlay of the images will determine the extent of TSL progression over time.
  - Digital measurements are more likely to provide accurate assessment of change.

Prevention

- Can be difficult due to the multifactorial aetiology and change over time.
- Prevention advice should be related to the probable cause of the tooth wear[7]:
  - Attrition: prevention of bruxism with the use of splints (soft bilaminar splint or hard such as Michigan splint).
  - Intrinsic erosion: referral to GMP or psychiatry. Full coverage splints for bulimia to prevent further damage.
  - Extrinsic erosion: diet advice.
  - Abrasion: oral hygiene advice and technique.
  - Habits: advice and corrective support.
  - Xerostomia: referral to oral medicine.
- Prevention of symptoms:
  - Fluoride applications.
  - Tooth Mousse™.
  - Dentine bonding agents.
  - GI restorations.

Diagnostic and management stages for TSL

Impression taking for TSL

- Alginate impressions in stock trays are usually adequate.
- Apply alginate material using a gloved finger to all occlusal and palatal surfaces, interproximal areas, and wear lesions prior to seating the stock tray with the remaining alginate and allow both to set simultaneously.
- This will ensure surface detail is picketed up with minimal air blows.

Facebow registration

- This will go over the use of a facebow for common semi-adjustable articulators. Check the individual model you are working with prior to use.

7 Hemmings K (2018). *Dent Update* 45, 3.

- A bite fork with record material such as beauty wax or polysiloxane material is applied.
- This is seated against the upper dentition.
- Once set, the patient should be requested to hold it in position with their index fingers or thumbs.
- The jig should be attached to the earbow. This should then be placed with the bite fork.
- The earbow should then be positioned to be parallel to the alar–tragal line.
- Secure in place.

Interocclusal registration

- In cases such as tooth wear, an is to aim to reorganize the occlusion rather than conforming to the existing one.
- This is due to the lack of interocclusal space meaning that the vertical dimension must be raised to accommodate the restoration.
- For this reason, the interocclusal registration must be in the retruded arc of closure (RAC). Other names used include retruded contact point or centric relation.
- This is regarded as the most reproducible interocclusal record as it is in the terminal hinge axis prior to the slide into Intercuspal position.
- For many patients it is adequate to ask them to roll the tongue back and ask them to slowly bring the teeth together.
- Some patients may not be able to achieve this and so a Lucia jig is helpful.
- This is constructed using greenstick composition which is melted into an approximate $8 \times 8 \times 8$ mm cube in a water bath.
- This is then carefully placed just over the incisal edges of the central incisor teeth with the bulk of the material over the palatal surface.
- A tongue spatula is placed against the palatal surface flat against the composition at a 45° angle to the occlusal plane of the upper teeth
- Once set this becomes the Lucia jig.
- The patient is then asked to slowly close onto the Lucia jig.
- Check that this is reproducible.
- Place record material between the remaining teeth and with the jig in place record the occlusion and allow to set. This and the Lucia jig becomes the RAC record.

Management

Management options for patients with tooth wear include the following[8]:
- Monitoring and advice.
- Fixed restorative rehabilitation:
  - Maintenance of the vertical dimension.
  - Increase in the vertical dimension.
- Removable restorative rehabilitation:
  - Maintenance of the vertical dimension.
  - Increase in the vertical dimension.
- Combination of options.

8 Hemmings K (2018). *Dent Update* 45, 11.

Indications for fixed restorative management
- Generalized/localized tooth wear.
- Sensitivity, pain, or discomfort.
- Functional disturbance.
- Dentoalveolar compensation with lack of interocclusal space.

Indications for removable restorative management
- Severe generalized tooth wear ± partially dentate/long edentulous spans.[9]
- Already wearing removable prosthesis.
- Unsuitable for fixed restorative options.

Planning treatment
- The final result must be anticipated prior to undertaking treatment with the risks and benefits conveyed to the patient, along with the implications of any restorative treatment and the long-term maintenance and repair that is likely to be involved.
- Assess how much remaining tooth structure there is and how much needs to be restored.
- Assess the space requirements for planned restorative materials.
- Does space need to be achieved by occlusal reduction; opposing tooth reduction; occlusal equilibration; orthodontics; Dahl approach; crown lengthening; elective devitalization; and/or an increase in occlusal vertical dimension with reorganization?[8]
- Use of diagnostic wax-up of the planned occlusion with any increase in the vertical dimension.
- Analysis of the diagnostic wax-up will determine the suitability of restorations and the size and material that would be most effective can be planned.
- Laboratory prescription with details on the proposed increase in vertical dimension. It is desirable to keep the build-ups 2 mm short of the gingival margin to maintain periodontal health. A decision on whether canine mutually protected occlusion with posterior disclusion in lateral excursion and protrusion is required as is the case in a lot of reorganized occlusion schemes.

Restorative materials
There are a wide range of materials used in restorative dentistry. These are some of the options to consider for restoration of the worn dentition:
- Direct resin restorations.
- Indirect resin restorations (e.g. composite veneers/palatal veneers).
- Ceramic veneers.
- Cast metal restorations (e.g. onlays/inlays, full coverage crowns, palatal veneers).
- Cast metal/ceramic restorations.
- All ceramic restorations.

The space requirements for these different types of restoration need to be considered when planning complex cases such as TSL and how this space will be created.[10]

9 Hemmings K (2018). *Dent Update* 45, 20.
10 Hemmings K (2018). *Dent Update* 45, 11.

Resin restoration of anterior teeth

This section will briefly go over a technique for build-up of teeth using composite resin. There are several different methods of achieving this and one will be described here:

- Construct a colourless silicone index using the wax-up.
- Using temporary crown and bridge material such as bis-acryl composite, place this into the putty index and seat over the patient's teeth.
- This will show the patient the anticipated end result. It is important to emphasize to the patient that this is merely an estimate of could be achieved rather than a precise outcome in terms of shape and size.
- Once agreed, section the colourless transparent silicone index though the incisal edges—this will leave a lingual and buccal section.
- When starting, apply a rubber dam as this will help with moisture control. Use a split dam if necessary.
- Start with the canine teeth first, then the central incisors, then lateral incisors, and then premolars if necessary.
- Composite is contraindicated for the use of building up posterior teeth.[11]
- Etch and bond the entire tooth surface.
- Apply the lingual/palatal part of the clear index firmly against the teeth.
- Use a translucent shade of composite and build up the lingual wall. Cure this layer, then apply the body or dentine shade building from the lingual wall.
- When built up at this stage, go as close to the contact as possible without actually touching it.
- Once the body has been built, go up to the incisal edge—a translucent shade would be best for this region.
- Repeat this with all the teeth that you wish to build in that session.
- Remove the index and what should now be built is the incisal edge, lingual and just short of the interproximal walls.
- Wrap a clear matrix band around the interproximal surfaces and pack composite against this, ensuring a tight fit with the matrix. This will ensure a lack of voids and help create a smooth interproximal surface with little need for polishing.
- Now all that is remaining is to build the labial surface. Some creativity could be shown here including staining to give the appearance of crack lines, building the mamelons, and varying degrees of translucency for the incisal edge and opacity for underlying dentine.
- Finish using polishing discs and pastes until the patient is happy and there are no plaque-retaining factors.
- Provide the silicone index to the patient so that future repairs can be done more easily.

11 Bartlett D (2006). *Int J Prosthod* 19, 613.

Further reading

Arkutu N, Gadhia K, McDonald S, et al. (2012). Amelogenesis imperfecta: the orthodontic perspective. *Br Dent J* 212, 485–489.

British Society for Restorative Dentistry: 🔊 www.bsrd.org.uk

Eliyas S, Vere J, Ali Z, et al. (2014). Micro-surgical endodontics. *Br Dent J* 216, 169–177.

Gulamali A, Hemmings K, Tredwin C, et al. (2011). Survival analysis of composite Dahl restorations provided to manage localised anterior tooth wear. *Br Dent J* 211, E9.

Malik K, Gadhia K, Arkutu N, et al. (2012). The interdisciplinary management of amelogenesis imperfecta—restorative dentistry. *Br Dent J* 212, 537–542.

McDonald S, Arkutu N, Malik K, et al. (2012). Managing the paediatric patient with amelogenesis imperfecta. *Br Dent J* 212, 425–428.

Patel M, McDonnell ST, Iram S, et al. (2013). Amelogenesis imperfecta—lifelong management. *Br Dent J* 215, 449–457.

RCS England. Restorative dentistry: Index of Treatment Need. Complexity assessment. 🔊 https://www.rcseng.ac.uk/-/media/files/rcs/fds/publications/complexityassessment.pdf

Restorative Dentistry UK: 🔊 www.restdent.org.uk

Siddall KZ, Rogers SN, Butterworth CJ (2012). The prosthodontic pathway of the oral cancer patient. *Dental Update* 39, 98–100.

Chapter 6

Oral and maxillofacial surgery

Introduction to oral and maxillofacial surgery

- Oral and maxillofacial surgery (OMFS) is one of the most diverse specialties in medicine.
- The scope of practice that is undertaken within an OMFS unit will vary from hospital to hospital, based on the interests and experience of the consultant surgeons who work there.
- OMFS can often be divided into subspecialties, including:
  - head and neck oncology
  - trauma
  - orthognathic
  - TMJ
  - dentoalveolar surgery
  - salivary gland
  - skin
  - CLP
  - craniofacial.
- Many OMFS surgeons will carry out operations across several of these categories, whereas others may have focused their practice, for example, almost exclusively managing oncology cases.
- As a result of the variety of case mix between units, the experience a Dental Core trainee will have in an OMFS unit also varies across the country, as do the duties that you will be expected to fulfil.
- It is worth researching a unit in advance of applying for a post or ranking options.
- Before starting a job, it would be wise to organise time to go and shadow the current trainees, as this can be invaluable in understanding exactly how a unit runs and what will be expected of you. This is often encouraged in each unit, with time allocation provided by HEE.
- Courses are also run nationwide which offer an introduction to the specialty and teach the basic skills that you will need before starting, such as cannulation, venepuncture, and suturing. These can be incredibly useful in allowing you to 'hit the ground running' when starting as a first-time OMFS Dental Core trainee.

Introduction to the ward

- Not all units will have an inpatient ward, although larger OMFS units will. They can sometimes be shared with other specialties.
- The amount of time a patient will remain an inpatient varies according to the operation they have had and their comorbidities/social circumstances.
- Many patients admitted for a postoperative overnight bed or with trauma will have few medical issues and only stay for a matter of days. Major head and neck cancer patients, however, are likely to be on the ward for 1–2 weeks and often have much more complex medical and postoperative requirements.
- In units with inpatients, the day-to-day running of the ward is the responsibility of the Dental Core trainees under the supervision of registrars and consultants.

Handover

- At the start/end of every shift, the on-call Dental Core trainee will 'handover' to the Dental Core trainee who is taking over duties. A comprehensive handover is an essential part of ensuring continuity of care between day and night teams.
- Most units will have a pre-existing handover sheet which is updated at the end of every shift and talked through with the next Dental Core trainee prior to the start of their shift.
- It will usually include a list of all inpatients on the ward with a short history of their reason for admission, details and dates of any operations, latest investigation results or issues, and any plan or jobs that currently need doing for them. It will also have details of any outstanding jobs on the ward, or patients who need reviewing in A&E/ are expected to attend.
- Prepare the handover in advance of ending your shift.
- Try your best to tie up loose ends before the end of your shift; however, sometimes it is impossible to get everything done and so you should not feel bad about handing jobs over that you have not had time to complete.
- Make sure you arrive on time for handover and do it in a quiet area away from the ward and other distractions. Keep it clear and concise and make sure nothing is missed off the list.
- Handovers will get more efficient as you get used to the process. In the beginning it can be worth going in early as they can take longer than the allotted time and you want to avoid keeping consultants waiting to start the morning ward rounds.

Ward round

- Ward rounds will be held daily, often first thing in the morning, and will normally be led by the Dental Core trainee who is on call that day, or who has been on call overnight.
- Your job on a ward round will be to:
  - lead the team (Dental Core trainees, registrars, consultants, and staff nurse) in a logical manner around all the current inpatients
  - introduce each patient, giving a brief summary of the reason for admission, history of stay and progress report for past 24 hours, as well as any plan currently in place or recent results (e.g. blood tests or scans)
  - record the notes from the ward round for each patient (Box 6.1)
  - record your list of jobs for the day.
- Following the ward round, it is often helpful to take 5 minutes to review and reconcile what has occurred and to clarify things in your mind, as well as prioritize the jobs you have for that day.
- Ward jobs can often include:
  - taking blood from patients (although some wards will have access to a phlebotomist)
  - cannulating
  - clerking for theatre and consent
  - prescribing or changing medications
  - requesting input from other specialties

> **Box 6.1 Example of a ward round notes**
> *31/01/23 OMFS ward round 08:15*
> **OMFS team:** [Initials or names of team present, i.e. consultant, registrar, Dental Core trainee.]
> **PCO:** [Patient complaints that day—nil if none.]
> **On examination:** [Brief details of any assessment of patient that day.]
> **Flap:** [If postoperative oncology patient, describe the flap appearance ± Doppler signal.]
> **MEWS:** [Record most recent score from chart and note if been stable or varied.]

* removing drains
* inserting nasogastric tubes
* clerking new admissions.

Results: [Any relevant results from past 24 hours, e.g. blood tests or scans.]
Plan: [Ensure clearly written at end of notes, e.g.:
1. Continue with IV antibiotics.
2. Remove drain PM (afternoon).
3. Review PM ward round.]
Sign: [Name, grade, GDC No.]

* In busier units, the list of ward jobs can at times be overwhelming, so it is important to keep organized and to prioritize things. Prioritizing jobs can be complex and confusing at times. It comes with experience and is best discussed with a senior in the early days until you get a feel for it.
* As a first-time Dental Core trainee you can sometimes feel a little out of your depth. Nurses are always an excellent source of help or advice especially early on in your post. They have frequently been working there for a number of years and have seen most things, as well as knowing how the hospital and department work so they can be an invaluable source of information.
* Preparing for the ward round can help things run smoother and here are some top tips to help:
  * Make sure you know the location of the patients who need to be seen, that is, which ward, bay, and bed they are in (this should be written on the handover sheet).
  * Ensure notes are easily available for each patient in advance, and even consider pre-writing a proforma ready to complete during the ward round to save time.
  * Have a pen torch, gloves, tongue depressors, marker pen, and stethoscope all to hand.
  * Consider printing out blood results or scan reports.
  * Go to ward rounds even when you're not on the ward that day. In the early days it helps you to get used to how things work, later you can keep on top of what's going on and your colleagues will always appreciate another pair of hands!
  * Never presume or try to make up an answer about a patient—if you don't know something, say so.

Observations

- All inpatients on a ward will have regular 'observations' recorded by the nurse team on an end-of-bed chart. Observations are the patient's vital statistics, most often comprising heart rate, blood pressure, temperature, oxygen saturation, and respiratory rate.
- Monitoring a patient's observations over time can show signs of deterioration in their condition, as a result the Early Warning Score (EWS) was created. The EWS is calculated using a specific chart which scores each of the individual observation results from 0 to 3. The scores are then totalled to give an overall EWS.
- Higher EWS indicates a more unwell or unstable patient, an escalating EWS overtime is an indication of a deteriorating patient. There is often a locally determined EWS threshold at which the medical emergency team (MET) is contacted if a patient is not responding to efforts to stabilize their condition.
- NB: some hospital trusts have developed their own Modified Early Warning Score (MEWS) system which works on the same principles but may include slightly different vital statistics or thresholds for scores.

Clerking patients

'Clerking' is the term given to admitting a patient to the ward or pre-theatre. It can involve the following:

- Taking a history of reason for admission.
- Medical history (MH), dental history (DH), and social history (SH).
- Confirming the procedure and theatre date.
- Clinical examination.
- Skin/location marking of surgical site.
- Consent.
- Check all relevant radiographs/scans have been completed and are available to view.
- Check if needs to be nil by mouth (NBM).
- Venous thromboembolism (VTE) assessment (➔ VTE assessments).
- Bloods?
- Cannulation?
- IV fluids (➔ IV fluids)?

Prescribing

- Once admitted, it is essential that a patient's normal routine medication is prescribed for them on the hospital computer system or paper drug chart, as well as any additional medication prescribed as part of their admission.
- As always when prescribing new medication, it is imperative that any allergies are recorded, and interactions checked.
- As a dentist working in hospital your prescribing privileges are not limited to the dental practitioner's formulary in the *British National Formulary* and you may therefore be prescribing drugs you are not familiar with. It is essential that time is spent researching any unfamiliar drugs prior to prescribing them.

- The *British National Formulary* app is very simple to use and can prove invaluable in checking doses and interactions, but many wards will have a ward pharmacist who is often very happy to help. Their role on the ward is to review patients' medications to ensure they are safe, at correct doses, and without interactions. Out of hours there should be on-call pharmacists available to take advice from when needed.
- Co-prescribing is often used with certain medications. This is where one medication is prescribed to counteract the undesirable effects of another. For example, laxatives are often prescribed with opiates, or proton pump inhibitors (e.g. omeprazole) may be prescribed alongside long-term non-steroidal anti-inflammatory drugs.
- Abbreviations used in prescribing:
  - *Route*: PO (oral), IV (intravenous), IM (intramuscular), SC (subcutaneous).
  - *Regimen*: STAT (immediately (once)), OD (once daily), BD (twice daily), TDS (three times daily), QDS (four times daily).
  - *Duration*: 1/7 (1 day), 2/7 (2 days), 1/52 (1 week), 1/12 (1 month).

VTE assessments

- VTE assessments are completed for every patient on admission. Often there is a proforma to follow and the assessment may be done by nurses but could be the responsibility of a Dental Core trainee depending on local arrangements.
- Questions are asked relating to the patient and the plans for their stay.
- This generates the patient's risk of VTE which in turn determines the precautions advised as VTE prophylaxis, such as TED (thromboembolic deterrent) stockings or low-molecular-weight heparin injections.

IV fluids

- Fluids are prescribed in many different scenarios, ranging from a simple dehydrated patient to a patient with significant blood loss in hypovolaemic shock. The three types of fluids that can be prescribed are crystalloids, colloids, and blood products.
- For OMFS patients, the most frequent prescribing of fluids you will need to undertake is for patients who are being kept NBM for theatre and therefore need IV fluid to keep them hydrated.
- For this, a simple crystalloid formulation is all that is needed. The most commonly used are:
  - 5% dextrose solution: isotonic, essentially just water as dextrose metabolized
  - 0.9% NaCl (saline): contains 150 mmol/L Na^+
  - Hartman's solution: isotonic, provides fluid and electrolytes, more physiological.

You will commonly need to prescribe IV fluids and so it is imperative that you understand the principles. The NICE guidelines 'Intravenous fluid therapy in adults in hospital'[1] provide a comprehensive summary.

---

1 🔗 www.nice.org.uk/guidance/CG174

In some patients (e.g. the elderly, kidney disease, cardiac failure, electrolyte disturbances) precise prescription of fluids is critical and advice should be sought.

Flap monitoring

- Monitoring free flaps on patients is a vital part of a Dental Core trainee's role within most OMFS oncology units.
- The 'flap' is an area of tissue (varying combinations of skin, muscle, and bone) which is harvested from a donor site (e.g. arm, leg, chest, shoulder, hip) and placed into the head and neck to fill the defect left following a resection (e.g. cancer or osteonecrosis).
- Flaps are raised with a pedicle of blood vessels which are anastomosed with the neck vessels using microscopes to re-establish a blood supply.
- Often initially, hourly monitoring of flaps is required to ensure that any signs of failure are picked up as early as possible.
- Delayed detection of a failing flap can be devastating for the patient and the surgical team.
- *You should be shown what a healthy flap looks like.* Flaps can vary in appearance from patient to patient, so it is helpful to see a flap that you will be monitoring for the first time with somebody who has already been looking after it to confirm how it looks and feels and what is 'normal' for that flap.
- Also bear in mind that flaps can look different in different light—some modern LED torches cast a bluish light and make flaps look paler, for example.
- A dark, firm, purple flap can be a sign of venous congestion, whereas a pale, soft flap with slow capillary refill can be a sign of arterial supply issues.
- Some flaps have no skin attached and are solely bone and muscle (e.g. scapula flap) which can be harder to monitor.
- Occasionally, internal or external Doppler ultrasound can be used on vessels supplying flaps to check for blood flow.
- Senior team members should be informed *immediately* if there is any concern regarding the health of a flap.
- Major head and neck oncology patients will often go to the intensive care unit immediately postoperatively and be kept there for the first 24 hours (and sometimes longer) until the consultants are satisfied that they are stable enough for the OMFS ward.

Tracheostomies

- Particularly on oncology wards, many OMFS patients can have tracheostomies in place.
- The majority of 'trachy' care will be done by specialist nurses on the ward who are very experienced in managing them.
- It is, however, essential that you familiarize yourself with what a tracheostomy is, what model is used in your unit, and how it is put together. You may be called to help manage a blockage, bleeding from around the area, or a displacement (Fig. 6.1).

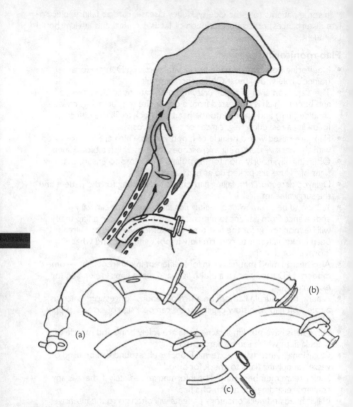

Fig. 6.1 Tracheostomy position and equipment. Reproduced from Corbridge R, Steventon N (2010). *Oxford Handbook of ENT and Head and Neck Surgery*, p. 241. Oxford University Press.

'DNACPR' and advance decisions

- Some patients may have a 'Do not attempt cardiopulmonary resuscitation' (DNACPR) order or advance decision in place. All members of the team should be aware of this as they can affect what treatments can be carried out for the patient, especially in the event of a medical emergency.
- A DNACPR is put in place when a patient has decided that should their condition deteriorate, they do not want any treatment carried out to resuscitate them.
- An advance decision (aka living will) can be put in place by patients to allow them to make decisions about or refuse treatments in the future even if their consciousness or ability to communicate deteriorates.

The MDT

- OMFS inpatients will often have input into their care from more than just your team.
- Within the hospital there are many specialized teams who visit patients on wards to help with specific needs such as:
  - dieticians
  - diabetic nurses
  - physiotherapists
  - SALTs
  - occupational therapists.
- You should be aware of what services are available and know the teams involved as you will be working with them from day 1.
- Communication is key within the MDT and clearly written notes in the patient's record help everybody to know what progress is being made with a patient.

Discharging patients

- When patients come to be discharged, you will likely be required to complete their discharge paperwork. This often consists of a discharge letter which will be sent to the patient's GMP and any to take out (TTO; aka to take home (TTH) or to take away (TTA)) medications that they could need to continue after their stay.
- Nurses will send the TTO prescription either to the main pharmacy or the ward pharmacist who will then issue the medications. This can sometimes cause delays in patients being able to go home so ensure TTOs are completed in a timely fashion.
- All patients require a discharge letter when leaving hospital. This should include:
  - the reason for admission and treatment completed
  - the findings of tests/scans/investigations during the hospital stay
  - the plan for the future/follow up appointments
  - any medications stopped or started—if either of these, for how long? Permanent? Repeat prescription needed by GMP?
  - any outlying jobs for the GMP, such as were the urea and electrolytes (U&E) abnormal during the stay? Do you want the GMP to repeat these? In how long?
- Any future OMFS review appointments asked for in the discharge letter will be made by the ward clerk.

Introduction to on-call and A&E

'On-call' shifts can take the form of long days, nights, and weekends where you will most often carry a 'bleep' (pager) or mobile phone. Through this, clinicians/nurses both within and outside the hospital can contact you to ask for OMFS advice or request a review of a patient.

Assessment of cases from A&E

- Most A&E departments are split into majors, minors, and paediatric departments and it is likely that you will regularly review patients in each with maxillofacial problems.
- When taking a call from A&E, or an outside practitioner wanting to refer a patient in, always make sure you take notes of the referral details and include:
  - name and grade of referring doctor/practitioner
  - their phone or bleep number
  - patient details—name, date of birth (DOB), hospital number
  - area where patient currently is
  - reason for referral/history of injury or problem
  - patient's condition (airway issues etc.)
  - known medical issues
  - any treatment already undertaken, or medication started
  - if they have been cleared of head injury.
- It is *ESSENTIAL* that any patient with a history of trauma to the head and neck has been cleared of head and spinal injury by the A&E doctors *prior to accepting any referral.*
- If you are unsure what advice to give over the phone or what to do with a patient, don't be afraid to tell the referrer that you will call them back after consulting a senior colleague.
- Occasionally, it can take a long time for imaging to be done in A&E, and so following their assessment, ensure the A&E doctors have ordered the appropriate radiographs before you go to review the patient as this can save you a lot of time.
- The mix and frequency of referrals you receive from A&E will vary from hospital to hospital based on the area in which the hospital is situated and the services on offer in surrounding units. In many cities there is a centralization of services around a single hospital designated a 'major trauma centre', meaning surrounding A&E departments will see less of the polytrauma cases such as road traffic accidents. Other units may have no paediatric department as a nearby specialist children's hospital may see all the patients.

Management of cases from A&E

- Many A&E departments have a lack of equipment for managing OMFS cases.
- It will often be of benefit to you and your colleagues to put together an 'A&E bag' with basics from the OMFS department such as:
  - LA and (dental) syringes
  - suturing instruments
  - sutures
  - saline pouches

- gauze
- composite
- wires
- composite bonding agent.
- At times when A&E is busy and pressures are mounting, triage staff may try to refer patients straight to you without them being seen by an A&E doctor first. This can be unsafe and also cause complications if the patient is then labelled as 'accepted by OMFS'. *You should insist that all patients are first seen by a member of the A&E team.*
- The most common OMFS conditions you will be called to see in A&E are listed in the following section (➲ Common A&E conditions).

Common A&E conditions

Dentoalveolar infections

- Assessment:
  - As for initial assessment of any patient, Airway, Breathing, Circulation, Disability, Exposure (ABCDE) primary survey—always check airway is patent, no breathing issues, and observations are stable. Check for signs of sepsis.
  - If any concerns over airway (e.g. raised floor or mouth, difficulty swallowing/speaking, spreading submandibular swelling, drooling, trismus) then request anaesthetic review and inform senior colleagues immediately.
  - Radiographs/computed tomography (CT) scan (discuss with a senior before ordering a CT scan).
  - Determine what the problem is. If pulpitis, *do not* give antibiotics. Patient needs to see an emergency dentist for appropriate treatment. (It is helpful to have the contact details of the local emergency dental services to pass on to the patient.)
- If a collection is present, determine the space which is being occupied (Fig. 6.2).

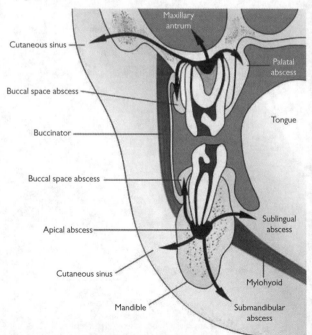

Fig. 6.2 Spaces of odontogenic infection. Reproduced from Sammut S et al. (2013). Facial cutaneous sinuses of dental origin – a diagnostic challenge. *Br Dent J* 215, 555–558, with permission from Springer Nature.

- Management:
  - No identifiable collection and not spreading: to see GDP for extraction/root canal treatment.
  - Collection present intraorally (e.g. buccal sulcus or canine space): drain under LA if possible and later GDP for extraction under LA and oral antibiotics.
  - Collection which cannot be drained under LA or is spreading/concerning: inform the registrar and if agreed, admit for GA extraction with incision and drainage and IV antibiotics.
  - *Note*: if you are unsure of how to safely drain an intraoral swelling, ask a senior to demonstrate the technique to you first before attempting.
- Admitting patient:
  - IV access (+ take bloods) and prescribe IV antibiotics.
  - Keep NBM.
  - Prescribe IV fluids.
  - Add to emergency theatre list and inform the on-call anaesthetist.
  - Consent for the proposed procedure.
  - Arrange a bed.

Lacerations

- Assessment:
  - Bleeding: if uncontrollable then large tacking sutures or staples sometimes required to stabilize before finer closure later in a theatre setting. Consider bipolar electrocautery to help stop bleeding vessels.
  - Structures involved: are any nerves (cranial nerve (CN) examination), blood vessels, ducts, or glands involved? If so, likely to need closure under GA with repair of involved structures.
  - Location: is particular care required in reapproximating the wound edges correctly (e.g. vermilion border of the lip, eyebrows)?
  - Compliance: is the patient compliant enough? If too drunk, attempt to wash and stabilize and bring back to close when sober. If too young or anxious, may need GA or sedation.
  - Debris: if very dirty wound or glass involved, may need exploration under GA to ensure all foreign bodies removed prior to closure.
  - Wound size: is it too large to anaesthetize with LA, too complex to be within your skillset, or significant tissue loss preventing primary closure? If so, senior review needed and likely GA to repair/reconstruct.
  - Through and through lacerations (communication through skin into the mouth) should always be closed intraorally first before skin closure.
  - Diagrams when recording in notes can often be helpful.
  - May need suturing (➜ Suturing).

Facial fractures and trauma assessment

- Facial fractures are a common occurrence in A&E and OMFS units. The vast majority are not life-threatening.
- The exception to this is any facial fracture which has resulted in uncontrolled bleeding, or an unfavourable bilateral mandibular fracture which is collapsing posteriorly and obstructing the airway.

- Initial examination:
  - First check ABCDE.
  - Take a thorough history of how the injury occurred, this will give an indication as to where the facial fractures may be located and the velocity of trauma can affect the pattern of fractures.
  - MH, drug history, and so on all need recording.
- Extraorally:
  - Palpate the full facial skeleton checking for any steps or asymmetry. This can sometimes be hard to detect in the presence of swelling or pain.
  - Standing above and behind a seated patient, and looking down as you assess can help you detect any facial asymmetry in the midface. Lacerations and bruising will be fairly evident.

CN assessment

Carry out a full or limited CN examination to check for any deficiencies, especially:

- CNs II, III, IV, and VI (eye signs):
  - Visual acuity: use a Snellen chart to check. If patient usually wears glasses, they should wear them if possible.
  - Range of movement: ask patient to follow your finger with head kept still. Move finger to draw a rectangle in the air and then an 'X' or cross from each corner to check they can move their eyes to the full extremities without tethering. Limited upward or lateral movements can be signs of orbital wall/floor fractures with muscle tethering.
  - Hypoglobus, proptosis, or enophthalmos: eye sitting lower, protruding out- or inwards more than the contralateral side. Best viewed from above and behind the patient.
  - Pupils: should be equal sizes and reactive to light.
  - Subconjunctival haemorrhage: an inferior subconjunctival haemorrhage without a posterior border (no visible edge to the bleeding) can be diagnostic of an orbital floor fracture.
- CN V (trigeminal nerve): sensory deficit in one of the three branches. If present, map out as accurately as possible on a diagram in notes and score out of 10 for sensation compared to normal side.
- CN VII (facial nerve): test all branches by asking patient to raise eyebrows, scrunch eyes tight shut, puff out cheeks, show teeth/grimace, and tighten platysma in neck.
- Intraorally:
  - Check occlusion and ask patient if it feels normal. If not, there could be a mandibular fracture although slight occlusal discrepancies can occur as a result of TMJ effusion post trauma even in the absence of a fracture.
  - Check for loose or damaged teeth, steps or new gaps in the dental arch, alveolar fractures, laceration to soft tissues, and bleeding or sublingual haematoma.
  - If a Le Fort I fracture is suspected (➔ Maxillary fractures), check for mobility between the maxillary teeth and the rest of the maxilla superiorly.
- Radiographing and managing facial fractures:
  - Radiographs may have been carried out prior to you being called to see the patient. If not, the type of radiographs you order will depend

on the fracture you suspect, guided by your clinical examination and history.
- As your experience grows, your aptitude for detecting fractures both clinically and radiographically, as well as recognizing the common patterns of facial bone fractures will improve.
- If facial fractures are suspected and the patient is having a CT head to check for brain injury, it might be worth asking the radiologists to include the facial bones in the CT scan. Otherwise, plain film radiographs are the first-line imaging for facial bone fractures.

Mandibular fractures

Investigations
- Radiographs: orthopantomogram (OPG) and PA mandible or CT if comminuted.

Management
- Most fractures will need open reduction and internal fixation (ORIF) with titanium plates and screws. Some fractures may be treated conservatively, for example, in elderly edentulous patients, high condylar fractures, or in non- or minimally displaced fractures with no change to the occlusion.
- Bridle wires are sometimes used instead of fixation with plates and are placed around teeth either side of the fracture line and tightened to hold the fracture in place.
- Patients with fractures requiring surgical intervention need to be admitted and worked up for theatre. The process when admitting a mandibular fracture may vary slightly from unit to unit, but usually you will need to do the following:
  - Inform your registrar.
  - Keep NBM.
  - Cannulate and prescribe IV fluids.
  - Bloods are often not required if the patient is fit and well and there is no infection.
  - Prescribe analgesia and any regular medicines the patient is on.
  - If an open fracture (communicates with the oral cavity) then prescribe IV antibiotics (refer to local trust guidelines).
  - Add to the emergency theatre list and inform the on-call anaesthetist.
  - Ask bed manager to admit to the ward.
  - Consent the patient.
- In some situations, intermaxillary fixation may be used, often in the form of arch bars. This effectively wires the top and bottom jaws together with the teeth in occlusion with the aim of ensuring that the jaw fractures heal in a position where the patient's normal bite is maintained.
- Having intermaxillary fixation can obviously be inconvenient for the patient in terms of eating/drinking and so a soft/liquid diet is essential. It can also be an airway risk for the patient if, for example, they vomit. As a result, it is always wise to have a pair of wire cutters at the patient's bedside to allow quick removal of the wires in an emergency.
- Bridle wires and arch bars are often removed under LA postoperatively which can be quite unpleasant for the patient. There is a technique to doing it well so ask a senior to demonstrate it first time around.

- For postoperative patients, or those being managed conservatively, the advice given is a soft diet for 6 weeks, analgesics, avoidance of contact sports, regular chlorhexidine mouthwashes (if appropriate), antibiotics (if an open fracture), and review in 1 week's time on the trauma clinic.

Zygomatic fractures
- Investigations: radiographs—two OM views or CT if complex.
- Management:
  - Zygomatic fractures are often managed conservatively unless there is an obvious cosmetic or functional issue. Most will be reviewed after 5–7 days to assess the situation after initial swelling has resolved. Any eye issues should be referred to ophthalmology for review.
  - If the decision is taken to ORIF the fracture, then the process is as described previously when admitting and listing. Postoperative eye observations must be undertaken on the ward to ensure no retrobulbar haemorrhage occurs.

Maxillary fractures
- Investigations: radiographs—OM views or CT.
- Management: Le Fort I, II, and III fractures are often associated with higher-velocity injuries, and many present in combination with other major trauma, but can occur in isolation. Fractures often require admission and ORIF (Fig. 6.3).

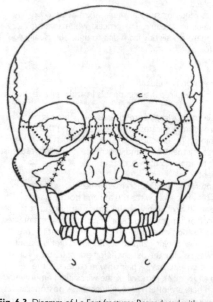

•••••• Le Fort III
+ + + + Le Fort II
——— Le Fort I

Fig. 6.3 Diagram of Le Fort fractures Reproduced with permission from Rushworth B, Kanatas A (2020). *Oxford Handbook of Clinical Dentistry* (7 ed). Oxford University Press.

Orbital floor fractures

- Investigations: radiographs—OM views (check for 'teardrop sign') or CT if likely to be operated on.
- Management:
  - Need for surgical intervention depends on the nature of the injury. Muscle entrapment in children is an absolute indication for early intervention (→ White-eyed blowout). Most patients, however, will be reviewed after a few days to determine if there is any aesthetic or functional indication for operating. Any patients with diplopia (double vision), decreased acuity, or other eye signs should have an ophthalmology review.
  - It is *ESSENTIAL* to check the eyes of patients with injuries in this area regardless of how swollen shut they are. Retrobulbar haemorrhage (→ Retrobulbar haemorrhage) can be catastrophic for the patient and so pupillary response and visual acuity must be checked in every patient.
  - If orbital floor repair is undertaken, regular postoperative eye observations must be undertaken on the ward to ensure that no retrobulbar haemorrhage does occur.

Nasal and frontal bone fractures

- Investigations: radiographs—nasal bone fractures often require no radiographs; however, nasoethmoidal and frontal bone fractures require a CT scan to confirm if suspected.
- Management:
  - Frontal bone fractures may need neurosurgical input if they involve the cranium.
  - Often surgery is only needed if the depression causes a cosmetic defect. Nasal bones may require manipulation under anaesthesia, which can be done under GA or LA; in some units these will often be managed by ENT.

Major trauma/pan-facial fractures

- Investigations: radiographs—most will have had a wide-field CT scan as part of the major trauma assessment.
- Management:
  - Many polytrauma patients will have multiple and often comminuted facial bone fractures. These patients, however, are often very unwell at first admission and have other much more serious injuries which need attention.
  - If the facial fractures are stable and causing no major bleeding or airway issues, then often these patients are reviewed in the days after initial admission once they are stabilized to determine how managing their facial fractures fits into the larger, multispecialty treatment plan.

Bleeding from the mouth

- History:
  - Any recent dental treatment, extractions, or trauma?
  - What has been done so far to try to stop it?
  - How long has it been bleeding for? Continuous or intermittent?
  - Ask to estimate total blood loss—cup full? Sink full?
  - Has the patient swallowed a lot of blood?
  - MH check—any anticoagulants/bleeding disorder?

- Clinical examination:
  - Good light, wide opening, and suction.
  - Swabs and mouth mirror/tongue depressor can help.
  - Source of bleeding must be visualized. If bleeding is significant, unlikely to be a tooth socket.
- Bloods:
  - Full blood count (FBC) may be necessary to check haemoglobin levels if significant blood loss suspected, particularly in elderly patients. Platelet levels should also be checked.
  - Coagulation screen can check for any coagulopathy.
- Management:
  - Tooth socket: most bleeding in the mouth if minor will stop with adequate sustained pressure—consider placing a pack accurately in the patient's mouth and clearly explaining the need to bite firmly without releasing/talking; leave the patient in A&E and return to check on them in 20–30 minutes. Tranexamic acid-soaked gauze can be considered but many believe offers little benefit.
  - If bleeding persists, pack and suture. If already done by GDP but appears loose/inadequate, consider removing and redoing. Pack with a cellulose matrix (e.g. Surgicel®) and place sutures tightly to compress the socket edges against the bone (horizontal mattress can often be a good option).
  - Laceration: if accessible to do under LA then close with resorbable sutures.
  - Postoperative bleed: occasionally bleeds can occur from a recent operative site (e.g. laser resection of a tongue). Pressure can sometimes stop but may require suturing or cauterization. Ask for a senior review if any concerns.
  - Lesions: if source is a firm mass with contact bleeding, always consider a sinister diagnosis.
  - IV tranexamic acid can be very helpful in stopping persistent bleeding if local measures are failing alone but should only be used with advice from medical or senior OMFS colleagues.

Dental trauma in OMFS
- When giving advice over the phone, avulsed permanent teeth should be re-implanted as soon as possible. If this is not possible, they should be stored either in the patient's own saliva, milk, or saline and emergency care sought immediately. The extra-alveolar dry time is critical for prognosis.
- Splinting teeth is notoriously challenging as a Dental Core trainee in A&E. Try to get good lighting, equipment, and assistance if possible. There are many ways to splint teeth, ask a senior to show you how it is best done with the equipment you have available in your unit.
- If a tooth is avulsed and unaccounted for, a chest X-ray must be carried out to rule out aspiration into the lungs.
- Any missing fragments of anterior teeth in combination with laceration to the labial mucosae should raise suspicion of loss of the fragment into the tissues and a lateral soft tissues X-ray may be useful in investigating this.

  See also ➔ Dental trauma.

Mandibular dislocation
- Assessment:
  - Patients are unable to close the mouth and may be drooling.
  - Establish how it occurred—yawning, post GA, trauma, dentistry.
  - Unless history of trauma, radiographs are often not necessary.
- Management:
  - Manual reduction is often needed.
  - Sit the patient in a chair with a high back or against a wall so their head can be supported at the back.
  - Wrap your thumbs in gauze or tape to protect them.
  - Stand in front of the patient and place your thumbs on their lower molar teeth and wrap your fingers beneath the lower border of the mandible.
  - With increasing and sustained pressure press the mandible *downwards and backwards* to move the condylar head down and over the articular eminence and back into the fossa.
  - Often one side will relocate first followed by a 'clunk' of the other side going back in. Relief for the patient is often instantaneous.
  - If manual reduction fails due to pain or spasm, LA, sedation, or GA may be needed. Place a Barton's bandage to help reduce chance of re-dislocation.

Sebaceous cysts
- Will present as a swelling in the skin, almost always with a punctum that releases foul-smelling discharge on pressure. When infected can be very painful and require drainage under LA.
- A small amount of LA into the overlying skin before incising should establish drainage. Following emptying of the cyst, irrigate with saline and either place a drain and dressing or pack with iodine-soaked gauze then review and change the pack regularly over the next week or so. Antibiotics may also be prescribed on discharge (usually flucloxacillin).
- Formal excision of the cyst will be required once the infection has settled.

Cellulitis
- Red, shiny, firm, and often tender swelling of the skin. Caused by infection either from a break in the skin (e.g. trauma, insect bite, etc.) or infection of a deeper structure beneath the skin (e.g. dental abscess).
- If you are unable to find a cause it is worth considering whether it could be related to underlying sinus pathology and an ENT review may be requested (particularly for periorbital cellulitis).
- Management of the infection will address it and usually antibiotics are the only treatment needed. Be aware of conditions such as erysipelas which can cause blistering and tissue necrosis if severe and necrotizing fasciitis which is a rare but extremely serious condition with high mortality.

Penetrating neck wounds
- Penetrating trauma to the neck can cause devastating damage to the structures beneath leading to airway loss, haemorrhage, or neurological deficits.

- Injuries can be caused by stabbings, impalement, or gunshot wounds. If a patient arrives with an object still in place, *DO NOT REMOVE*.
- Management of these patients needs to be carefully assessed and your senior should be informed and involved from the start.
- The patient may simply need to be monitored if the wound is clear of vital structures. If there is any concern however it may need exploration ± intervention under GA.
- The specialty called to manage penetrating neck wounds may vary between ENT and OMFS from unit to unit.

Bites

- Dog, cat, and human bites can present in A&E.
- Cat and human bites are particularly prone to infection.
- Treat with a thorough wash out, prophylactic antibiotics (refer to local trust guidelines), and closure. Delayed closure can be an option if significant concerns over infection.

Salivary gland diseases

- Most salivary swellings will be related to acute infections or blockages. The presence of any local lymphadenopathy or nerve palsy should raise suspicion of a more sinister underlying cause, particularly if the swelling is painless.
- Infection:
  - *Bacterial*: acute sialadenitis presents as a firm, very tender, erythematous swelling of the affected gland. Often related to dehydration and more common in elderly patients. Pus can sometimes be expressed through the ducts via 'milking' of the gland and a swab should be taken for culture and sensitivity testing. Treatment is antibiotics, IV if severe.
  - *Viral*: mumps is relatively rare following widespread vaccination in the UK but can present as bilateral (and rarely unilateral) swelling of the parotid glands as well as malaise, myalgia, headache. HIV, cytomegalovirus (CMV), and Epstein–Barr virus (EBV) can also cause sialadenitis.
- Obstruction:
  - *Sialoliths*: salivary gland stones are most commonly found in the submandibular ducts. Patients often report 'meal-time syndrome' where their swelling and symptoms occur around mealtimes as saliva production increases and then settle afterwards. They can sometimes be seen on a plain film occlusal radiograph or ultrasound scans.
  - *Mucoceles/mucous retention cysts*: occur on the labial mucosa or floor of mouth. Painless and often caused by trauma. When in the floor of mouth referred to as a 'ranula'. Mucoceles can often be excised under LA, ranulas may need removal under GA with the associated gland.

Paediatric patients

- Management of OMFS injuries in paediatric patients can be challenging and will vary from patient to patient based on their ability to cooperate.
- Injuries to the teeth and face are common in children, but jaw/facial fractures are not. Most injuries in children will have an obvious and innocent explanation, but always be suspicious of non-accidental

injury with any child whose injury does not fit the story being given. Be aware of *red flags* with changing/inconsistent stories, or the child's demeanour/behaviour. Keep up to date with safeguarding training and get to know referral pathways individual to the unit you are working in.

- Dental trauma is managed according to guidelines (➜ Dental trauma) which differ according to whether deciduous or permanent teeth are involved and their level of root development.
- Avulsed primary teeth should never be re-implanted.
- Parents of children with intrusion, concussion, or subluxation injuries should be warned of the possible consequences to the permanent successor tooth including abnormal crown morphology, delayed eruption, or dilaceration of the root.
- Dental infections can spread quickly in children and so swellings should be managed cautiously. Often admission for IV antibiotics and extraction under GA ± incision and drainage is required.
- One other injury to look out for is a 'white-eyed blowout' (➜ White-eyed blowout'). This is an injury which needs treating urgently or can lead to major complications for the child.
- Suturing of lacerations in children can be possible under LA if the child is cooperative. Often behaviour management techniques and the use of topical anaesthetics (e.g. lidocaine, adrenaline, and tetracaine (LAT) gel) can help significantly. Wherever possible use resorbable sutures, especially if closing lacerations under GA, to prevent the need for further distress in the future with suture removal.

Transferring patients

- Depending on the local set-up, transfer of patients from an outside hospital into your unit may be a regular or an infrequent event. Regardless, it is of the upmost importance that it is done safely and only when appropriate.
- Often patients will need to be transferred by ambulance and the referring team will arrange this.
- Trauma patients with possible head injury should only be transferred once cleared as safe to do so. Any patient under neurological observations ('neuro obs') should be left where they are until cleared.
- Patients with swellings must be deemed to have a stable airway before they are transferred between hospitals and in severe cases anaesthetic review may be required prior to agreeing to move the patient.
- Patients who are medically unwell, but have reasonably minor maxillofacial injuries, are often better managed without transferring them. An example of this in the hospital could be an elderly patient who has fallen out of their hospital bed and fractured their zygoma. Rather than move them to the OMFS ward, it can be arranged for a member of the OMFS team to visit the patient and assess them on their medical ward. The patient's safety and best interests are always paramount and must be fully considered before deciding to transfer them.
- Transfer of patients will need to be agreed with a senior first—check your department's local protocol.

Senior advice/approval

- As a Dental Core trainee you will always have a senior colleague in the form of a registrar or consultant to turn to for advice. You should never decide to carry out a treatment you are unsure of.
- It is expected when you first start that you are inexperienced and will be asking a lot of questions. As you gain experience, you will be trusted to carry out more tasks and make more decisions independently.
- Some decisions, however, will always be 'above your pay grade' and must be run past a senior colleague. You should never feel pressured into making a decision or carrying out a procedure you are not comfortable with.

Surgical skills

Venous access/venepuncture skills

- Depending on local arrangements, it may be your responsibility to cannulate and take bloods on patients who you are admitting. Both taking blood and cannulating are practical skills that you can only really learn through experience and doing it on real patients. With practice, it becomes a routine part of your skillset and with most patients you will have no trouble.
- Some patients with poor venous access (e.g. high BMI, IV drug abuse) may prove difficult. A&E colleagues, phlebotomists, or anaesthetists can always be approached for help with difficult cases but will likely want to see that you have at least attempted it yourself first. There is a difference, however, between attempting to gain venous access and simply stabbing in the dark repeatedly and so for the patient's safety, know when to seek help.
- Cannulas come in different colours based on the size of the lumen in the cannula tip. Larger cannulas may be needed in situations where high flow rate into the veins is needed (e.g. major trauma, shock); however, most of the time pink cannulas (20 gauge) will be sufficient and are more straightforward to insert.
- Bloods can be taken from a cannula as soon as it has been inserted prior to it being flushed through with saline and can save the patient having to be stabbed twice. *Once a canula has been flushed through, blood should not be taken from it.*
- If taking blood from a patient who already has a cannula in place, or who does not need cannulation, then either a vacutainer needle and holder or butterfly system can be used.
- Note: if the patient has an infusion underway (e.g. saline, medication) through a cannula, do not take bloods from that arm as it can interfere with results.
- When ordering bloods, the printed label should tell you which coloured blood bottle needs to be filled. These are vacuum sealed and when pressed onto the bell housing on the vacutainer will fill with the required amount of blood before stopping. This can be double checked by ensuring the blood level in the vial reaches the marked black line on the vial label.

Suturing

Suture techniques

Suture technique is something that really must be taught in a practical tutorial and so is outside of the scope of this handbook. You should, however, be aware of the various suturing techniques and situations in which they can become useful:

- *Simple interrupted*: most commonly employed suture for intraoral and extraoral wounds. Easy and effective.
- *Continuous*: can be more time efficient for closing longer linear wounds, but more technique sensitive and if part of suture is cut or pulled through, the whole thing can come loose.
- *Horizontal mattress*: good for areas where compression is needed (i.e. around a socket), can be modified to include cross-over X-pattern.
- *Vertical mattress*: most often used to take the tension out of a wound or to provide strength when closing.

- *Deep sutures*: buried beneath the skin surface with knot at the deeper aspect. Used to take tension out of a wound before superficial closure, resorbable suture must be used.

Suture materials
- Choice of suture material and size will vary depending on the task in hand.
- You should understand the difference between the materials you have available to you and experiment with them as the handling characteristics can vary significantly.
- Understand the difference between the needle types:
    - *Round bodied*: circular cross section, no cutting surface, only sharp tip. Dilates tissue rather than cuts and so less likely to 'pull through' tissues, although can be harder to pass through in some situations. Good for friable tissues.
    - *Taper pointed*: as for round bodied, but with sharper point to make cutting through tissues easier.
    - *Cutting*: has cutting surface on the upper aspect of the needle curve. Easier to pass through tissues, but 'surface seeking' and higher risk of pulling through or 'cheese-wiring'.
    - *Reverse cutting*: cutting surface on the back of the needle curve. Still passes through tissues well but 'depth seeking' and so much less likely to pull through. A good choice for most situations, especially for inexperienced clinicians.

Tips
- Good light and set-up of instruments essential before starting. Try to find a quiet side room to take the patient into so you can take your time and concentrate.
- Don't be afraid to ask for an assistant if you need it. A&E nurses or clinical support workers may be free to come and help.
- Most wounds should be closed within 24 hours.
- If a wound has partially closed, once anaesthetized, open it up to explore, wash out, and ensure no foreign body present before closing.
- Consider regional blocks with LA for larger wounds (e.g. supraorbital block).
- Always oppose corners or landmarks of a laceration first to ensure edges sutured in correct position (e.g. vermilion border of lip).
- Deep wounds should be closed in tissue layers where possible (e.g. for scalp lacerations, close pericranium, aponeurosis, connective tissue, and skin).
- Situations where there has been tissue loss can be very difficult to manage and will likely need a senior review.
- For ear or nose lacerations, never leave exposed cartilage.
- 3-0 or 4-0 sutures work well intraorally.
- 5-0 sutures are good for most skin work, however 6-0 is better for finer suturing (e.g. around eyes).
- Vicryl Rapide® sutures are resorbable and work well in most situations intraorally and on skin and means the patient doesn't have to return for removal (particular benefit in children with low compliance); however, consultants in some units may have other preferences and choose non-braided sutures for skin work.
- Suture removal (if needed) can often be arranged at their local GMP's practice or in the community to save the patient a trip back to hospital.

Theatre

Clerking patients for theatre

- When you are on theatre duties, it will be one of your responsibilities to 'clerk' the patients prior to the list beginning. The purpose of clerking is to carry out all necessary checks prior to the patient being taken to theatre to ensure that the operation planned is still appropriate and that it is safe to proceed.
- When clerking patients, the following checklist should help:
  - Confirm patient's name and DOB.
  - What operation do they believe they are having done? Does this match what is written on the theatre list and consent form?
  - Does the patient have any new complaints or has anything changed in relation to the intended operative site?
  - Check the operative site is as previously documented (e.g. is the tooth that is planned to be extracted still present?).
  - Are any new investigations or radiographs required?
  - Check MH and if changed record the details.
  - Check consent form is present, rediscuss it with patient and sign confirmation section (➔ Consent).
  - Has VTE assessment been completed and appropriate prophylaxis prescribed (➔ VTE assessment)?
  - Has the operative site been marked (skin marker indicating site and side)?
  - Is the patient starved?
  - Does the patient require a bed for an overnight stay, and if so, is one booked and available?
  - If a day case, does the patient have an escort and transport home arranged?
  - Any final questions from the patient?

Document the above checks briefly in the notes. If there are any issues discovered that may change the planned operation or mean the operation can't go ahead, it is important you inform your senior colleagues as soon as possible.

Consent

- Consent is more than just a piece of paper; it is a process that clinicians go through with patients to ensure that they are fully informed before agreeing to undergo a procedure.
- Consent, wherever possible, should be a two-stage process, that is, the initial discussion and signing of the form is done at assessment when surgery is planned (in clinic) and it is rediscussed and confirmed on the day of surgery once the patient has had time to digest information and reflect.
- We are now governed by Montgomery consent—patients should be told what any reasonable person in their situation would expect to know. This includes the advantages and disadvantages of the planned operation, as well as any alternatives that are available and all material risks that are involved.

- A clear and honest conversation with a patient, ensuring they fully understand what is being discussed and giving them the opportunity to ask questions, will make for fully informed and valid consent. Simply asking them to sign a form does not.
- You should not consent a patient for a procedure that you yourself cannot carry out, unless you have received training on how to consent a patient for that particular procedure.
- There are four types of consent forms within the hospital:
    - Consent form 1: patients with capacity undergoing treatment under LA, sedation, or GA.
    - Consent form 2: consent for paediatric patients.
    - Consent form 3: consent for procedures under LA only.
    - Consent form 4: for patients who lack capacity.
- You should be aware of the law and principles involved in assessing and managing patients who may lack capacity. You should be familiar with and apply the legislation and guidance, including the Mental Capacity Act 2005 (MCA) and the Children's Acts 1989 and 2004. The MCA has five underpinning principles (**⇄** Mental Capacity Act 2005 (MCA)).
- You should become comfortable in assessing a patient's capacity to consent. The *CURE* test can be helpful, the patient must be able to do all the following in order to be deemed to have capacity:
    - *Communicate*: can the person communicate their decision to you (even if not verbally)?
    - *Understand*: can the person understand the information you have given to them?
    - *Retain*: can the patient retain the information in order to make the decision?
    - *Evaluate*: can the patient reflect on the information to make the decision effectively?

Scrubbing and gowns

- When operating in theatre, we attempt to keep the surgical environment as sterile as possible. Patients are therefore draped with sterile towels and the operating team and scrub nurse will all wear hats, masks, surgical gloves, and sterile gowns.
- 'Scrubbing' or 'gowning up' for theatre is done in a regimented way which ensures that below the elbows is sufficiently clean, and that the gown and gloves are put on without touching anything non-sterile. An assistant will help in tying the back of the gowns.
- You should ask a member of theatre staff or a senior colleague to demonstrate the proper scrubbing technique.

WHO checklist

- The WHO preoperative checklist is read out in every theatre prior to an operation being started. The purpose of this is to try to prevent wrong-site surgery.
- Among other things, the patient's identity, planned operation, consent form, marking of the site, instruments, and anaesthetic elements are checked with all theatre staff present. Once all have confirmed they are in agreement, the operation can begin.

- Many units now also use modified WHO checklists during their minor oral surgery lists under LA as well.

Assisting during GA lists

- You will be required to assist senior colleagues operating. This will often involve aspirating, retracting, or holding things in place to enable them to carry out the procedure.
- Assisting in theatre is often a Dental Core trainee's favourite part of the job. You will get to see a vast mix of operations close up and appreciate the anatomy and complexity of OMFS first hand.
- While it can be exhilarating it can also be exhausting. Particularly in major cancer operations you can be stood for many hours without a break. These tips should help out:
  - Eat a good meal before theatre, if you are in theatre all day, have lunch already planned as you don't know when you'll get a lunch break or how long it will last.
  - Take breaks when you get the opportunity, don't try to be a hero.
  - If you tire while retracting, tell the consultant before you slip or make a mistake through fatigue. Simply taking a few seconds' break and repositioning yourself can make all the difference.
  - If you start to feel faint, say something straight away. Do not try to fight it or ignore it as before you know if you'll be being picked up off the theatre floor which is much more embarrassing than asking if you can take a 5-minute break to sit down.
- Depending on the procedure being undertaken, your competence, and previous experience, you may be given the opportunity to do parts of an operation yourself. Make the most of these opportunities as they will not only give you a sense of accomplishment but are a chance for you to demonstrate your abilities to your seniors.

Post-theatre ward round

- Many consultants will wish to go and visit their patients after the operating list has finished to check on their condition and handover any special instructions to the nurses in charge of their care.
- You should handover patient-specific instructions to the on-call Dental Core trainee after the post-theatre ward round to inform them:
  - who is on the ward
  - what operation they have undergone
  - any specific concerns that there might be or jobs that need doing.

Discharging patients

Theatre patients who are not admitted to the ward but are treated as day cases will still need discharge paperwork completing. This includes discharge letters and TTOs (➔ Discharging patients).

Outpatient operating

- In many units, the majority of operating is carried out in the outpatient department under LA or with sedation.
- Sometimes you will be allocated to these lists as an assistant to help and learn from a senior carrying out more complex surgery. Other times Dental Core trainees have their own minor oral surgery lists in which

you will be given the opportunity to do procedures on your own with assistance from either a dental nurse or a colleague.

- The kinds of procedures likely to be undertaken on a Dental Core trainee's list include:
  - simple extractions
  - surgical removal of roots/teeth
  - straightforward wisdom teeth removal
  - incisional/excisional biopsies of benign lesions.
- A Dental Core trainee's confidence and competence in these procedures will vary based on your previous experience. As with anything, if you do not feel confident in carrying out a procedure that is listed for you to complete, always ask a senior for help or guidance. As you progress you may have the opportunity to move on to more complex procedures.
- There is less of a need for formal clerking as there is for GA theatre, however you should still confirm the patient's identity, MH changes, planned operation, and consent.

Ordering investigations or histopathology

- Always ensure investigations or histopathology requests are ordered immediately to make sure they do not get forgotten.
- When ordering, there will always be an opportunity to provide clinical information. This is vitally important in allowing the person receiving the sample, or reporting on the scan, to contextualize what they have in front of them (Box 6.2 and Box 6.3).

Box 6.2 Example of a poor histopathology request
Specimen description: biopsy tongue.
Clinical information: ulcer left tongue.
Urgent: yes.

Box 6.3 Example of a good histopathology request
Specimen description: incisional biopsy of ulcerated lesion left lateral tongue. ?Malignancy.
Clinical information: painful non-healing ulcer left tongue. Present 5 weeks. Smoker 30/day, excess alcohol intake. Suspected oral cancer.
Urgent: yes

Introduction to outpatient clinics

- How much responsibility you will be given as a Dental Core trainee during outpatient clinics may vary between units, but in most hospitals, you will be expected to see patients on clinics.
- Clinics may be solely new patient referrals, review appointments, or a combination of the two.

Assessing patients in outpatient clinics

- For new patients you will be expected to read the referral, take a history, assess the patient, and order any further tests that may be required such as plain film radiographs, blood tests, and so on.
- If you are able, come up with a diagnosis and treatment plan before presenting the case to a senior colleague to confirm the plan. As you settle into units you will likely be able to treatment plan and list patients for straightforward procedures without seeking prior approval.
- When taking a history, be systematic and targeted. You need to ensure you don't miss things, but at the same time don't spend time on things that are not relevant to the clinical condition the patient has been referred for.
- Your notes should be clear and comprehensive but concise. A useful template when writing up your notes for new patient assessments is provided in Box 6.4 but get comfortable using your own.

> **Box 6.4 Example of an outpatient note**
> **Date and clinic:**
> **Ref by:** [e.g. GDP for surgical removal LL8.]
> **CO:** [Complaining of—patient's complaint in their words.]
> **HPC:** [History of the patient's complaint.]
> **MH:** [MH including medications and allergies.]
> **SH:** [Smoking, alcohol, work circumstances, living conditions, etc.]
> **OE:** [On examination.]
> - **E/O** [Extraoral—TMJs, lymph nodes, muscles of mastication, CNs? Facial symmetry, glands, etc.]
> - **I/O** [Intraoral—soft tissue and hard tissue examination.]
> **Radiographs/investigations:** [Results/reports of investigations carried out.]
> **Diagnosis:** [Provisional or definitive.]
> **Discussion:** [Options, pros, cons, and risks discussed with patient.]
> **Treatment plan:** [Plan agreed with patient.]
> **Review arrangements or discharge?:**
> **Sign, print name, and GDC No.:**

- Review patients will either be attending for postoperative checks following a procedure, results of a biopsy, or to monitor progression of a condition. Before seeing the patient make sure you read the notes and understand the patient's history and any recent results that might be available.

- *Tip*: clinic letters can often be a good summary to read through and get up to speed with a case quickly (and are often more legible than written clinic notes!).
- Clinics can often be very busy and can easily run behind if patients take longer than expected. Being organized and time efficient will help things keep to time. If (and when) you do run late, always apologize to patients and make sure they don't feel rushed when they come in for their consultation.
- Never feel pressured to make any decisions you are not comfortable with. You are seeing patients in the clinic on behalf of the consultant in charge of their care, and it is they who ultimately have responsibility for them and will make the decisions regarding their treatment.

Further tests
- Patients with more complex problems may be sent for further testing from the clinic to be reviewed later with the results.
- These may include more complex imaging such as:
  - MRI scans: good for soft tissue imaging (e.g. oral cancers)
  - CT scans: better images of hard tissues (e.g. bones)
  - CBCT scans: different from medical CT and lower dose of radiation. Often used for impacted teeth or jaw lesions (e.g. cysts)
  - ultrasound scans: no radiation and non-invasive (unless ultrasound-guided needle aspiration of a lesion), often used for investigation of salivary gland or neck swellings as first line
  - sialography: cannula inserted into salivary duct and radiopaque dye injected before plain film radiographs taken to show gland and duct.
- CT and MRI can sometimes require patients to be injected with contrast medium for which they need to have healthy functioning kidneys. Some radiology departments will require the patient to have blood tests before the scan to provide up to date estimated glomerular filtration rate figures and you may need to arrange this.
- Blood tests may sometimes be ordered either to check for causes of certain conditions (e.g. oral medicine-related lesions) or prior to listing a patient (e.g. coagulation screen prior to surgery).

Dictation/letter writing
- All patients seen on clinic, whether new or review, will require a letter written to update the referring clinician and anybody else who may need to be kept in the loop (e.g. GMP if referred by GDP) as to their progress. You may be asked to dictate letters for the patients that you see.
- As with your clinical notes, keep your letters clear and concise.

Introduction to emergencies

- Fortunately, genuine emergencies in OMFS are few in number. There are situations, however, that you must be aware of, and if faced with, be prepared to act to prevent serious harm or death to patients.
- In the event of any emergency situation, you should always follow the Royal College of Surgeons Advanced Trauma Life Support® (ATLS®) guidelines when initially assessing the patient with a primary survey (ABCDE):
  - **A**irway: clear or obstructed? Can the patient speak? Is there a foreign body, raised floor of mouth/tongue, bleeding, etc.?
  - **B**reathing: is the patient breathing? Any stridor or wheeze? Respiratory rate and O_2 sats?
  - **C**irculation: heart rate, blood pressure, central/peripheral perfusion, signs of bleeding/haemorrhage?
  - **D**isability: Glasgow Coma Scale (GCS) or AVPU? Pupil response?
  - **E**xposure: consider removing/loosening clothing to allow further examination of neck/elsewhere on body if relevant.

Airway loss

- Significant swelling causing occlusion of the airway can result in a total or partial loss of the patient's ability to breathe. This could be as a result of a spreading dental abscess, a postoperative bleed into the neck, or postoperative swelling.
- The airway can also be lost in situations such as a blocked or displaced tracheostomy or facial fractures where the base of tongue collapses posteriorly (e.g. unfavourable bilateral mandibular body fractures).
- In almost all cases with accurate and timely assessment, diagnosis, and initiation of treatment, possible causes of airway loss can and should be addressed before the situation becomes an emergency.
- In cases of severe dental abscess or neck swellings, early anaesthetic review to secure an airway, if necessary, can be the priority over dealing with the swelling itself.
- Airways can be secured electively either via intubation or a tracheostomy. Emergency cricothyroidotomies are rare but may need to be employed in some circumstances. There will most likely be somebody more senior than you who can be called upon to perform an emergency cricothyroidotomy, but you should be familiar with the procedure just in case.

Ludwig's angina

Presentation

- A true Ludwig's angina is a bilateral infection of the submandibular and sublingual spaces. It originates as a floor of mouth infection (often of dental origin) which rapidly spreads as a cellulitis into the submandibular spaces.
- There is often no abscess formation but instead a 'woody' firm bilateral cellulitis of the submandibular tissues which can raise the tongue and restrict/occlude the airway.

Management
- Primary survey (ABCDE).
- Your senior should be informed immediately as should the on-call consultant anaesthetist as securing the airway is of paramount importance.
- A CT scan may be needed to determine if there is a collection present which requires surgical drainage.
- In cases where a collection is present, surgical incision and drainage is undertaken as a matter of urgency. If the swelling is purely cellulitis, then medical management only is undertaken in the form of IV antibiotics.
- A surgical airway may be required (tracheostomy) and the patient may be admitted to the intensive therapy unit.

Retrobulbar haemorrhage

This emergency is caused by bleeding behind the eye and can lead to patients going blind. It is thankfully rare but should be looked out for in patients who have received trauma to the orbit or surrounding structures, or who have been operated on in this area (e.g. orbital floor repair).

Signs (5 Ps)
- **P**ain/pressure—behind eye.
- **P**roptosis.
- **P**erception—deterioration in vision (loss of colour/visual acuity).
- **P**aralysis—ophthalmoplegia (inability to move the eye).
- Di**P**lopia.

Management
- Call your senior immediately.
- Surgical lateral canthotomy to release the pressure as soon as possible.
- ± Medical treatment with IV mannitol (20 mL of 20%), hydrocortisone (100 mg), and acetazolamide (500 mg).

White-eyed blowout

Presentation
Can occur in paediatric orbital floor fractures. Due to elasticity of bones, the orbital floor breaks, the inferior contents of the orbit herniate through the fracture, and the 'trapdoor' bone fracture springs back up to entrap the tissues.

Signs
- Loss of upward eye movement on affected side.
- No subconjunctival haemorrhage (hence white eyed).
- Possible oculo-cardiac reflex (bradycardia, hypotension, nausea, and vomiting).

Management
- Urgent surgical release of trapped tissues to prevent necrosis and long-term problems.
- Orbital floor repair.

Sepsis

Sepsis is a life-threatening complication of infection and can be triggered by OMFS infections (including dental abscesses). It must be detected and managed early to give patients the best chance of recovery and survival.

Signs
- Temperature <36°C or >38.3°C.
- Tachycardia (>130 bpm).
- Hypotension (systolic ≤90 mmHg).
- Hypoxic (O_2 sats <92% on room air).
- Confusion/decreased responsiveness.

Management
'Sepsis Six' (BUFALO):
- **B**lood cultures.
- **U**rine output (measure).
- **F**luid challenge.
- **A**ntibiotics (IV).
- **L**actate (measure).
- **O**$_2$ to keep sats >94%.

If you suspect a patient has sepsis, you should initiate a call to the hospital medical emergency team (MET call).

Facial aesthetic complications

Introduction

- Facial aesthetics, medical aesthetics, and non-surgical aesthetic treatments are terms used to describe a wide range of procedures designed to improve a patient's appearance.
- These may be to reduce the signs of ageing, by smoothing lines and wrinkles, restoring and providing support to soft tissues of face, enhancing facial features, stimulating collagen production, or treating the deeper layers of the skin to improve hyperpigmentation, scarring, and surface texture.
- At the time of writing, facial aesthetics in the UK is almost entirely unregulated, meaning that it is legal for non-medical or non-dentally trained practitioners to perform treatments.
- Non-medical or non-dentally trained practitioners have no regulatory body (e.g. General Medical Council, GDC, Nursing and Midwifery Council, or General Pharmaceutical Council) which recognizes medical aesthetics as part of registrant scope of practice and no professional obligation to use regulated pharmacies, provide emergency care, or have proper indemnity/insurance in place. The issue this presents is that there are larger numbers of procedures being undertaken without a safety net of patient aftercare, with practitioners not being contactable or unable to manage a complication or emergency.
- Complications can and will happen to all practitioners, regardless of training, experience, or location. However, patients are less likely to attend hospital emergency departments and walk-in-centres after being treated by clinicians with more robust safety standards in place (appropriate training, CPD, professional regulation, safe techniques, informed consent and working within the medical model, use of regulated pharmacies supplying CE-marked products and equipment, out-of-hours aftercare, complication management training, and having an appropriate emergency kit).
- Unsatisfactory results from non-surgical aesthetics are vastly different to complications and in the worst case, emergencies resulting from treatments. In all instances of unsatisfactory aesthetic results, patients should be encouraged to return to their original practitioner to manage or seek independent advice from alternative clinicians (see ➔ Further reading for help with signposting patients to appropriate providers).
- Often, other specialities would be contacted before OMFS to assess patients presenting with facial aesthetics complications.
- However, if you are asked to see a patient presenting with complications requiring emergency management arising from non-surgical aesthetic treatments, this may well be an area less comprehensively covered by dental undergraduate and postgraduate training pathways.
- In all cases, upward consultation with your senior (after having taken a full history) is important and timely onward referral to relevant specialities as needed (including ophthalmology, ENT, or plastic surgery).

- In all cases, in addition to a standard presenting, medical, and dental history, an aesthetically relevant history should be taken ideally including the following:
  - Date and time of initial treatment.
  - Type of treatment (e.g. hyaluronic acid (HA) filler, botulinum toxin, etc.).
  - Name of product(s) used.
  - Areas of face and neck treated (e.g. cheek, jawline, lips, nose).
  - Copies of any treatment documentation the patient may have brought.
  - Name of original practitioner and clinic (to contact if the patient doesn't have the above information). It is also worth recording if the patient states they have contacted/tried to contact the original clinician.
  - Onset of problem (number of hours/days/weeks since treatment).
  - Duration of complaint and changing nature of problem.
  - Any photographs of how the presenting complaint started for useful comparison (worsening size, colour change, swelling, etc.).
  - Any problems noticed during treatment itself (sudden pain, numbness, etc.).
  - Has any remedial/emergency treatment already been tried?
  - Document which structures have been clinically affected. This can include visual field checks, eye movements, and assessment of muscles affected.
  - Always document that you have advised the patient not to undertake any activity carrying increased risk due to the symptoms (e.g. no driving or operating heavy machinery if eyesight is impaired). This protects you, the patient, and the public.
  - Always take a full MH as patients, on occasion, can associate a presenting symptom (e.g. drooping eye or cheek) with having treatment but consideration of the timeframe, onset, and ensuring there is no underlying medical cause is also important.
  - History of allergies (to wasp and bee stings), cold sores (HSV), autoimmune conditions, and neurological history are all important.

Botulinum toxin A

Background

- Botulinum toxin, often referred to as Botox®, is a naturally occurring protein produced by the bacterium *Clostridium botulinum*.
- The toxin blocks the transition of chemical messages sent from the nerve to cause the muscle to contract. Without these messages, the muscle stays in a resting state until the 'messengers' recover.
- This recovery takes ~ 8–12 weeks on average. Licensed brands of botulinum toxin A include, Botox®, Azzalure®, and Bocouture®.

Potential complications

- Treatments are generally very safe with emergency/serious adverse events being incredibly rare.
- The overall risk of allergy to botulinum toxin is very low and would usually present within the first 48 hours.

- Common side effects include bruising, swelling at injection sites, redness at injection sites, flu-like symptoms, and a headache or a sensation of 'tightness' or 'heaviness'. These are usually very transient lasting on average 24–48 hours.
- Adverse effects including asymmetry of expression and drooping of the brow or eyelid ('ptosis') usually occur within a few days of treatment and are expected to be temporary, usually resolving spontaneously within weeks. These can be distressing for patients but have minimal risk of longer-lasting damage.

Management
- Eyelid ptosis:
  - Usually lasts 4–6 weeks and will lessen in severity over this time.
  - You can assess baseline severity and recovery of eyelid ptosis by measuring the margin reflex distance by using a pen torch and measuring the distance in millimetres to the eyelid margin from the corneal light reflex. This is usually >2.5 mm in health.
  - Management and monitoring recovery of a severe ptosis would be in the scope of ophthalmology/orthoptics and onward referral if deemed necessary is prudent.
  - Initial management if the eyelid ptosis, if severe, includes prescription of apraclonidine 0.5% eyedrops or Iopidin® eyedrops (off-label) which can open the eyelid 1–2 mm for up to 4 hours which can be really helpful for patients.
  - Eyedrops are supportive, not curative, but eyelid ptosis will recover fully with time.
  - You do not have to prescribe eyedrops as they have their own side effects to be aware of.
- Lip, cheek, and brow ptosis:
  - No emergency management although some brow positions can be improved by further botulinum toxin injections to combat adverse muscle pull.
  - Ptosis usually lasts 4–6 weeks and will lessen in severity over this time.
- Periorbital swelling:
  - Can be due to trauma but more commonly due to reduced lymphatic drainage due to the relaxation of the orbicularis oculi muscle (to reduce the appearance of lines around the eyes) in predisposed patients.
  - This tends to present between 7 and 14 days when muscles start to relax and fluid builds up and usually resolves quickly after this.
  - Advising patients to massage/compress the area in the morning and whenever swelling occurs and to try and use any muscles using facial expressions as much as possible to encourage drainage will speed recovery and lessen symptoms.

Thread lift procedures
Background
- Thread lift procedures use dissolvable sutures to tighten and lift the skin across any part of the face, including the forehead, cheeks, jowls, jawline, and neck.

- They are considered minimally invasive and have some advantages over full face lift surgery.
- The main three types of sutures are made from polydioxanone (PDO), polylactic acid (PLA), or polycaprolactone (PCA). Both PLA and PDO have collagen-stimulating properties and dissolve over time leaving tighter remodelled/repaired tissue instead as they often produce type 3 collagen tissue behind to prolong the result.
- The threads are either smooth ('monos') for improving skin texture or consist of barbs, cogs, anchors, or screws to reposition the tissue.
- Thread lifts are a regulated procedure. Clinics where thread lifts are performed by nurses, doctors, and dentists are required by law, to be registered with the Care Quality Commission.
- A typical treatment ranges from placing from a single thread per side but can involve 50 threads or more to treat the full face and neck.

Potential complications

Known complications include:

- Pain
- Thread extrusion/visible sutures (especially in people with thin skin)
- Minor bruising
- Infection
- Snapping of threads
- Haematoma
- Swelling
- Migration
- Bulging
- Dimpling
- Hair loss
- Salivary gland injury
- Sensory abnormality
- Foreign body reactions
- Facial asymmetry.

Management

- Upward consultation with a senior colleague is advised as management of thread lifts is likely to be out of a Dental Core trainee's scope of practice.
- Dependant on the individual training and experience of thread lifts within your OMFS team, onward referral (with full history and management thus far) to the plastic surgery team is the most recommended course of action.
- Overall, it is more likely that the plastic surgery team have greater experience, exposure, and training in thread lifting and are best placed to manage emergency complications arising from them.
- Further aesthetic treatments to correct unaesthetic outcomes or in some cases, removal of threads, are sometimes indicated.
- It would always be appropriate to initially manage signs and symptoms of pain and infection with analgesia and antibiotics (if indicated) until specialist input is sought.

Hyaluronic acid dermal fillers

- Dermal fillers are soft, gel-like substances that are injected under the skin.
- They can address several common concerns including smoothing of deep under-eye circles, lifting of cheekbones, restoring volume of the lips, smoothing of facial lines/folds, and enhancement of features (e.g. non-surgical rhinoplasty and jawline contouring).
- Dermal fillers can be composed of a variety of naturally occurring or synthetic substances.
- The most common component in dermal fillers in recent times is HA. HA is a naturally occurring complex sugar in your body that helps to provide volume, structure, elasticity, and moisture to your skin.
- As you age you lose your natural HA. The bones, muscles, and fat pads also change, affecting your facial shape. This leads to the signs of ageing as seen by facial volume loss, reduced skin elasticity, folds, and wrinkles. HA fillers can last from 6 months to 18+ months before being gradually absorbed by the body.
- Common HA filler brands include Juvederm®, Teosyal/Teoxane®, Restylane®, Belotero®, Revolax®, and EPTQ® but there are many available on the market.
- HA fillers are the most commonly used fillers as they can be 'reversed' in emergency situations and electively if needed.
- Hyalase® (hyaluronidase) is a soluble protein enzyme that is typically used to break down the HA found in dermal filler.
- Hyalase® is reconstituted form a 1500 IU vial using bacteriostatic saline in varying strengths dependant on its use in emergency or elective reversal situations.
- The injectable solution works by breaking up the bonds that hold the HA molecules together and encourages the body to reabsorb those molecules in a natural process that it knows how to do on its own.
- It is a prescription only medication and not all hospitals/clinics hold regular stock.
- Patients should be fully consented before the use of Hyalase® as administration carries its own risks and considerations; however, in an emergency situation most are outweighed by the risk of the HA filler requiring reversal.
- There are some patients who have an increased risk of allergy to Hyalase® (those having allergies to wasp and bee stings).

Alternative dermal fillers

- There are other types of dermal filler available including:
  - calcium hydroxyapatite (CaHA)
  - poly-L-lactic acid (PLLA)
  - polymethyl methacrylate
  - autologous fat transfer (fat transplanted from another part of your body).
- CaHA:
  - A mineral-like compound naturally found in human bones.
  - It has been used in dentistry and reconstructive plastics surgery for years with a long track record of safety.

- PLLA:
  - A synthetic filler that helps to stimulate collagen production.
  - This filler is different from other fillers because its results are gradual.
  - Restoration of soft tissue volume occurs over several months as it stimulates the body to produce collagen.
- Polymethyl methacrylate:
  - A semi-permanent filler.
  - While it is more durable compared to other more readily biodegradable fillers, it has potential complications such as forming lumps and being visible under the skin.
- All of these are less commonly used than HA, but an awareness of their use is important as they are not reversible and complication management can often mean surgical involvement.
- Hyaluronidase is ineffective on non-HA-based fillers like Sculptra® (PLLA) and Radiesse® (CaHA).

Potential complications of HA dermal fillers
- Known complications of HA fillers:
  - Ophthalmic emergency: visual disturbance and risk of blindness.
  - Vascular occlusion: causing soft tissue damage and necrosis.
  - Inflammatory lesions (infection, delayed-onset nodules, allergy, and hypersensitivity reactions).
  - Bacterial infection.
  - Nerve injury.
  - Haematoma formation.
  - Salivary gland injury.
  - Lumps of filler or fluid (non-inflammatory lesions).
- There are other emergencies (e.g. stroke that can occur at the time of dermal filler injection); however, these would be directly referred to emergency departments and the stroke team.
- There are a number of organizations that have regularly updated emergency protocols and flowcharts for the management of complications relating to dermal fillers (→ Further reading).
- These are usually membership based but have emergency contacts for members of the public to find clinicians trained to administer emergency treatment and offer guidance.
- The scope of this handbook is to assist Dental Core trainees with appropriate guidance, referral requirements, and awareness of clinical features rather than detailed clinical outlines to treat more advanced complications.

Management
- Generally, for all complications relating to dermal fillers, upward consultation with a senior colleague is advised as management of dermal fillers are likely to be out of a Dental Core trainee's scope of practice.
- Dependant on the individual training and experience of dermal fillers within your OMFS team, onward referral (with full history and management thus far) to the plastic surgery team is the most recommended course of action.
- Overall, it is more likely that the plastic surgery team have greater experience, exposure, and training in non-surgical aesthetics and are

best placed to manage emergency complications arising from them. It is important to ensure that whatever treatments you provide are within your scope of practice.

Ophthalmic emergency

- It would be incredibly rare for OMFS to be presented with primary visual disturbance resulting from dermal fillers as an emergency.
- These cases should be directed directly to ophthalmology/emergency eye departments. However, having an awareness of the causes and management is useful.
- Blindness from dermal filler injections is extremely rare but arguably the most significant complication.
- Blood supply to the eye could be affected if dermal filler enters or compresses any branches of the arterial supply including:
  - central retinal artery (primarily supplying blood to the retina)
  - supratrochlear artery
  - supraorbital artery
  - lacrimal artery
  - posterior ciliary arteries
  - ophthalmic artery itself.
- The ophthalmic venous network is via the superior and inferior ophthalmic veins and vorticose veins into the cavernous sinus and affecting this drainage can have an adverse effect on retinal function.
- The highest-risk injection sites associated with ophthalmic emergencies are glabellar (lower forehead/between eyebrows), nasal, nasolabial fold, forehead, temple, and the periocular area itself. The glabellar and the nasal regions have significantly higher risk.
- Symptoms of visual disturbance and blindness usually occur immediately/within minutes of injection and can come from a variety of aetiologies including:
  - complete vascular occlusion
  - emboli (where filler or clot breaks away and travels further up the vascular network)
  - vessel injury
  - compression injuries (from filler on the external wall of the vessel)
  - stroke.
- To save retinal blood supply, effective treatment is needed within 60–90 minutes (maximum).
- Logistically, it is unlikely from time of injection to effective treatment in a hospital setting that vision can be completely saved.
- Primary treatment would be with Hyalase® (hyaluronidase) by an appropriately trained clinician to dissolve the HA using several injection techniques.
- It takes 45–90 minutes to dissolve with Hyalase® even when a clinician has it to hand, so immediate treatment at the time of injury is the best chance a patient has of improved visual outcomes.
- Other methods can subsequently be used to increase intraocular pressure and reduce vessel resistance, reducing secondary chances of blood clot/emboli and moving emboli away from ocular system.
- It is possible to worsen the clinical situation with inappropriate treatment, therefore the key advice is to ensure direct and emergency ophthalmology input is organized if you were to be called about any such patient.

Vascular occlusion

- It would be unusual for OMFS to be presented with suspected vascular occlusion and skin necrosis resulting from dermal fillers as an emergency.
- These cases would usually be sent directly to plastic surgery or dermatology teams. However, the remit of head and neck teams and on-call arrangements nationwide means having an awareness of the causes and management is useful.
- Soft tissue necrosis occurs when dermal filler enters and blocks (or partially blocks) a blood vessel, reducing oxygen supply to cells and soft tissue.
- This will cause cell death, soft tissue death, and necrosis. Tissue necrosis over days leads to infection, scarring, and loss of the soft tissue itself.
- Reduced blood flow can occur by complete and direct intra-arterial blockage, embolus (where filler or clot breaks away and travels further up the vascular network), or compression on an artery, capillaries, or vein.
- Presenting symptoms (usually within minutes–hours of injection) of vascular occlusion include:
  - pain
  - change in skin colour/pallor (pale, dusky grey/purple)
  - skin mottling
  - swelling.
- After 24 hours, colour change can worsen and evolve with the development of darker tissue and small pustules appear on the surface of skin where necrosis and bacterial injection are occurring.
- At all stages, capillary refill time (CRT) will be reduced. CRT should be <2 seconds after firm pressure (for a minimum pressure of 5 seconds) returning the tissues to a pink colour. Presenting CRT should always be documented in your notes.
- Primary treatment would be with Hyalase® (using an emergency strength concentration) by an appropriately trained clinician to dissolve the HA filler in and around the injection site and wider area of vascular occlusion and branches of arterial supply.
- Additional measures include:
  - reducing chance of blood clots worsening the clinical picture by using aspirin (where MH allows)
  - reducing vessel resistance to blood flow including use of heat and nitrates
  - sildenafil (where MH allows)
  - reducing risk of secondary infection with antibiotics and increasing oxygen delivery (emergency onward referral for hyperbaric oxygen).
- Management needs to be quick and well organized to reduce scarring and volume of tissue loss.

Inflammatory lesions

Delayed onset nodules ± biofilm reactions, granulomas, microbial, allergy, and type IV hypersensitivity reactions:

- Active clinical monitoring in mild cases (or known cause, e.g. systemic viral infection).

- Dependent on suspected cause (where swelling is more significant or underlying infection is also suspected), in moderate–severe cases management may involve:
  - blood tests (erythrocyte sedimentation rate and C-reactive protein), biopsy, and swabs for histopathology
  - antihistamines
  - ± steroids
  - ± antibiotics
  - ± antifungals.
- Antibiotics are indicated where cardinal signs of infection are present.
- If secondary HSV (cold sores) are suspected, systemic and topical antivirals ± antibiotics (if secondary infection is present) should be offered.
- Always seek advice from senior colleagues before considering prescribing steroids as immunosuppression in any patient who is systemically unwell can be problematic.
- The Aesthetic Complications Expert (ACE) Group suggests antibiotics for 2 weeks, adding an additional antibiotic for another 2 weeks before using Hyalase® (hyaluronidase) to reverse or reduce lumps.
- Treatment with Hyalase® can be repeated every 2–4 weeks.
- Type I hypersensitivity reactions would have occurred and been managed at the time of injecting (would have occurred in minutes).

Bacterial infection

- Treat early as per your trust or department guidelines.
- If skin infection appears superficial and impetigo-like, a topical antibiotic (e.g. fusidic acid) is indicated.
- First line antibiotics often include flucloxacillin or clarithromycin (if allergic to penicillin).
- The ACE Group guidelines suggest if these are not effective, second-line medication includes adding penicillin, amoxicillin, or co-amoxiclav (or clindamycin if allergic to penicillin).
- If a patient presents with signs of severe systemic infection or sepsis, admission for inpatient management is indicated.
- Similarly, as with any other infection, fluctuant abscesses may need surgical incision and drainage alongside antibiotics.

Nerve injury

- Rule out more severe causes of facial weakness/paralysis and asymmetry such as stroke (using standard FAST assessment tool).
- Assess which nerves are affected using CN and facial function tests, think about timing/onset if considering concurrent Bell's palsy with viral aetiology.
- Treatments to consider include:
  - steroids
  - antiviral treatment
  - recovery exercises could be considered and referral to a specialist for rehabilitation.
- Actual nerve damage (neuropraxia and axonotmesis) cannot be treated with any success.
- Protective, symptomatic, and functional management of nerve deficit (e.g. avoidance of trauma, ophthalmic protection (eye patch, drops))

should be given along with reassurance that the areas should recover within months.
- Review is advised and referral to ophthalmology if ocular symptoms are significant.
- If pressure from the placement of dermal filler is suspected to be causing pressure/compression to a motor nerve, consideration must be given to treating with steroids to reduce inflammation or with Hyalase® to reduce direct pressure from the filler.

Haematoma
- Rarely needs active treatment.
- If haematoma is large ± symptomatic, it may be possible to aspirate blood from a haematoma after injecting with hyaluronidase but this is not often undertaken and rarely in an emergency setting and not without specialist/senior guidance.

Salivary gland injury
- Often presents as swelling over the angle of the jaw/neck and/or parotid gland with minimal pain and minimal bruising.
- Swelling can worsen around mealtimes and fluctuates during the day related to saliva leaking from traumatized gland fascia.
- There is minimal active management needed:
  - Advise against foods causing excessive saliva production.
  - And on occasion, a pressure dressing to reduce the risk of sialocoele formation and leakage of saliva into tissues.
- Review as the problem should resolve within a week.

Non-inflammatory lumps and bumps
- Massage.
- Saline injection into lump and massage.
- Mechanically extrude material if filler or reversal with Hyalase® (hyaluronidase).

Medical micro-needling, deep chemical skin peels, and medical-grade skin treatments
- Medical micro-needling and deep skin peels are used most often in clinical environments to improve skin quality, texture, and appearance.
- These are usually very safe but adverse outcomes which may present to secondary care include:
  - pain
  - swelling
  - redness beyond that expected
  - infection and skin breakdown (ulceration etc.).
- It would be unusual for OMFS to be contacted regarding a patient presenting with skin damage resulting from skin treatments as an emergency.
- These cases would usually be directed directly to plastic surgery or dermatology teams. However, the remit of head and neck teams and on-call arrangements nationwide means having an awareness of the causes and general wound management is useful.

Further reading

Aesthetic Complications Expert (ACE) Group: www.acegroup.online
British Association for Medical Aesthetic Complications (BMAC): ℅ www.bmac.co.uk
British Associations of Aesthetic Plastic Surgeons (BAAPS): ℅ www.baaps.org.uk
British Association of Dermatologists (BAD): ℅ www.bad.org.uk
British National Formulary: ℅ www.bnf.org
Complications in Medical Aesthetics Collaborative (CMAC): ℅ www.cmac.world
Dental Trauma Guide: ℅ www.dentaltraumaguide.org
National Tracheostomy Safety Project: ℅ www.tracheostomy.org.uk
Moore UJ (2011). *Principles of Oral and Maxillofacial Surgery* (6th ed). Wiley-Blackwell.
NICE (2013, updated 2017). Intravenous fluid therapy in adults in hospital. ℅ www.nice.org.uk/guidance/CG174
NICE (2016, updated 2017). Sepsis: recognition, diagnosis and early management. ℅ www.nice.org.uk/guidance/NG51
Save Face (register of appropriately trained clinicians): ℅ www.saveface.co.uk

Chapter 7

Oral medicine

Introduction to oral medicine

Definition

Oral medicine is a specialty within dentistry which involves the diagnosis and non-surgical management of chronic, recurrent, and medically related disorders of the oral and maxillofacial region. The scope of the specialty includes diagnosis and management of mucosal disease, salivary gland disease, and non-dental causes of orofacial pain.

Oral medicine services

The majority of oral medicine consultants are employed as NHS consultants or academics, the latter holding honorary consultant contracts. In some areas, access to oral medicine services is not readily available. In these situations, oral surgery and oral and maxillofacial units in peripheral hospitals may provide these services.

Education and training in oral medicine

Traditionally, entry to specialty training in oral medicine required dual qualification in dentistry and medicine. However, in 2010, the GDC approved a curriculum for oral medicine training, whereby a medical degree was no longer a prerequisite for entry into specialist training. The current training pathway is 5 years. However, this may be reduced in recognition of previous training or if the trainee has completed a medical degree. In order to be admitted to the specialist list trainees are required to complete specialist training, pass the intercollegiate specialty fellowship examination (ISFE) in oral medicine, which is normally undertaken during the last 6 months of training, and have obtained an outcome 6 in their final ARCP.

Entry into specialist training in oral medicine is very competitive and many applicants will have completed a Dental Core trainee placement in oral medicine or worked as a specialty doctor/dentist in oral medicine. In addition, many will be members of the British and Irish Society for Oral Medicine (BISOM) and will have presented at oral medicine conferences, have publications in peer-reviewed journals, and participated in audit/quality improvement and research projects.

Assessing the oral medicine patient

Setting the scene

Presenting complaint

History of presenting complaint

Assessing the oral medicine patient

- Often the history alone reveals the diagnosis and listening to the patient is an important step in this process: 'If you listen carefully to the patient, they will tell you the diagnosis' (Sir William Osler).
- A good history is one which explores the patient's ideas, concerns, and expectations. The following is a guide to assessing the oral medicine patient.

Setting the scene

- Ensure privacy.
- Read correspondence/review notes.
- Introduce yourself and determine how the patient may like to be addressed.
- Note the referrer details in case you may need to clarify something in the patient's history with them and for future correspondence.
- Observe ethnicity, occupation, and spoken language.
- The consultation should begin with a series of open-ended questions, then use closed questions to focus on key areas of the consultation.

Presenting complaint

- Although you may have a referral letter or a previous clinic letter, it is often good practice to start by asking the patient an open-ended question such as 'Why have you attended today?' This can help them feel involved and may identify hidden agendas or cues, for example, 'I am worried I may have oral cancer'.
- Additionally, some patients use this as an opportunity to express all their symptoms and concerns which can appear disjointed and irrelevant. Try not to interrupt the patient as this information may aid in the diagnosis and save you time later on.

History of presenting complaint

As a general guide the following information should be determined:
- Duration—when and how did the complaint start?
- Onset—sudden or gradual, can you recall what you were doing at the time?
- Sites affected—intraoral versus extraoral and associated symptoms.
- Precipitating, exacerbating, and relieving factors.
- If there were previous episodes, were any investigations undertaken, can they recall the diagnosis, and what treatments were initiated?
- Impact on quality of life?

A useful mnemonic what taking a pain history is SOCRATES:
- **S**ite.
- **O**nset.
- **C**haracter.
- **R**adiation.
- **A**ssociated symptoms and signs.
- **T**iming.
- **E**xacerbating/relieving factors.
- **S**everity usually quantified on a linear analogue scale ranging from 0 to 10 where 0 is no pain and 10 is the worst pain imaginable.

Increasingly, medical schools are using the mnemonic ICE to acquire an understanding of patients' understanding and expectations about their condition:
- **I**deas about their condition and what may be causing it.
- **C**oncerns about the condition.
- **E**xpectations about the condition and treatments.

Medical history

This should include the following:
- Details of any medical admissions/surgery.
- Recent or ongoing attendances with GMP/hospital consultant(s).
- A review of all systems with focused questions.
- Enquiries about allergies (food, drugs, animal, household).

Drug history

Enquire about current and past treatments. This section should include the following:
- Why was the drug indicated?
- Response to treatment.
- Are they undergoing regular monitoring because of the medication?
- Dosage and frequency.
- Are they compliant with the medication?
- Details of self-prescribed or herbal remedies.
- Use of illicit drugs.

Social history

Often poorly done but important in oral medicine. It is important to ask about:
- Marital status and health and well-being of family/friends
- Occupation
- Habits such as smoking (type and pack years) and alcohol consumption (type and average units per week)
- Recent travel if appropriate
- Diet.

Dental history

- Dental attendance patterns.
- Dental anxieties.
- Dental hygiene and use of toothpastes and mouth rinses.
- Any recent significant dental treatment.

Closure

At this point it is useful to summarize the information that was acquired during the history taking and clarify any outstanding issues.

Dealing with challenging situations

The angry patient
- It is generally best to let the patient vent their anger but acknowledge the situation in the process, be empathetic, and, if appropriate, apologize.

- If possible, attempt to resolve the situation and never be afraid to involve another member of staff if you feel the consultation is getting out of control.

The reserved patient
- Be patient, use open questions, and actively engage the patient.

The poor historian
- In this situation it is best to limit your questioning to closed questions and, where possible, summarize.
- Learn how to interrupt politely.
- Signposting allows the consultation to be directed.

General examination

General examination

- Should begin the moment the patient walks through the door.
- In particular:
  - Dress.
  - Behaviour.
  - Habits.
  - Movements.
  - Speech.
  - Assessment of visible skin.
- Some units will record weight and blood pressure as a routine part of the consultation.

Extraoral head and neck examination

- The face should be examined for swellings, pallor, pigmentation, CN abnormalities and erythema.
- Eyes should be examined for exophthalmia, corneal arcus, jaundice, redness, or scarring.
- The neck should be examined from the front. All regional lymph nodes should be palpated, and this is best achieved by standing behind the patient.
- The TMJ, masseter, temporalis, and salivary glands should be palpated, and any discomfort noted.
- Mandibular opening and closing paths should be recorded noting any clicks or crepitus.
- The extent of mandibular opening should be recorded.
- CNs should be assessed, particularly movement and sensation in appropriate situations.

Neck swellings

- Local causes such as infections usually do not last beyond 3 weeks.
- Viral infections usually present as multiple small (<2 cm) cervical lymphadenopathy.
- Bacterial infections are usually unilateral with large (3–4 cm) cervical lymphadenopathy.
- Systemic causes include malignancy such as lymphoma/leukaemia, Kawasaki disease, *Mycobacterium* infections, sarcoidosis, systemic lupus erythematosus, and juvenile idiopathic arthritis.
- Non-lymph related neck swellings:
  - Goitre, dermoid cyst, thyroglossal cyst, and laryngeal swelling affect midline.
  - Submandibular and parotid gland pathology and brachial cysts present in the anterior triangle.
  - Carotid artery aneurysm, carotid body tumours, cystic hygroma, and cervical ribs present in the posterior triangle.

Intraoral examination

- Should be performed in a systematic order ideally using a double mirror technique to retract the tissues under good lighting.
- Comment on appearance of all hard and soft tissues, oral hygiene, and lubrication of the oral mucosa.

- All mucosal surfaces should be examined, and abnormalities recorded appropriately in terms of size, site, shape, surface consistency, colour, margins, and whether pain is elicited on palpation.
- All lesions of concern should be photographed for monitoring purposes.

Normal anatomy often referred as pathology or anatomical variants of normal

Fordyce spots

- Small, painless, raised white or yellow swellings which are sebaceous glands normally seen on the buccal or labial mucosa and vermilion borders of the lips.
- Numbers increase with advancing age.
- Can sometimes be confused with thrush and lichen planus.
- They do not require treatment unless of cosmetic concern.

Fissured tongue

- Affects 5% of the population and prevalence increases with advancing years.
- Affects males and females equally.
- Sometimes seen in combination with erythema migrans.
- Usually asymptomatic but further investigation may be required if patient reports symptoms.

Tori

- Developmental benign exostosis affecting midline of the hard palate (most common) or lingual to the lower premolar teeth.
- No treatment is generally indicated unless patients are symptomatic or if the tori are causing difficulties with denture construction or wear.

Varicosities

- Most commonly seen on ventral tongue and floor of mouth. They tend to become more prominent with increasing age.
- Commonly present as blue/purple spots, nodules, or ridges which are usually asymptomatic.
- Frequently blanch with diascopy.

Circumvallate papillae.

- Circumvallate papillae are 8–12 mushroom-shaped swellings which are arranged in a V distribution at the junction of the anterior 2/3 and the posterior 1/3 of the dorsal aspect of the tongue.
- They are supplied with taste buds responsive to bitter flavours.

Lingual tonsils

- Lingual tonsils are collections of lymphoid tissue forming part of Waldeyer's ring located on the lateral border of tongue below the foliate papillae; these collections of lymphoid tissue can vary in size and may enlarge in response to a local infection.
- These are considered normal when they are soft, appear symmetrical, and are covered with intact mucosa. If one side is significantly larger than the other side, or if one is firm or ulcerated, then this should be further evaluated.

Stenson's duct
- Stenson's duct is the intraoral opening of the parotid salivary gland; the opening can be flat or polyp shaped and is situated adjacent to the second molar tooth.
- Milking saliva from this confirms that this is Stenson's duct.

Leukoedema
- Leukoedema is a white-grey translucent appearance which is often noted on the buccal mucosa but disappears when the mucosa is stretched.

Linea alba
- Linea alba is a white horizontal line along the buccal mucosa at the level of the occlusal plane. Commonly seen in those with a parafunctional habit.

Investigations used in oral medicine

Clinical photography
- Clinical photography is an essential tool in oral medicine practice particularly with the introduction of affordable, high-quality, easy-to-use digital cameras.
- Its main uses in oral medicine include the monitoring of disease progression and treatment outcomes over time.
- It can also be used as part of the planning process for biopsies and in patient and professional education.

Radiology—intraoral views

PA radiographs
- PA radiographs show all of the tooth, root, and surrounding PA tissues.
- These are useful for confirming pathology in PA regions such as cysts and abscesses.
- Additionally, they may be useful in confirming the presence of a foreign body as is the case on an amalgam tattoo.

Radiology—extraoral views

OPG
- Good as a screening view to access dentition and periodontal status.
- Can be useful as an initial screen for investigating suspected pathology of the antrum, mandible, and TMJs.
- It is a 2D image and ghost images can result. Furthermore, images can be susceptible to distortion.

CBCT
- Modification of CT which uses a cone-shaped X-ray beam which rotates around the patient's head creating multiple images which can be used to create a 3D model.
- It is becoming widely used for imaging of bony/dental pathology of maxilla and mandible and delivers a much-reduced dose of radiation compared to conventional CT.

Other imaging techniques

MRI

- MRI is a form of imaging that utilizes strong magnetic fields and radio waves to produce detailed images of the soft tissues.
- In oral medicine, it is useful for imaging the meniscus, soft tissues in the facial unit, and intracranial pathology which may be a cause of facial pain or altered sensation.
- The cost involved with such scans, coupled with long scanning times, patient factors including claustrophobia, and movement, are some of the problems associated with this type of investigation, although open scanners are now available in some hospitals.
- Furthermore, it can be contraindicated if patients have metal implants or foreign bodies so it is always important to ask about this.
- In addition, if contrast is to be used, it is important to check renal function.

Sialography

- Sialography is a technique of imaging the architecture of the major salivary glands and their associated ducts by injection of an iodine-based contrast medium which is then visualized using either conventional X-rays or CT scanning.
- This technique traditionally was used to detect causes of obstruction such as calculi or strictures.
- The technique is contraindicated in those individuals with an allergy to iodine and during episodes of acute infection.
- Interventional sialography is sometimes used for calculi removal.

Ultrasonography

- Ultrasound imaging uses high-frequency sound waves which are >20,000 Hz and not audible to the human ear.
- The resulting image, referred to as a sonogram, is generated by sending pulses of high-frequency waves into a tissue by means of a probe.
- The sound waves then are reflected to varying extents by different tissues and are recaptured and displayed as an image.
- Ultrasound is one of the most frequently used investigations in oral medicine and is used to image the salivary glands, lymph nodes, and thyroid and to investigate soft tissue swellings such as cysts, abscesses, vascular lesions, and foreign body inclusion.
- Ultrasound is frequently undertaken in combination with fine needle aspiration.
- Its main advantages include real-time imaging, portability, low cost, and not involving the use of ionizing radiation.
- The main disadvantage is that it is operator dependent.

Other investigations used

Mucosal biopsy

- This process involves removal of a tissue sample (incisional) or all of a lesion (excisional) for histological examination and definitive diagnosis.
- Indications:
  - When there is unexplained ulceration persisting for ≥3 weeks.

- Lesions such as fibroepithelial polyps and mucoceles which interfere with function.
- Unexplained red patches or white patches, especially if speckled or non-homogeneous in appearance.
- Lesions which have malignant signs such as induration, fixation, ulceration, bleeding, rapid growth, and as an aid in diagnosis (e.g. labial gland biopsy in Sjögren syndrome).

Sialometry

- Sialometry is a measure of saliva flow and therefore a measure of dysfunction of the salivary glands.
- Many different techniques have been devised to assess this. The technique most commonly used is a measure of whole unstimulated saliva production.
- This involves asking the patient to sit quietly without talking and chewing and expectorating any saliva that accumulates in the mouth during a 15-minute period into a container which may be pre-weighed.
- Alternatively, a blunt needle and syringe can be used to draw up and measure the amount of saliva produced in the container during this time.
- An unstimulated whole saliva flow rate in a normal person is 0.3–0.4 mL/minute, and <0.1 mL/minute is significantly abnormal.

Microbiology

- A microbiological swab is sometimes used to detect the presence of bacteria, fungi, or viruses.
- There are many different types of swabs. Gel or charcoal medium swabs are used for the recovery of aerobes, anaerobes, and fastidious organisms.
- Where a viral aetiology is suspected, swabs should be placed in an appropriate transport medium.
- Some oral medicine units quantify the oral microflora using the concentrated oral rinse technique. This is particularly useful if one wants to evaluate response to, for example, antifungal treatment.

Haematological investigations

- Haematological investigations in oral medicine are used not only for diagnosis but also for work-up before commencing certain medications, monitoring for disease activity, and complications of some of the medications used in treatment.

Common oral medicine conditions

Diagnosis and management

Oral medicine practice can be divided into three main areas: mucosal disease, conditions affecting the salivary glands, and facial pain.

Mucosal disease

Oral ulceration

Oral ulceration may be defined as a discontinuity in an epithelial surface. This can be caused by local causes such as trauma, idiopathic conditions such as aphthous ulceration, drugs such as nicorandil, a malignant process such as squamous cell carcinoma, and systemic causes such as inflammatory bowel disease.

Recurrent aphthous ulceration

- Recurrent episodes of one or more round or ovoid-shaped ulcers which recur at intervals ranging from days to months.
- Males and females are equally affected with an incidence of ~20% in the population.
- Onset usually in childhood with decreasing severity and frequency with age.
- Familial expression.
- Three types:
  - Minor aphthae are the most common (80%) and consist of small multiple ulcers 2–4 mm in diameter which heal within 7–10 days without scarring. Tend to affect buccal, labial mucosa, lateral borders of tongue, and floor of mouth.
  - Major aphthae are less common (10%) and typically present as large ulcers >1 cm. They can affect any part of the oral mucosa. Healing may take several months and scarring often results.
  - Herpetiform ulceration is uncommon, affecting 10% of the population. They present as multiple pinpoint ulcers which enlarge and coalesce to produce irregular-shaped ulcers which heal with 1–3 weeks. They can affect any part of the oral mucosa, but the ventral tongue is the most common site.
- Management of recurrent aphthous ulceration involves the identification of predisposing factors such as stress and genetic and dietary factors.
- Treatment should aim to control symptoms, reduce duration, increase disease-free intervals, and prevent long-term complications. Many treatments used in oral medicine for management of oral ulceration are used off-licence.
  - These include covering agents, analgesic, antiseptic mouthwashes such as benzydamine hydrochloride and chlorhexidine, topical corticosteroid preparations such as hydrocortisone hemisuccinate pellets, and mouth rinses such as betamethasone.
- Ideally, topical agents should be used in the first instance. However, if these are unsuccessful then a short course of systemic steroids may be advocated. In extreme cases, treatments with systemic modulating agents such as colchicine, azathioprine, or thalidomide may be necessary.

Traumatic ulceration
- Usually related to a known event.
- Single ulcer of variable size and not site specific.
- If long duration may have a keratotic halo.
- Systemic upset uncommon.
- Managed by identification and elimination of predisposing factors and symptom relief using topical agents such as covering agents or antiseptic mouthwashes. Patients should be reviewed to ensure resolution of the ulcer.
- If the area of ulceration persists for ≥3 weeks following elimination of trauma, the area should be biopsied.

Infectious causes of oral ulceration—bacterial

Tuberculosis
- Tuberculosis is a re-emerging infection caused by *Mycobacterium tuberculosis*.
- Intraorally, it can affect any mucosal site, but is typically seen on the postero-dorsal aspect of the tongue as a deep painful ulcer.
- Biopsy reveals necrotizing granuloma with Langerhans giant cells and epithelioid cells. *Mycobacterium* can be identified using Ziehl Nielsen stain.
- Patients should be referred urgently for management.

Gonorrhoea
- Gonorrhoea is a sexually transmitted diseases caused by the Gram-negative bacteria *Neisseria gonorrhoea*.
- Although oral mucosa involvement is rare, patients may present with multiple ulcers and a fiery red appearance of the oral mucosa with a white pseudo-membrane.
- Patients with oral gonococcal infection may be asymptomatic or present with severe oral symptoms and a painful pharyngitis. Lymphadenopathy may be present. The lesions of oral gonorrhoea are not specific and may mimic a wide variety of other oral conditions such as erythema multiforme (EM; ➔ Erythema multiforme).
- Confirmation requires isolation of the offending organism via culture.
- These patients should be referred to a genitourinary medicine specialist and are usually managed with a short course of high-dose penicillin.

Syphilis
- Caused by the spirochete *Treponema palladium*. In the head and neck region it can present as chancres, mucous patches, ulcers, gumma, pain particularly if there is neural involvement, leukoplakias, lymph node enlargement, abnormalities of teeth (notching of incisors, moon-shaped molars), oronasal fistulas, saddle nose appearance, frontal bossing, and sensory neural deafness.
- Can cross placenta to infect fetus and cause congenital infections (Hutchinson's incisors—notching of incisor teeth), mulberry molar teeth, interstitial keratosis, bone sclerosis, arthritis, and deafness.
- There are ~9000 cases each year in England and four stages have been identified.
    - *Primary syphilis* presents as a papule which ulcerates to form the chancre (flat, dull red, indurated, painless ulcer which exudes serous

fluid). There may be painless enlargement of the local lymph nodes. Healing occurs within 3–8 weeks.
* *Secondary syphilis* presents within 2–8 weeks after the primary infection heals. This is characterized by generalized infection with a maculopapular rash involving the skin and mucous membranes. These highly contagious lesions may fuse to form wart-like condyloma accumulata. There is generalized lymphadenopathy in 50% and about 1/3 of affected individuals get snail-track mucosal ulcers. Rarely may see periostitis, arthritis, hepatitis, or glomerulonephritis.
* *Tertiary syphilis* usually presents 3–10 years after the primary lesion and is characterized by gummata or granulomatous nodules in the skin, mucous membranes, bones, liver, testes, CVS, and CNS. If the oral cavity is involved, shallow punched-out ulcers are noted.
* *Quaternary syphilis* may present as long as 10–15 years after the primary infection and may affect the cardiovascular system to produce a dilated aorta and aortic valve regurgitation, aortic dissection, aortic stenosis/aneurysms/incompetence. Neurological involvement produces tabes dorsalis—degeneration of spinal dorsum tracts with ataxic gait, and trophic changes in joints, general paralysis of the insane, and meningovascular syphilis.
* Diagnosis was traditionally by demonstration of treponemes by dark-ground microscopy. However, this has now largely been superseded by more sensitive techniques which utilize the polymerase chain reaction technique and antibody testing.
* If syphilis is diagnosed, patients should be referred to a genitourinary medicine specialist and are usually managed with a short course of antibiotics.

Infectious causes of oral ulceration—viral

Herpes group of viruses
* Eight viruses which can be further classified into three groups:
  * Alpha herpesviruses (HSV-1, HSV-2, VZV).
  * Beta herpesviruses (CMV, HHV-5, HHV-6, HHV-7).
  * Gamma herpesviruses (EBV, HHV-4, HHV-8).
* Cause oral and perioral ulceration which is usually self-limiting. HHV-8 has been implicated in Kaposi's sarcoma and EBV in hairy leukoplakia.
* Herpes simplex virus (HSV-1, HHV-1) is a DNA virus, transmitted in saliva, which is neurotoxic with a tendency to remain latent.
* The primary infection occurs normally in childhood (2–4 years) with ~50% having subclinical symptoms which may be confused with teething. If the primary presentation occurs in adulthood, it is usually characterized by pharyngotonsillitis.
* Symptoms of the primary infection include fever or malaise, sore mouth or oropharynx, and gingivitis followed by formation of vesicles 2–3 days later which rupture giving rise to painful ulcers covered with a yellowish membrane.
* Cervical node enlargement.
* Diagnosis largely clinical. If the presentation is atypical, blood tests should be undertaken to exclude conditions such as leukaemia.
* Management is symptomatic control and involves a soft diet, good fluid intake, antiseptic mouth rinses, and analgesics such as paracetamol.

If the infection is detected early (within 72 hours) or the patient is immunocompromised, some benefit may be gained through use of aciclovir 200 mg tablets taken five times daily for 5 days.

- The secondary infection presents as herpes labialis or recurrent intraoral herpes. This affects 15% of the population and is due to reactivation of HSV which lies latent in the trigeminal ganglion. Typical factors which cause reactivation include fever, sunlight, trauma, hormonal changes, and immunosuppression.
- Areas of ulceration occur on upper or lower lip (mucocutaneous junction), occasionally nares, and conjunctiva and may be preceded by prodromal symptoms (tingling, burning, and itching). The characteristic clinical picture is erythema followed by papules which progress to vesicles which rupture to form pustules which scab and heal within 7–10 days.
- Management usually involves the use of topical agents such as topical 5% aciclovir. In severe or recurring cases, systemic aciclovir 200 mg five times daily for 5 days or valaciclovir 1000–2000 mg twice daily can be used.
- Recurrent intraoral herpes presents as unilateral painful ulcers localized to the keratinized gingiva and hard palate. Ulcers appear as crops usually over the greater palatine foramen which may be the result of trauma (LA).
- Ulceration normally resolves in 7–10 days. In immunocompromised individuals may appear as chronic, dendritic ulcers, frequently on tongue.

Zoster (shingles)

- Painful unilateral rash in a dermatome (distribution of a sensory nerve) due to reactivation of VZV.
- In ~1/3 of cases the maxillary or mandibular branch of the trigeminal nerve is affected resulting in a rash extraorally accompanied by pain which can be confused as toothache and ulceration affecting various mucosal sites. There is often accompanying lymphadenopathy when the mandibular branch is involved.
- Management aims to limit severity of pain and reduce complications. Analgesia is frequently prescribed in addition to high-dose antivirals such as 400–800 mg aciclovir, five times daily for 5 days, valaciclovir 1000 mg three times daily or famciclovir 500 mg three times daily for 7 days.
- If treatment is delayed or inadequate, post-herpetic neuralgia may develop. This is commoner in the older age group and is treated with tricyclic antidepressants or gabapentinoids.

Ramsey Hunt syndrome type 2

- Complication of shingles which results in reactivation of the VZV in the geniculate ganglion of CN VII. This presents as facial nerve weakness, pain, a rash, or blister formation affecting the external auditory meatus, with impaired taste and dryness.
- In addition to antivirals, corticosteroids are sometimes prescribed.

HHV-4 (EBV)

- Common among young adults and transmitted via saliva.

- Primary infection usually presents as infectious mononucleosis which is characterized by an exudative tonsillitis.
- Cannot be diagnosed on clinical grounds as similar symptoms caused by CMV, seroconversion in HIV, rubella, HHV-6, adenovirus, HSV, *Streptococcus pyogenes*, and toxoplasmosis.
- Diagnosis is by the Paul Bunnell test for heterophile antibodies to sheep erythrocytes which are diagnostic for infectious mononucleosis.
- HHV-4 also implicated in hairy leukoplakia and Burkitt's lymphoma.
- Management is symptomatic relief.
- Amoxicillin should not be given to patients with suspected infectious mononucleosis as complications including rashes and anaphylaxis have been reported.

Coxsackie virus
- Enteroviruses RNA viruses transmitted by faecal–oral route.
- Coxsackie A causes aseptic meningitis, herpangina (vesicular pharyngitis, a painful eruption of vesicles in the mouth and throat), and hand, foot, and mouth disease (vesicular stomatitis with lesions on hand and feet).
- Differs from herpetic stomatitis as it spares the gingiva. The condition is self-limiting with resolution normally within 10–14 days.

Systemic causes of oral ulceration
- Many systemic conditions have oral ulceration as a consequence.
- In these situations, recurrent episodes of ulceration are termed recurrent oral ulceration.
- Features which are suggestive of a systemic cause of oral ulceration include:
  - gastrointestinal symptoms
  - weight loss
  - fever
  - lymphadenopathy
  - organomegaly
  - late onset of ulcer presentation
  - severity
  - limited response to treatment
  - other accompanying oral lesions.
- Examples of systemic conditions which have oral ulceration as a presenting feature include:
  - inflammatory bowel disease such as Crohn's disease and ulcerative colitis
  - haematological causes such as anaemia, leukaemia, cyclic neutropenia, and myelodysplastic syndromes
  - autoinflammatory conditions such as Behçet's disease, and rheumatological conditions such as Reiter's syndrome and Sweet's syndrome.

Drug-induced oral ulceration
- This can occur locally, such as application of an irritant preparation (e.g. aspirin).
- It can also be a complication of systemic medications, such as:
  - antihypertensives
  - vasodilator/venodilator medications
  - antimetabolites

- non-steroidal anti-inflammatory drugs
- cytotoxic and disease-modifying antirheumatic drugs.
- Depending on the severity, management may involve symptomatic control or it may involve liaising with the relevant medical specialist.

Blistering disorders

- A vesicle is a blister <5 mm.
- A bulla is a blister >5 mm.
- Blisters often break down to leave erosions or ulcers.
- Seen in a variety of cases such as:
  - burns
  - angina bullosa haemorrhagica (ABH)
  - infections (e.g. Coxsackie, HSV, VZV)
  - mucocutaneous conditions such as lichen planus, pemphigoid/pemphigus, linear immunoglobulin (Ig)-G disease, EM, epidermolysis bullosa, and dermatitis herpetiformis.

Angina bullosa haemorrhagica

- ABH is a condition characterized by acute, benign, subepithelial oral mucosal blisters filled with blood that are not attributable to a systemic disorder or haemostatic defect such as thrombocytopenia.
- This condition is characterized by rapid onset of blisters which break down to produce ulcers, which occur spontaneous or following trauma. Blister formation may be preceded by a sharp prickling sensation.
- This condition is uncommon and generally affects older people. The soft palate is the commonest site. However, blisters have been reported affecting the buccal mucosa, anterior 1/3 of the tongue, and occasionally the pharynx.
- The lesions may be confused with other more serious disorders (e.g. mucous membrane pemphigoid, epidermolysis bullosa, linear IgA, dermatitis herpetiformis); however, the isolated nature, rapid healing, and rare recurrence of ABH blisters and the absence of areas of ecchymosis, epitasis, or gingival bleeding are helpful in excluding a coagulopathy or vesiculobullous condition such as pemphigus or pemphigoid.
- The condition is managed by confirming haemostasis and, if the appearance or symptoms are atypical, biopsy to exclude a vesiculobullous process.
- Analgesics are used to manage pain. Individuals generally suffer five to ten episodes over 2–3 years. In some cases, the condition remits spontaneously.

Pemphigus

Group of potentially life-threatening chronic autoimmune diseases characterized by intraepithelial blistering disorders and resulting in flaccid blisters and erosions of the skin and mucous membranes.

Pemphigus vulgaris

- Uncommon, typically affects middle-aged and elderly patients of Ashkenazi Jewish, Asian, or Mediterranean descent.
- Female predisposition.
- May be associated with other autoimmune diseases such as systemic lupus erythematosus and myasthenia gravis.

- Clinically presents as chronic desquamative gingivitis with fragile blisters which appear on the mucosa of mouth (soft palate, posterior hard palate, buccal mucosa, lips, and gingiva), pharynx, larynx, oesophagus, nose, conjunctiva, anogenital region, rectum, and skin which rupture to produce widespread erosions.
- Confirmed on clinical examination accompanied by perilesional biopsy and direct and indirect immunofluorescence. Desmoglein 3 is the main antibody involved in oral lesions and desmoglein 1 is the main antibody involved in skin lesions.
- The aim of management is to induce disease remission using corticosteroids followed by the introduction of maintenance treatments which are steroid sparing such as azathioprine or mycophenolate mofetil and, in extreme cases, rituximab with monitoring of disease activity and for complications of medication.

Paraneoplastic autoimmune multiorgan syndrome (PAMS)

- Mucocutaneous condition that resembles pemphigus vulgaris but usually occurs in association with malignant disease such as non-Hodgkin's lymphoma, chronic lymphocytic leukaemia, Hodgkin's lymphoma, thymoma, and solid organ tumours.
- First described by Anhalt in 1990 as paraneoplastic pemphigus, it was renamed as PAMS in 2001 due to the binding of antibodies to other organs including lung, kidney, smooth muscle, intestine, colon, and thyroid.
- Presents with mucocutaneous findings which frequently are confused with other conditions such as pemphigus vulgaris, lichen planus (⊃ Lichen planus), EM (⊃ Erythema multiforme), and graft-versus-host disease (⊃ Graft-versus-host disease).
- Oral mucosal lesions are often resistant to treatment prompting further investigations.
- Diagnosis is confirmed on biopsy with direct immunofluorescence and indirect immunofluorescence on rat bladder.
- This condition is managed by identification and management of the underlying malignancy in combination with immunosuppression therapy.
- Prognosis is poor unless associated with a benign tumour.

Pemphigoid

- Subepithelial immunologically mediated vesiculobullous disorders which affect stratified squamous epithelium.
- Mucous membrane pemphigoid (cicatricial pemphigoid) in which mucosal lesions predominate, rarely skin lesions.
- Oral mucosal pemphigoid where only oral lesions. Does not involve a progressive ocular scarring process and negative serology to bullous pemphigoid antigens.
- Bullous pemphigoid which involves mainly the skin.
- Ocular pemphigoid which affects mainly conjunctiva and may cause scarring.

Mucous membrane pemphigoid

- Chronic autoimmune disease of the mucous membranes and/or skin.
- Relatively common with a female predominance; affects the fifth to sixth decades.

- Characterized by desquamative gingivitis, tense bullae, and persistent irregular erosions or ulcers which may heal with scarring.
- Untreated ocular involvement may lead to scarring and blindness (entropion, symblepharon, ankyloblepharon). Nasal lesions may bleed and scar, laryngeal scarring may lead to stenosis.
- Oral lesions easily confused with other bullous conditions.
- Diagnosis is confirmed with biopsy and direct immunofluorescence.
- Indirect immunofluorescence is usually negative in this condition.
- Management involves maintenance of good oral hygiene, and an ophthalmological assessment as ocular manifestations in 20% which if untreated could lead to blindness. Mild mucosal disease can be managed with a topical steroid. In severe cases may need immunosuppression (e.g. dapsone, azathioprine, and/or systemic corticosteroids).

Erythema multiforme

- EM is a mucocutaneous condition mediated by IgM immune complexes in the superficial microvasculature of skin and mucous membranes.
- Uncommon and typically affects young adults in the 20–30 age group with females slightly more susceptible compared to males.
- May involve the mouth alone. Often accompanied by prodromal symptoms which include malaise, fever, and myalgia.
- Oral lesions precede lesions on other mucosal sites and present as macules that progress to widespread erosions. The lips are commonly involved and swell, crack, and bleed, followed by crusting.
- Skin lesions present as target lesions and follow a symmetrical distribution in the acral extremities including the extensor surfaces of the arms, legs, elbows, knees, and dorsal aspect of the hands and feet.
- Ocular symptoms include lacrimation, photophobia, and symblepharon. Genital lesions are painful and can present as balanitis, urethritis, and vulval ulcers.
- A number of triggers have been implicated. These include infections such as HHVs and *Mycoplasma pneumoniae*; drugs including antimicrobials, anticonvulsants, and protease inhibitors; food additives such as benzoates; nitrobenzene; perfumes; terpenes; and immune disorders such as GVHD and sarcoidosis.
- EM minor is the commonest presentation affecting ~80% and involving one mucosal surface. Onset is acute and self limiting and can be episodic or recurrent. Typical target lesions symmetrically cover <10% of the body surface area.
- EM major occurs in ~20% of cases and at least two mucosal sites are involved. Cutaneous involvement is <10% but more extensive that the minor variant.
- An infective cause is thought to be the trigger in EM major. Steven–Johnson syndrome similar to EM major. However, skin lesions are atypical and not localized to acral areas and the likely cause are drugs.
- Toxic epidermal necrolysis affects 10–30% of the body surface area. It has a poor prognosis with fatality reported in ~1/3 of those affected. This condition tends to affect older individuals.
- Drugs are the likely triggering factor.
- Diagnosis of EM is clinical with emphasis on history taking and exposure to recent infections and commencement of drugs.

- Serology can be undertaken for HHVs and *M. pneumoniae*. Biopsy is usually not necessary unless there is no response to treatment, or the clinical appearance of the lesions is atypical.
- Management is usually supportive.
- Prophylactic aciclovir 400 mg once or twice daily for 6 months has been used in recurrent cases where HSV has been implicated.

Patches affecting the oral mucosa

White patches

There are many causes of white patches affecting the oral mucosa. These may be inherited or acquired. Acquired white patches are traumatic, inflammatory, or neoplastic. White patches are usually painless unless there is associated ulceration.

White sponge nevus

- White sponge nevus is an example of an inherited white patch which was first described by Cannon in 1935, and which is also known as familial white folded mucosal dysplasia or leukoderma exfoliative mucosae oris.
- It is a benign, uncommon, autosomal dominant disorder that involves a point mutation in the genes coding for the keratin proteins 4 and 13, that predominantly affects non-keratinized stratified-squamous epithelium.
- The onset is in early childhood. Lesions of white sponge nevus appear as white-to-grey, diffuse, painless, spongy folded plaques that are typically found on the buccal mucosae. Other common sites include the labial mucosae, tongue, floor of the mouth, and alveolar mucosae. Less frequently, the mucous membranes of the nose, oesophagus, genitalia, and rectum are involved.
- White sponge nevus may be confused with other white lesions of the oral mucosa, including cheek biting, lichen planus (➔ Lichen planus), lupus erythematosus, hereditary benign intraepithelial dyskeratosis, tobacco-induced keratotic lesions, pachyonychia congenita, keratosis follicularis, and candidiasis (➔ Oral candidiasis).
- No treatment is required. Progression of the disorder stops at puberty and there is no malignant transformation.

Frictional keratosis

- Acquired, painless white patch which affects any oral mucosal site although the buccal mucosa, lateral borders of tongue, and edentulous ridges are the most common sites due to chronic irritation (e.g. fractured tooth).
- Diagnosis is made on history of the lesion and clinical examination, response to removal of the irritant, and, if necessary, with biopsy to confirm the diagnosis and exclude dysplasia.

Smoker's keratosis

- Hyperkeratosis of the epithelial secondary to smoking.
- Commonly affects buccal mucosa, commissures, and palate.
- Clinically presents as epithelial thickening with pigment changes.
- Diagnosis is clinical and confirmed on biopsy.

Oral candidiasis

- Infection of the oral and/or perioral tissue by *Candida* species implies pathogenic rather than commensal status.
- Very common, often multifactorial clinical problem with a variety of clinical presentations. It may indicate a serious underlying systemic disease.

Acute pseudomembranous candidiasis

- Confluent white-yellow creamy plaques on surface of oral mucosa and tongue which are usually asymptomatic and may be wiped off to reveal an erythematous surface which may bleed.
- Associated with antibiotics or corticosteroid use, hyposalivation, immune defects, leukaemia and other malignancies, HIV, and immunosuppressant therapy.
- Commonly caused by *C. albicans* but *C. krusei* and *C. glabrata* may also be implicated. Diagnosed clinically.
- Swab of the area can detect organism involved and determine sensitivity to antifungal therapy.
- Management involves identification and elimination, if possible, of predisposing factors. Treatment involves the use of polyenes such as nystatin or azole antifungals such as miconazole or fluconazole, provided they are not contraindicated.

Chronic hyperplastic candidiasis (candidal leukoplakia)

- Well-demarcated slightly elevated adherent white lesions of the oral mucosa which range from small translucent lesions to large dense opaque plaques which commonly affect the vermilion border, buccal mucosa, palate, and tongue.
- Associated with smoking, iron and folate deficiencies, and defective cell immunity.
- Diagnosis is confirmed on biopsy. Management involves elimination of risk factors such as smoking and systemic antifungal therapy provided it is not contraindicated.

Chronic mucocutaneous candidiasis (CMC)

- CMC refers to a group of disorders characterized by recurrent or persistent candidal infections of the skin, mucous membranes, and nails with *Candida* species, usually *C. albicans* due to impaired cell-mediated immunity against *Candida* species.
- Several classifications exist. CMC may occur as part of autoimmune polyendocrinopathy candidiasis ectodermal dystrophy (APECED) which is characterized by at least two of the following: CMC, hypoparathyroidism, and Addison disease.
- Other autoimmune disorders may be associated, such as type 1 diabetes, autoimmune thyroiditis, Graves's disease, alopecia areata, vitiligo, hypogonadism, biliary cirrhosis, hepatitis, idiopathic thrombocytopenic purpura, and pernicious anaemia.
- CMC may be seen in patients with hyperimmunoglobulin E syndrome. Recurrent oral candidiasis is not uncommon in patients with HIV infection.

Lichen planus/lichenoid lesions

- Common CD-8-mediated immunologically mucocutaneous disorder which affects the stratified squamous epithelium.
- Oral lichen planus may occur in isolation, or it may affect the nails, skin, scalp, and genital mucosa.
- Clinical picture is mainly of white lesions, but atrophy, erythema, and ulceration frequently encountered and not uncommon to see a mixture of presentations which can vary in degree of symptoms.
- Malignant potential of 1–3% in non-reticular lesions.
- In contrast, lichenoid reactions are often linked to an identifiable cause such as drugs, or dental filling materials. Patch testing can be helpful in determining the causative agent.
- In both cases, biopsy is indicated to confirm the diagnosis. Management involves patient education, particularly a discussion on the potential malignant nature of the condition, meticulous oral hygiene, and symptom control using various combinations of corticosteroid preparations and, in extreme cases, immunomodulators such as azathioprine.

Leukoplakia

- 'White plaques of questionable risk having excluded other known diseases or disorders that carry no increased risk for cancer.'
- Note this is a clinical diagnosis only.
- Affects 0.1% of the population.
- Middle-aged to elderly patients.
- Males > female.
- Homogeneous plaques are usually flat, corrugated, or wrinkled.
- Non-homogeneous plaques are either verrucous, proliferative and verrucous, nodular, or erythroleukoplakia.
- Malignant potential overall is 3% over 10 years.
- Features suggesting malignant potential include clinical appearance, site, and histological findings.
- Proliferative verrucous leukoplakia is a diffuse, white, and/or papillary lesion seen in older patients often associated with HPV; slow progression to verrucous or squamous cell carcinoma.
- Candidal leukoplakia/speckled leukoplakia at commissures may respond to antifungal therapy and smoking cessation.
- Syphilitic leukoplakia, especially of dorsum of tongue, is a feature of tertiary syphilis, rarely seen, with high malignant potential.
- Hairy leukoplakia caused by EBV. Corrugated surface and affects margins of the tongue. Seen in immunocompromised patients and is a complication of HIV infection. Diagnosis is confirmed on biopsy.

Red patches

May be traumatic, inflammatory, or neoplastic. Most are symptomatic and are usually widespread.

Erythematous or atrophic candidiasis

- Examples include denture-related stomatitis and antibiotic- or steroid-induced candidiasis.

- These conditions are characterized by widespread erythema and soreness of the oral mucosa commonly occurring on the dorsum of the tongue and on the palate.
- They are diagnosed clinically and confirmed microbiologically which may guide treatment.
- Management involves identification and elimination of causative factors and appropriate antifungal therapy.

Median rhomboid glossitis

- A rhomboid-shaped area of depapillation affecting the central dorsal aspect of the tongue anterior to circumvallate papillae. Occasionally it may present as a hyperplastic or lobulated exophytic growth.
- This condition is thought to occur as a result of atrophy of filiform papilla due to candidal infection.
- Predisposing factors include smoking, denture wearing, corticosteroid sprays/inhalers, and HIV infection.
- Diagnosis is clinical and confirmed microbiologically with swabs of the area. Biopsy is warranted if there is doubt about the diagnosis or poor response to treatment.
- Management involves identification and elimination of predisposing factors, appropriate antifungal therapy, and follow-up to ensure resolution.

Candida-associated angular cheilitis

- An infection, which has developed at the angles of the mouth as a result of spread of organisms from the oral cavity.
- This common condition presents as inflammation at the angles of the mouth. It is diagnosed clinically and managed by identification and elimination of predisposing factors and appropriate therapy.

Linear gingival erythema (LGE)

- LGE is a periodontal disorder diagnosed based on distinct clinical characteristics.
- It was originally thought that LGE was directly associated with HIV, and it was thus called HIV-associated gingivitis (HIV-G).
- Later research confirmed that LGE also occurs in HIV-negative immunocompromised patients, and it was thus renamed.
- LGE is limited to the soft tissue of the periodontium, appearing as a red line 2–3 mm in width adjacent to the free gingival margin. Unlike conventional periodontal disease, though, LGE is not significantly associated with increased levels of dental plaque.
- The prevalence of LGE remains unclear and there is no known treatment.

Plasma cell gingivitis

- Rare usually asymptomatic condition characterized by erythema and oedema of the attached gingiva which may occasionally be seen as a solitary lesion or accompanied by lip and tongue swelling.
- The mucosa has a red and often granular appearance.
- Plasma cell gingivitis is thought to be a hypersensitivity reaction to components (cinnamaldehyde and cinnamon) of toothpaste, chewing gum, mints, and so on.

- Diagnosis is confirmed on biopsy which reveals abundant plasma cells. Leukaemia and multiple myeloma must be excluded.
- In some cases, a good response is achieved with topical corticosteroid preparations.

Erythema migrans
- Also known as benign migratory glossitis or geographic tongue, this condition affects 1–2% of the population and is often an incidental finding on clinical examination although a proportion of patients complain of irritation or tenderness when consuming spicy foods and alcohol.
- Erythema migrans presents as atrophic patches surrounded by elevated keratotic margins, the pattern of which varies from day to day.
- Other sites that can be affected include the ventral aspect of tongue, buccal mucosa, floor of mouth, and gingiva.
- Often the tongue is heavily fissured. Treatment is often not indicated if the area is asymptomatic.
- In those individuals who are symptomatic, it is important to exclude an underlying haematinic deficiency.
- Management of the symptomatic patient is challenging. Antifungals, topical steroid preparations, lidocaine gel, vitamin B, and zinc preparations have been used with limited success.

Erythroplakia
- 'Any lesion of the oral mucosa that presents as a bright red velvety plaque which cannot be characterized clinically or pathologically as any other recognizable condition.'
- Erythroplakia is a potentially malignant disorder which affects the soft palate and ventral aspect of the tongue.
- Biopsy is mandatory to identify the degree of dysplasia which is almost always present.
- Management involves surgical excision, elimination of risk factors, and long-term monitoring.

Oral mucosal swellings
- There are many causes for oral mucosal swellings.
- Important features to note include:
  - whether the swelling is single or multiple
  - colour
  - temperature
  - size
  - shape
  - consistency
  - whether it is tender
  - whether it discharges
  - its anatomical relationships
  - surface texture
  - margins
  - whether it is fixed or mobile
  - superficial or deep.
- Mucosal swellings may be normal anatomical variants as in the case of the folate or circumvallate papillae which are often mistaken for

pathology (❷ Normal anatomy often referred as pathology or anatomical variants of normal), or they may be acquired.
- Acquired swellings include developmental anomalies such as:
  - unerupted teeth, tori, cysts, and hamartomas
  - infective inflammatory lesions such as dental abscess or salivary gland infections
  - non-infective inflammatory lesions such as fibrous lumps, Crohn's disease, sarcoidosis or sialosis, allergy in angioedema
  - traumatic (e.g. haematoma), hormonal as in pregnancy and hyperparathyroidism, medication induced as in phenytoin and ciclosporin, benign and malignant neoplasms, haemangiomas, fibro osseous lesions, and deposits.

Oral pigmentation

- Oral pigmentation may be a physiological or a pathological process.
- If the lesion is focal, the colour can provide clues to the diagnosis.
- If the lesion is red, blue, or purple and blanches with diascopy, it is likely to be a varix or haemangioma. If it is non-blanchable, it may be a thrombus or haematoma. Amalgam tattoos, foreign bodies, or blue nevus tend to present as blue/grey lesions.
- Melanotic macules, pigmented naevi, melanoacanthoma, and melanoma usually present as brown lesions with the latter showing variation in colour, asymmetry, and with irregular borders.
- If the lesion is diffuse and bilateral, it is important to ask about onset.
- Early onset (i.e. in childhood) may suggest physiological pigmentation or an underlying systemic condition such as Peutz–Jeghers syndrome.
- Diffuse and bilateral pigmentation which is of adult onset, and which does not have systemic symptoms include medication, post-inflammatory, and smoker's melanosis.
- If there are generalized pigmentation and systemic signs and symptoms, consider heavy metal poisoning, Addison's disease, Kaposi's sarcoma, small cell carcinoma, and inappropriate adrenocorticotropic hormone secretion.

Oral cancer

Potentially malignant oral disorders

Actinic cheilitis
- Also known as actinic keratosis, solar keratosis, and solar cheilosis.
- Variable clinical presentation depending on stage.
- Typical sites include nose, temple, forehead, and lower lip.
- Early lesions tend to be red and oedematous. Long-standing lesions may be dry, scaly, and warty, with white to grey changes on the lower lip.
- Diagnosis is based on a history of sun exposure and clinical examination. If there is uncertainty regarding diagnosis, a biopsy should be undertaken. Management involves patient education and, depending on the extent, may warrant a referral to dermatology.

Erythroplakia, leukoplakia, lichen planus, and candidal/syphilitic leukoplakia
See ➥ Patches affecting the oral mucosa.

Submucous fibrosis
- Chronic disorder affecting those individuals who chew betel nut, pan masala, or gutka.
- Results in tightening of buccal, palatal, and lingual mucosa causing trismus. Other reported symptoms include a burning sensation or intolerance to spicy foods, ulceration, and dryness of the mouth.
- If fibrosis affects nasopharynx or oropharynx, may get referred pain to ear, nasal voice, or dysphasia (these usually indicate severe disease). Carcinoma may develop in up to 8%.
- Management involves patient education, symptomatic management, and surveillance for malignant transformation.

Graft-versus-host disease
- Allogeneic haematopoietic stem cell transplantation is a potentially curative option for many haematologic malignancies.
- Graft-versus-host disease occurs when donor T cells respond to proteins on host cells.
- In the oral cavity, this can present as erythema, lichenoid striae, leukoplakias, ulceration, mucoceles, limited opening, and a Sjögren syndrome-like condition affecting the salivary glands.
- Squamous cell carcinoma is a late complication. These patients require long-term surveillance.

Management of premalignant lesions
- Accurate record of site ideally with photography.
- Patient education.
- Surveillance with biopsy if change in appearance of the lesion.
- Depending on comorbidities, degree of dysplasia, and size of lesion, consider referral for excision.

Malignant lesions
- Approximately 90% of oral cancers are oral squamous cell carcinomas.
- Other malignant tumours include:
  - epithelial malignancies such as other carcinomas, arising from a surface (e.g. melanoma, maxillary antrum tumours)

- salivary gland tumours, lymph reticular neoplasms which affect the upper jaw, mandible, palate, vestibule, and gingiva
- sarcomas which although rare can present at any age and are characterized by rapid growth and may arise in connective tissue, bone, muscle, and blood vessels and metastatic tumours (i.e. within a lymph node, within bone, or soft tissues).
- Risk factors for oral cancer include tobacco, alcohol, genetic factors, and viruses (e.g. EBV, HPV).
- Patients complaining of an unexplained sore throat, hoarseness, strider, difficulty in swallowing, a lump in the neck or unilateral ear pain, red or speckled patches, swellings, mobile teeth, unexplained oral ulceration, or CN palsies persisting for ≥3 weeks should be referred urgently for further assessment.
- Treatment requires a multidisciplinary approach using a combination of surgery, radiotherapy, and chemotherapy.

Conditions affecting salivary glands

- Saliva is involved in lubrication, has an antibacterial role, and is involved in digestion and mineralization.
- There are three groups of paired salivary glands:
  - The parotid glands are the largest and produce ~20% of the daily saliva which is a thin serous saliva.
  - The submandibular glands produce ~70% of the daily saliva which is 80% serous and 20% mucus.
  - The sublingual glands are the smallest of the major salivary glands and produce ~5% of the daily saliva which is mucous in nature.
- Scattered throughout the mouth are ~600 minor salivary glands which contribute ~5% of total daily saliva. These are located mainly in the labial mucosa but can also be seen in the soft palate, tongue, and buccal mucosa.
- These frequently mirror disease processes affecting the major glands and are easily harvested from the labial mucosa for confirmation of a suspected diagnosis.

Hypersalivation

- Also known as sialorrhoea, this describes a condition where there is excess saliva produced.
- Local causes for this include trauma or infection. It may also be caused by a number of neurological conditions such as amyotrophic lateral sclerosis, Parkinson's, and stroke.
- Other factors that have been attributed to hypersalivation include medication such as risperidone and clozapine.
- Management may involve behavioural management programmes or the use of anticholinergic agents, such as hyoscine hydrobromide whose use is limited by the side effects produced which include constipation, excessive oral dryness, urinary retention, blurred vision, and tachycardia.
- In extreme cases, botulism toxin serotype A, a neurotoxin which inhibits the release of acetylcholine, may be used or surgical redirection, ligation, or removal of the salivary glands may be undertaken.

Xerostomia

- Also known as dry mouth. This is the subjective sense of dryness which may be related to reduced salivary production or a change in the composition of saliva.
- There are many causes for this including anxiety, mouth breathing, salivary gland aplasia, systemic conditions, head and neck radiation, and drugs.
- Clinically this may present with dry mouth and eyes, but other sites may be affected such as the skin and nasal, laryngeal, and genital mucosa particularly when a systemic condition such as Sjögren syndrome is suspected.
- In addition, there may be difficulty speaking, swallowing, and controlling dentures.
- Generalized oral soreness and inflammation with an unpleasant taste.

- Frothy saliva, dental mirror sticking to the oral mucosa, and lack of saliva pooling in the floor of the mouth are good indicators of xerostomia.
- The Challacombe scale is a quick method of screening for oral dryness.
- Sialometry is a simple chairside test for xerostomia or hypersalivation. Normally unstimulated saliva flow is 0.5 mL/minute; <0.1 mL/minute suggests hyposalivation.
- Having established there is xerostomia, a review of medications may identify a number of contributory drugs.
- Blood tests should be carried out if there is a high index of suspicion for a systemic cause.
- Management involves patient education and a combination of salivary sialagogues, substitutes, and oral lubricants.
- Stimulants such as pilocarpine 5 mg three times daily may be used but compliance is often poor due to side effects, and it is contraindicated in cardiovascular and pulmonary disease.

Halitosis

- Also known as oral malodour. This condition affects up to 30% of adults over the age of 60 years.
- While it may be a normal physiological process such as halitosis on waking, a number of other causes have been implicated.
- These include poor oral hygiene, local infection, smoking, alcohol, consumption of members of the durian group of vegetables which include garlic, onion, spices, cabbage, cauliflower, and radish, ovulation, drugs, and systemic disease.
- Consideration must also be given to psychogenic causes particularly when there is no evidence of a cause.
- Diagnosis is based on a concise history including dietary analysis and clinical examination.
- If there is an obvious cause such as poor oral hygiene, plaque retentive sites, or an infection this should be treated.
- Patients with halitophobia may benefit from a specialist mental health assessment.

Trimethylaminuria (fish malodour syndrome)

- Trimethylamine is produced by intestinal bacterial breakdown of choline- and carnitine containing foods such as eggs and fish.
- This then undergoes oxidation in the liver to produce trimethylamine oxide which is odourless and excreted in the liver.
- In some individuals, oxidation of trimethylaminuria is impaired.
- The unoxidized trimethylamine is excreted in urine, sweat, vaginal secretions, and saliva. This results in a characteristic oral and body malodour which is often described as resembling 'rotten fish or faeces'.
- Trimethylaminuria is diagnosed with a urine test that measures the ratio of trimethylamine (the fishy-smelling chemical) to trimethylamine N-oxide (the odourless version). This is usually carried out the day after a 'choline load'.
- This involves eating a suggested meal including foods high in choline, such as saltwater fish, eggs, baked beans, or soya beans.

- There is currently no cure or approved drugs to treat trimethylaminuria, but symptoms can be improved by making lifestyle changes such as avoiding choline- and carnitine-containing foods.

Dysgeusia

- Dysgeusia is defined as persistent abnormal taste which may be attributed to part of the normal ageing process.
- However, it is also associated with upper respiratory infections particularly viral; following head trauma; may be a complication of surgical procedures affecting CNs V, VII, IX, X; or a consequence of radiotherapy or chemotherapy or use of certain medications.
- Dysgeusia is frequently reported by patients with burning mouth syndrome.
- Management involves identifying and eliminating any underlying causes. Where an endocrine or psychogenic cause is suspected, these patients should be referred for appropriate investigations.

Salivary gland swellings

Inflammatory causes

Sialadenitis

- May be acute or chronic.
- Acute infection results in pain and swelling. Mumps caused by the paramyxovirus is the most common cause in children resulting in bilateral parotid swelling with systemic upset (➔ Mumps).
- Acute bacterial infections are more common in the elderly or in individuals who are dehydrated or have undergone head and neck radiotherapy. In this case, the swelling is usually unilateral with redness of the overlying skin and associated tenderness.
- Abscess formation may result with discharge of pus to the skin surface.
- Treatment is symptomatic measures including analgesia and hydration.
- Where the cause is bacterial, appropriate antibiotics should be prescribed. Usually, flucloxacillin or amoxicillin are prescribed.
- In the case of penicillin allergy, erythromycin can be used as an alternative.
- In chronic cases, the affected gland is swollen but not painful.
- Clinical examination and imaging help to confirm the diagnosis. In some cases, treatment involves surgical removal of the gland.
- Recurrent parotitis of childhood presents as recurring episodes of parotid swelling which are usually non-tender and resolve after 3 weeks.
- Diagnosis is clinical with characteristic findings on imaging (sialectasis). Sjögren syndrome should be excluded. Management involves massage of the affected gland and the use of sialogogues. This condition usually remits around puberty.

Sarcoidosis

- Multisystem non-caseating granulomatous disorder of unknown cause which can affect any organ but typically presents with bilateral hilar lymphadenopathy and/or pulmonary infiltrations, skin lesions, and eye involvement.
- This condition typically affects young and middle-aged adults.

- Heerfordt's syndrome is an acute presentation of sarcoidosis and consists of a triad of fever, uveitis, and parotid gland ± other salivary and lacrimal glands enlargement. In addition, a facial nerve palsy may occur in addition, although it is not needed to make the diagnosis.
- Sarcoidosis is confirmed through a combination of history, biopsy, chest radiograph, and bloods—serum angiotensinogen-converting enzyme.
- If sarcoidosis is suspected, these individuals should be referred to a respiratory physician for management.

Sjögren syndrome

- Sjögren syndrome is a chronic systemic autoimmune disease of the exocrine glands resulting in dryness of the mucosal membranes.
- It is an uncommon condition, affecting any age but commonly seen around menarche and menopause.
- It is nine times more common in females compared to males.
- There are two major types:
  - Primary Sjögren syndrome presents as dry eyes and dry mouth.
  - Secondary Sjögren syndrome in addition presents with a connective tissue disease such as rheumatoid arthritis or systemic lupus erythematous.
- Clinically Sjögren syndrome can present with keratoconjunctivitis sicca (red and infected conjunctivae), dry, gritty painful eyes with reduced visual acuity, and photosensitivity.
- The lips are cracked and dry with evidence of angular cheilitis and there is frequently salivary gland swelling due to ascending infection.
- Intraorally there is evidence of xerostomia resulting in difficulty chewing, swallowing, and talking with an associated taste disturbances and burning sensation in mouth. Dental caries is common.
- The tongue is heavily fissured and there are often signs of chronic erythematous candidiasis affecting mainly the tongue and palate.
- Over 1/3 of individuals with primary Sjögren syndrome have extra glandular associated conditions.
- The most serious is low-grade marginal zone lymphoma which occurs in ~5% of cases.
- Predictors of lymphoma development in this group include lymphadenopathy, parotid gland enlargement, leucopenia, hypergammaglobulinemia, cryoglobulinemia, hypocomplementemia, palpable purpura, skin vasculitis, anaemia, and peripheral neuropathy.
- There are several diagnostic criteria for Sjögren syndrome which measure a number of objective and subjective symptoms.
- Management of the oral symptoms is similar to that previously described. These patients are often managed in combination with other specialties such as ophthalmology and rheumatology.

IgG4 disease

- Previously called Mikulicz disease. This fibroinflammatory condition is rare, tends to be more prevalent in the seventh decade among Japanese men, and presents in the head and neck region with enlargement of one or more salivary and/or lacrimal glands with accompanying dry mouth, dry eyes, and arthralgia, although to a lesser degree than what is reported in Sjögren syndrome.

- Patients are antibody negative for Ro and La but rheumatoid factor and anti-nuclear antibody positivity have been reported.
- IgG4 disease responds to immunosuppression and when suspected these individuals should be referred to rheumatology for management.

Non-inflammatory causes of salivary gland swelling

Sialosis

- Sialadenosis (sialosis) is a common, benign, non-inflammatory, non-neoplastic, bilateral, symmetrical, and painless enlargement of the parotid salivary glands, although the submandibular glands can also be affected.
- The underlying pathology is acini hypertrophy.
- Causes include drugs, alcohol, diabetes, pregnancy, malnutrition, anorexia, and bulimia.

Adenomatoid hyperplasia of the minor salivary glands

- This presents as an asymptomatic tumour-like mass with localized hyperplasia of the minor salivary glands.
- The palatal mucosa is the most common site, and the aetiology of this condition is unknown.
- As the clinical appearance can often mimic a malignancy, biopsy is undertaken to confirm the diagnosis.

Necrotizing sialometaplasia

- Uncommon, benign, self-limiting condition which presents as a swelling which ulcerates and may be preceded by paraesthesia.
- This condition commonly affects the minor salivary glands of the palate and is thought to be due to ischaemia of the minor salivary glands through trauma (e.g. dental injections, smoking, or vascular disease).
- Clinically this can resemble a malignancy, so a biopsy is undertaken to confirm diagnosis.

Mucocele

- These appear as blue, fluctuant, dome-shaped cystic lesions of minor salivary glands thought to be caused by trauma to the minor salivary gland duct.
- The commonest site of presentation is the lower labial mucosa, buccal mucosa, or ventral aspect of tongue, although they can be seen on the palate, where they may discharge to give a painful erosion.
- If spontaneous resolution does not occur, surgical excision may be required.

Ranula

- A ranula is a retention cyst usually observed on the floor of the mouth and thought to be due to obstruction of the sublingual gland.
- It presents as a blue, dome-shaped, fluctuant swelling.
- It is classified as simple if confined to sublingual space or deep if it dissects through mylohyoid and presents as a central neck swelling (plunging ranula).
- Treatment is surgical and may involve gland removal.

Sialoliths

- Sialoliths are calcified structures that develop in salivary ductal systems.
- The submandibular gland is most commonly affected although minor salivary glands can also be affected.
- Patients usually present with episodic pain or swelling of affected gland especially at mealtimes.
- A radio-opacity may be noted on X-ray in either the gland or duct.
- Management involves removal of the stone and sometimes the gland.

Pneumoparotitis

- A process whereby pressurized air from the mouth is introduced into the parotid duct.
- This condition is frequently seen in those individuals with raised intraoral pressure such as those individuals who play wind instruments or balloon or glass blowers.

Neoplasms of the salivary glands

- Most common neoplasm of mouth after squamous cell carcinoma with ~600 registered every year. They are epithelial in origin and usually present with painless unilateral swelling.
- The parotid gland is the most common site, followed by the submandibular and minor salivary glands. Tumours of the sublingual gland are rare.
- The smaller the gland, the more likely the tumour is malignant.
- Features suspicious of malignancy include facial palsy, sensory loss, pain, difficulty swallowing, trismus, and rapid growth.
- A number of factors have been implicated in development of salivary gland tumours. These include smoking, infections, occupational exposure to chemicals, and those exposed to radiation.
- Benign tumours include pleomorphic salivary adenomas and Warthin's tumours.
- Malignant tumours include mucoepidermoid carcinomas, adenoid cystic carcinomas, and polymorphous low-grade adenomas.

Pleomorphic salivary adenoma

- Most common salivary gland tumour which is largely benign.
- About 75% of these tumours arise in the parotid gland. Intraorally, they may be seen at the junction of the hard and soft palate.
- They are slow growing, rubbery, or lobulated.
- Usually, benign can recur if incomplete excision (3% recur in 5 years).
- Treatment involves wide excision as there is a tendency to seed and recur in incision scar if opened at surgery or incomplete excision.
- Carcinoma ex pleomorphic adenoma is defined as a carcinoma arising in a pre-existing pleomorphic adenoma and tends to recur and metastasize.

Warthin's tumour

- Usually presents as a painless, slow-growing, soft or fluctuant parotid mass.
- These benign tumours are commoner in males and found in smokers, those with autoimmune disease, and those exposed to radiation.
- They respond to enucleation.

Adenoid cystic carcinoma
- Rare, slow-growing, and malignant tumour which infiltrates, spreads perineurally, and metastasizes to distant sites.
- On histopathology it has a 'Swiss cheese' appearance.

Mucoepidermoid tumours
- Most common childhood neoplasm which is slow growing. It usually presents as a slow-growing, painless, firm, encapsulated swelling which can be low grade and high-grade malignant tumours.
- Treatment involves wide excision but may recur.

Polymorphous low-grade adenoma
- Arises in minor glands, usually palate and is slow growing.
- Invasive and can spread along nerve sheaths.
- Rarely metastasizes.

Management of salivary neoplasms
- Benign parotid tumours managed by partial or complete parotidectomy.
- Malignant tumours are managed by wide local excision and adjuvant radiotherapy.

Facial pain

May be dentoalveolar, mucosal, musculoligamentous, or neurovascular in origin. This section will focus on musculoligamentous and neurovascular causes of orofacial pain.

Musculoligamentous

Temporomandibular disorder

- A group of conditions that affect the TMJs, muscles of mastication, and associated tissues.
- This condition typically occurs in the second to third decade and is twice as common in females compared to males.
- It is often seen in combination with other chronic pain conditions such as irritable bowel syndrome and fibromyalgia.
- The aetiology is multifactorial.
- Clinically, this condition may present with pain in the TMJ or muscles of mastication with radiation, joint noise on movement, and, in extreme cases, episodes of jaw locking.
- Headache, otalgia, and tinnitus are frequently reported in addition.
- Diagnosis is clinical and confirmed on elicitation of pain on provocation. Be vigilant for history of previous malignancy, lymphadenopathy, neck masses, sensory or motor function, trismus, unexplained weight loss or pyrexia, age at presentation, and occlusal changes as these suggest a more sinister cause.
- Temporomandibular disorder is managed using a combination of patient education, self-management skills, physical therapies, and psychological and medical interventions.

Neurovascular

Primary headaches

Migraine

- Neurological condition characterized by attacks of headache; hypersensitivity to visual, auditory, olfactory, and cutaneous stimuli; with accompanying nausea and vomiting.
- Migraine is episodic if it occurs <15 days per month and chronic if it persists more frequently than this.
- Attacks normally last for 4–72 hours and are characterized by unilateral frontotemporal pain which is provoked by physical activity, foods, odours, sleep deprivation, and so on and relieved by resting and medication.
- Onset is usually in childhood with a reduction in incidence after the fourth decade.
- Management includes treating the acute symptoms using a combination of analgesics and/or triptans.
- Prophylactic treatment is used when attacks occur more than twice weekly and there is interference with quality of life.
- This includes the use of beta-blockers, calcium channel blockers, and antiepileptics.
- Second-line treatments include use of tricyclic antidepressants.
- Imaging is indicated if the headache pattern changes, in late-onset presentation, or there are accompanying features such as seizures.

- Migraine can present as facial pain. This is rare and attacks typically last for ~60 minutes.
- The second and third branches of the trigeminal nerve are involved. Patients present with a throbbing mid to lower facial pain which may be accompanied by autonomic features and nausea. These individuals appear to respond to conventional migraine treatments.

Tension headaches

- May be acute or chronic, bilateral, and present as a mild to moderate squeezing sensation which has no accompanying features and are not aggravated by physical activity.
- Tension headaches may last from minutes to days and are thought to be provoked by stress and are relieved by stretching, exercise, and medication such as analgesics.

Trigeminal autonomic cephalgias

Unilateral headache accompanied by ipsilateral cranial autonomic features including lacrimation, conjunctival injection, epistaxis, and nasal symptoms.

Cluster headache

- This is the most common of the trigeminal autonomic cephalgia group of headaches and is characterized by severe boring pain affecting the retro-orbital or temporal areas with accompanying autonomic features which lasts between 15 and 180 minutes.
- During attacks, patients are restless and the pattern of attacks demonstrates a circadian rhythm occurring at predictable times over a 24-hour period for a period of time before going into remission and then recurring.
- Unlike paroxysmal facial hemicrania, this condition does not respond to indometacin.
- Acute attacks respond to high-flow oxygen and triptans.

Paroxysmal hemicrania

- Differs from cluster headache in that it does not normally occur at night.
- This condition is characterized by unilateral short attacks (2 30 minutes) of pain with autonomic features typically localized to the first branch of the trigeminal nerve without a circadian pattern.
- These headaches respond to indometacin with gastric protection.

Hemicrania continua

- Unlike paroxysmal hemicrania, this is a continuous headache which varies in intensity and may be accompanied by ipsilateral autonomic features.
- Like paroxysmal hemicrania, hemicrania continuum also responds to treatment with indometacin with gastric protection.

Short-lasting unilateral neuralgiform headache attacks with conjunctival injection and tearing (SUNCT)

- Rare headache condition characterized by short episodes of recurring unilateral headache with accompanying autonomic features often triggered by cutaneous stimuli.
- Patients may experience up to 100 stabbing attacks per day which may present in three patterns. Lamotrigine is effective in around 2/3 of patients.

Giant cell arteritis
- Also known as temporal arteritis, this condition is a result of an immune-mediated attack on elastin resulting in a chronic vasculitis of large and medium-sized arteries and the arch of the aorta.
- In the head and neck region, the superficial temporal artery is the main site affected.
- This condition is a medical emergency and if untreated can result in blindness in 20% of cases.
- Aortic aneurysms and thoracic dissections are late complications.
- This condition typically presents as a new persistent headache in those aged >60 years which is usually unilateral but may be bilateral and throbbing in nature which is worse on lying down.
- In addition, patients frequently report scalp pain, jaw and tongue claudication, polymyalgic symptoms (pain, stiffness, and tenderness in the proximal muscles of the arms and legs), repeated attacks of visual loss, and constitutional symptoms including fever, weight loss, and tiredness.
- Examination may reveal the presence of tenderness in the region of the superficial temporal artery in addition to neurological and ophthalmic changes.
- Diagnosis is confirmed on biopsy, imaging, and blood investigation (erythrocyte sedimentation rate >50).
- Management in the first instance is initiation of high-dose corticosteroids with bone and gastric protection which is tapered depending on symptoms and levels of inflammatory markers.
- Affected individuals should have a chest radiograph every 2 years to monitor for the development of aortic aneurysm.

Neuropathic pain

Neuropathic pain affecting the head and neck region may be episodic as in the case of trigeminal neuralgia or glossopharyngeal neuralgia or continuous as in trigeminal neuropathic pain and burning mouth syndrome.

Trigeminal neuralgia
- The International Association for the Study of Pain describes trigeminal neuralgia as sudden, usually unilateral, severe, brief, and recurrent stabbing pain in the distribution of one or more branches of the trigeminal nerve.
- Trigeminal neuralgia may be idiopathic, the most likely cause being compression of the nerve at the root entry zone caused by atherosclerotic changes in the superior cerebellar artery.
- Alternatively, and less commonly, trigeminal neuralgia may be caused by intracranial space-occupying lesions, multiple sclerosis, or infections such as HIV.
- Trigeminal neuralgia is rare and when it occurs the right side is most commonly reported, rarely affecting the first branch of the trigeminal nerve.
- Onset is often memorable and spontaneous and characterized by severe episodes of shooting pain which lasts for seconds but recurs.
- A trigger point may be identified and there may be autonomic features or sensory changes.

- Diagnosis is based on a combination of history taking, screening questionnaires such as the Magill Pain Questionnaire, imaging, and serology to exclude infective causes.
- Medical management involves use of the anticonvulsant carbamazepine with baseline and regular blood monitoring.
- Ideally a low dose should be started and escalated every 3–7 days to determine best pain control with lowest side effects.
- Oxcarbazepine, a keto derivative, is used second line and has a similar efficacy but fewer side effects. Baclofen, pregabalin, and lamotrigine is used as add-on therapy in severe cases.
- Often affected individuals have associated fear, loneliness, and depression and psychological interventions and support groups help to overcome some of these concerns.
- Surgical options include palliative destruction procedures such as radiofrequency, glycerol rhizolysis, balloon compression, and stereotactic radiotherapy (Gamma Knife®).
- There is at least a 50% recurrence rate with these procedures and additional complications such as numbness.
- Posterior fossa procedures include microvascular decompression with an 80% chance of being pain free with a recurrence rate of 4%.
- Complications of this procedure include the risks associated with a GA, hearing loss, stroke, and meningitis.

Glossopharyngeal neuralgia

- Sudden onset of short episodes of severe pain in the distribution of the glossopharyngeal nerve.
- Pain is most common in the posterior pharynx, soft palate, base of tongue, ear, tonsil, and angle of mandible.
- Triggering factors may include coughing, swallowing, talking, chewing, and yawning.
- Cardiac syncope may be an accompanying feature. Diagnosis is based on a combination of history and imaging.
- Management is pharmacological and similar to management of trigeminal neuralgia. If cardiac syncope is a feature, pacing may be needed.

Post-herpetic neuralgia (PHN)

- Pain that persists 3–6 months after a herpetic skin eruption is referred to as PHN.
- Patients describe a severe often burning pain with associated allodynia and hyperalgesia.
- Management of PHN is very difficult and involves the membrane stabilizing anticonvulsants such as oxcarbazepine, gabapentin, and pregabalin.

Trigeminal neuropathic pain

- This condition describes facial pain resulting from unintentional injury to the trigeminal system through, for example, dental infections, trauma (extractions or root canal treatment), or stroke.
- This pain is described as tingling, burning, stinging, or pins and needles. Often there is associated allodynia.

- Management involves a combination of medical interventions such as tricyclic antidepressants and anticonvulsants and psychological interventions.

Persistent idiopathic facial pain (PIFP)

- Previously known as atypical facial pain, PIFP refers to variable chronic persistent pain within the distribution of the trigeminal nerve which may be continuous, of varying intensity, and often described as deep and poorly localized.
- Pain has often been present for years, frequently crosses anatomical boundaries, and radiates to areas not supplied by the same sensory nerve.
- The pain is often described as severe, crushing, or burning with no identifiable cause and does not waken affected individuals from sleep. A significant proportion of these patients have psychiatric findings including depression.
- A combination of psychological interventions and medical treatments including use of tricyclic antidepressants and anticonvulsants are used in the management of these individuals.

Burning mouth syndrome

- Also known as glossopyrosis, glossodynia, and oral dysesthesia. Burning mouth syndrome is a benign condition that presents as a burning, scalded, or tingling sensation affecting the oral mucosa in the absence of any detectable mucosal changes and abnormal blood tests.
- It affects ~2% of the population with females seven times more likely to be affected compared to males.
- In 20% of cases it may be associated with a psychogenic cause such as anxiety, depression, cancer phobia, and concerns about a sexually shared infection.
- The current theory is that it is a neuropathic disorder with reduced pain and sensory thresholds. It frequently affects the anterior tongue, followed by the palate, lips, and lower alveolus.
- Three types have been recognized:
  - Type 1: comes on as the day goes on, unremitting.
  - Type 2: on waking and throughout the day.
  - Type 3: no regular pattern.
- Eating and drinking are reported as relieving factors and there is no reported sleep disturbance. Patients also frequently report dry mouth and taste disturbances.
- Management involves eliminating potential causes of oral burning and utilizes a combination of patient education and reassurance, topical analgesics such as benzydamine hydrochloride and lidocaine gel, psychological interventions such as cognitive behavioural therapy, and medical treatments in the form of tricyclic antidepressants and anticonvulsants.

Further reading

British Dental Journal (2017). Oral medicine themed edition. *Br Dent J* 223.

Hassan N, Dasgupta B, Barraclough K (2011). Giant cell arteritis. *Br Med J* 342, d3019.

Osailan S, Pramanik R, Shirodaria S, et al. (2011). Investigating the relationship between hyposalivation and mucosal wetness. *Oral Dis* 17, 109–114.

Houghton AR, Gray D (2010). *Chamberlain's Symptoms and Signs in Clinical Medicine: An Introduction to Medical Diagnosis* (13th ed). CRC Press.

Lewis MAO, Lamey PJ (2019). *Oral Medicine in Practice* (4th ed). Springer.

Primary Dental Journal (2016). Oral medicine themed edition. *Prim Dent J* 5(1).

Zakrzewska J (Ed) (2009). *Orofacial Pain*. Oxford University Press.

Chapter 8

Special care dentistry

Introduction to special care dentistry

Definition

Special care dentistry (SCD) is a specialty that focuses on the delivery of oral care for people with an impairment or disability and is defined broadly as: 'The improvement of oral health of individuals and groups in society who have a physical, sensory, intellectual, mental, medical, emotional or social impairment or disability or, more often, a combination of a number of these factors' (Joint Advisory Committee for Special Care Dentistry, 2003).

Special care services

The majority of special care dental services are located within community dental clinics in primary care, with a smaller proportion in secondary care trusts. While GDPs contribute to the overall picture of SCD, only a small number of practitioners currently have a specialist interest in this field. The ideal model is to provide services via managed clinical networks that focus on collaboration between various stakeholders with the aim of improving patient outcomes and access to specialist care when required. The case mix and complexity of patients (Table 8.1) should determine which setting is most suitable for treatment.

Table 8.1 Treating special care patients

GDP	Community dental services	Hospital
ASA I and II	ASA I–III	ASA I–IV
Can sit in dental chair	Requires a hoist/domiciliary care	Requires bariatric chair/stretcher
Able to cooperate with treatment under LA	Requires inhalation sedation/IV sedation/intranasal sedation	Requires inhalation sedation/IV sedation/intranasal sedation/multidrug sedation/GA
No medical input required	Liaison with GMP	Liaison with multidisciplinary medical/dental teams
Care provided by GDP/dentist with special interest	Care provided by dental officers and specialists	Care overseen by consultants/specialists

Education and training in special care

The specialty is growing and there is an increasing need to recruit dentists on the approved 3-year training pathway, which leads to specialist registration. Entry requirements vary depending on region, but generally applicants should demonstrate the following: experience post primary dental qualification within community and secondary care; publications in peer-reviewed journals; participation in audit and research; and experience of treatment under LA/sedation/GA.

Assessing the special care patient

History

Presenting complaint

It may be difficult to ascertain an accurate pain history from a patient who has communication difficulties or a learning disability. The following may indicate a potential dental problem:

- A change in behaviour: aggression, biting, sleep disturbance.
- Refusing to eat.
- Finger in the mouth, hitting of the face, night-time crying.
- Swelling of the face.

Medical history

Establishing an accurate medical history is paramount to the provision of dental care:

- Ask thorough questions regarding all health systems.
- Record current medications and any medications used to control behaviour that are prescribed to use when required (e.g. lorazepam, promethazine).
- Pay particular attention to patients who may have a bleeding condition that may be physiological or related to prescribed drugs.
- Ask the patient or carer when the last annual health check with the GMP was.
- Record the names of all medical physicians involved in the patient's medical care as you may need to liaise with them. Include community teams such as learning disability teams and community psychiatry.
- For patients with challenging behaviour, identify type, triggers, and methods of de-escalation to reduce risk of harm/injury to the patient and everyone involved in their care.
- If a GA is planned, this is an ideal opportunity to find out if other medical procedures/investigations are outstanding and whether these can be undertaken at the time of the dental GA.
- Although this multidisciplinary approach takes a lot of coordination, it will provide the most holistic outcome for the patient.
- Establish an accurate GA/sedation history, making note of dates, anaesthetic difficulties, premedication used/routes of administration, and complications. It is worth noting what worked well previously and any work-up that was required.

Social history

For an accurate social history, the following information should be gathered:

- Elicit place of residence. Types include: residential home with 24-hour care; supported living where carers visit a patient living independently at home; private residence with family; homeless.
- Determine who the patient's next of kin is, and in the absence of a next of kin, whether the patient has a close friend (➔ Consent).
- Does the patient attend a day centre, and has anyone in the day centre noticed any change in behaviour?
- Ask whether the patient is known to social services or special teams such as the learning disability or safeguarding adults team.
- Identify the following social habits (➔ Substance misuse):

- Alcohol consumption: maximum limit of 14 units a week spread over 3 days or more.
- Smoking: cigarettes, betel nut, or loose tobacco.

Substance misuse is common among some special care groups. Commonly misused drugs include depressants (e.g. heroin, benzodiazepines), stimulants (e.g. cocaine), and amphetamines. Cannabis is more commonly consumed, so identify form and frequency. While some drugs are taken orally, IV administration will increase risk of blood-borne viruses (hepatitis B/C, HIV), make IV access difficult, and interfere with treatment under sedation.

Dental history
- Previous dental treatment and treatment modality.
- What treatment has been successful in the past and measures that have facilitated this (e.g. morning appointments).
- Where does the patient have their regular dental treatment or reviews, if at all (e.g. domiciliary, community dental services)?

Examination

Extraoral
- Check for any obvious facial swellings.
- Signs of self-harm are commonly seen on the hands or face and an indication of excessively challenging behaviour in patients with a learning disability.
- Check the patient's BMI (weight(kg)/height (m²)). You may have to estimate this if there is a lack of patient cooperation or if the patient is wheelchair bound.
- Look at the patient: do they look well? Note abnormalities in skin, scars from surgery, hearing aids, tracheostomies, abnormal facial features, and use of walking aids.

Intraoral
- This may not always be possible due to challenging behaviour and lack of cooperation. Using distraction, bite blocks, finger props, or a toothbrush may aid brief examination.
- Make a note of the oral hygiene which may be poor in patients with behavioural problems. Calculus deposits can be heavy in percutaneous endoscopic gastrostomy (PEG)-fed patients.
- Check for intraoral pathology and soft tissue swellings. Make note of any carious teeth and which teeth are functional as you may decide to extract non-functional molar teeth under GA (e.g. 8s).

Investigations

- Radiographs: if the patient has multiple carious lesions, then a DPT may be more useful than multiple intraoral radiographs. Radiographs may only be possible under sedation or GA.
- Endodontic assessment of teeth showing signs of irreversible pulpitis or PA periodontitis (i.e. percussion, mobility, vitality, periodontal probing depths).
- Preoperative blood tests if possible and medically indicated.
- Capacity assessment (➔ Consent).

Baseline readings
- BMI (kg/m²): normal = 18–25; overweight = 26–30; obesity 1 = 31–35; obesity 2 = 36–40; obesity 3 = >40.
- Blood pressure: as hypertension is a silent disease, you may be the first health practitioner to identify it. If high (>200/110 mmHg), retake two more times. If still high, then defer treatment and advise patient to seek treatment from GMP.
- Palpate appropriate veins (in antecubital fossa or dorsum hand) to identify any potential problems with cannulation.
- Baseline SpO_2 should be between 95% and 100%; patients with respiratory problems may have low baseline SpO_2 of <94%.

Legislation relevant to special care

Assessing capacity to consent

Obtaining valid consent is often one of the most challenging tasks in SCD. While patients with severe learning disabilities may obviously lack capacity, those with mild to moderate learning disabilities may be more difficult to assess depending on the treatment involved.

For consent to be valid, a two-stage capacity assessment should be undertaken:

- *Stage 1*: does the patient have a disturbance or impairment in the functioning of the mind?
- *Stage 2*: does this disturbance affect the patient's decision-making ability for a specific treatment or task, that is, can the patient understand, recall, and weigh up the information presented, and are they able to communicate a decision?

Mental Capacity Act 2005 (MCA)

For those who lack capacity, health professionals need to follow the five principles of the MCA:

- Principle 1: patients should be presumed to have capacity unless proven otherwise.
- Principle 2: patients' decision-making should be enhanced through additional communication aids if applicable (e.g. sign language).
- Principle 3: patients are entitled to make unwise decisions.
- Principle 4: treatment must be in the patient's best interest.
- Principle 5: the treatment should be the least restrictive option. For example, if a patient requires excessive restraint to carry out treatment and the risk of harm under sedation/LA is high, then GA would be the least restrictive option.

Involving other parties

All attempts should be made to involve family members and consider their opinions. There are occasions when involvement of a third party becomes necessary:

Independent mental capacity advocate (IMCA): IMCAs should be consulted if a patient has no relatives or friends who can aid decision-making for serious medical treatment—whether this includes dental treatment, sedation, or GA is controversial and remains at the discretion of the dentist and the IMCA. Dentists should refer to local service guidelines and policies regarding involving IMCAs.

A lasting power of attorney (LPA): allows patients to appoint an adult to make decisions and manage finances, health, and welfare on their behalf should they lack capacity in the future (e.g. dementia). Dentists should make enquiries about the attorney's involvement in the patient's life and the extent to which they can make decisions (e.g. is the LPA limited to finances or does it include health?).

Advanced directives: allows competent adults (18 years+) to make advanced decisions and set out particular types of treatment they do not want should they lack the capacity.

Best interest meetings

A best interest meeting can be arranged to discuss the treatment plan for a patient who lacks capacity and may involve carers, the next of kin, IMCAs, LPAs, anaesthetist, and other healthcare professionals.

In urgent circumstances where the patient is at risk of rapid deterioration, the best interest decision may be made on the day,

Either way, involvement of those with an interest in the patient's care is necessary to comply with best practice, and documentation of how a best interest decision was made is essential.

Restraint

The MCA allows physical restraint, but only in situations where it is necessary to prevent harm to the patient.

Any restraint must be reasonable and in proportion to the potential harm. In SCD, the term 'clinical holding' is used to describe situations where it may be necessary to support the patient in accepting treatment. For example, a member of staff may support the head of a patient who has involuntary movements in order to extract a tooth.

In situations where high levels of clinical holding are needed, the clinician should re-evaluate the situation and consider alternatives to providing treatment such as the use of sedation or GA.

Use of excessive restraint could result in harm to the patient so should be approached with caution.

Disability laws

Disability discrimination laws were enforced in 1995. Current legislation gives disabled people the right to bring a civil claim against a practice that they consider has discriminated against them.

The Disability Discrimination Act 1995 was introduced in phases:
- 1996: it became unlawful for service providers to treat disabled people less favourably for a reason related to their disability.
- 1999: service providers were required to make reasonable adjustments in the provision of services for disabled people (e.g. domiciliary visits, texting appointments, or emailing information to people with a hearing impairment).
- 2004: service providers were required to make reasonable adjustments to the physical features of their practices to overcome physical barriers to care (e.g. lifts, ramps, improving signage).
- The Equality Act 2010 has now taken over from the Disability Discrimination Act to guarantee equality to all. Under the Equality Act, disabled people should be treated equally and should have access to health, education, employment, services, facilities, and transport.

Access

Innovative approaches need to be employed in order to improve access to dental services, especially for special care patients who might encounter financial, organizational, and sociocultural barriers. Access is more complex than just offering patients a reasonable supply of services. The following domains should be considered when assessing access and are based on the Penchansky and Thomas' model of access blended with Maxwell's dimensions of healthcare quality (effectiveness, efficiency, equity, access, acceptability, and appropriateness).

The 'six As' of access

1. *Availability*: refers to the number and type of services in the area. Is there a GA or sedation service available for patients with a learning disability?
2. *Accessibility*: the way in which patients reach the clinic (inter- and intra-building), such as distance from home, lift access, ramps, transport services, and other requirements of the Equality Act 2010.
3. *Accommodation*: the ease with which a patient can get an appointment. Is the service flexible enough to see the patient if they are late due to carer support or transport issues? Is there a walk-in service for special care patients who are in pain?
4. *Acceptability*: patient satisfaction with the service but also includes acceptance criteria for referrals, such as whether the practice accepts ASA III patients and those exempt from NHS charges.
5. *Appropriate to need*: is the service user obtaining what s/he requires from the profession?
6. *Affordability*: refers to the ability to pay for costs of dental healthcare. This includes hidden costs of travel, parking, and oral hygiene aids.

Case mix tool

This British Dental Association-developed tool[1] serves as an aid for the complexity assessment regarding treatment provision for patients with disability. It takes into account a number of patient factors and not just the complexity of treatment but those of access. Furthermore, case mix can serve as a tool for commissioning services, though it can be very subjective. Contracts should therefore reflect the nature of the patients seen and the additional resources that are needed to deliver treatment (e.g. hoists). Its use, however, has been limited to the community dental services and is utilized minimally in secondary care.

---

1 ஃ https://bda.org/dentists/governance-and-representation/craft-committees/salaried-primary-care-dentists/Pages/Case-mix.aspx

Communication

Communication is a cornerstone of modern dentistry and can significantly improve patient experience. This process can be disrupted in SCD in patients with hearing, visual, or intellectual impairments. Anxiety can also impact communication by making the retention and comprehension of information more difficult—a prime reason why consent for conscious sedation should be taken on a separate visit to the treatment.

Hearing impairments

Hearing impairments may be congenital or acquired as a result of trauma, pathology, and ageing. It affects 2% of young adults and 55% of those aged 60+ years. It may be mild (quietest sounds heard 25–39 decibels) to severe (quietest sounds 70–90 decibels), warranting use of sign language.
- *How to recognize*: hearing aids, hearing dogs.
- *Ways to communicate*: note which method the patient uses to communicate; ensure that hearing aids are switched on during conversation (these can be switched off when using high-speed drill); face the patient so they can lip read, minimize background noise, use visual aids, lower pitch of voice rather than shouting, use textphone/ type talk aids to communicate.

Visual impairments

Refers to visual acuity that cannot be corrected with lenses. Partially sighted patients will not be able to visualize the number of fingers held up at 6 metres, while those who are blind cannot visualize at <3 metres even with glasses, although only 4% cannot distinguish between light and dark. Aetiology includes trauma, glaucoma, diabetic retinopathy, macular degeneration, and cataracts.
- *How to recognize*: special glasses, white stick, guide dog.
- *Ways to communicate*: use tactile feedback (e.g. supporting the arms), face the patient during conversation, be descriptive about the procedure and sensations they may feel, ensure Ariel font is used in size 14 on leaflets in mixed case.

Speech impairments

Communicating with someone who has a speech impairment can make it difficult to understand a patient's needs. Aetiology includes stroke and muscular disorders (e.g. multiple sclerosis (MS)), which can result in aphasia (decreased speech production and understanding) and dysarthria (decreased phonation and articulation) respectively (➲ Movement disorders).
- *Ways to communicate*:
  - Ask closed questions for which the answers are yes/no.
  - Check that you have understood by repeating back the conversation.
  - Use the following alternative augmentative communication aids: text to speech software, talking mats, pen and paper, e-mail, voice recognition software.

Domiciliary care

What is domiciliary care?

For patients who are unable to attend the dental clinic, most community dental services offer dental treatment in the patient's residence. Domiciliary visits are a good way of understanding the difficulties a patient may face in daily living and oral hygiene maintenance.

Domiciliary care groups include patients who are *bed bound*:

- Have physical disabilities extensive enough to make access difficult.
- Refuse to leave their residence due to social phobia (e.g. agoraphobia).
- Have dementia.
- Are inpatients and are unable to attend a dental clinic (e.g. geriatric patients).

Preparation for the domiciliary visit

- Ensure each patient knows approximately what time you will arrive to avoid clashes with other health visits and carer support.
- Read through patient records to plan your treatment and ensure you have the suitable materials available.
- Check your emergency drugs bag and expiry dates. You must carry all the drugs that dentists are expected to use in an emergency.
- Update your clinic staff of your whereabouts regularly.
- Carry an alarm.
- Never attend a residence alone—always have a chaperone.
- Ensure you are positioned closest to the door.
- If you feel unsafe at any point, leave the patient's premises.

Treatment planning for domiciliary patients

A definitive treatment plan is not always possible and is dependent on the cooperation of the patient and the availability of equipment and materials. Here are a few points to consider:

- If at all possible, try and arrange a single visit to dental surgery where high-quality, low-maintenance dentistry is carried out along with any surgical treatment.
- Dentures are often the easiest dentistry to carry out in a patient's home as the materials are easily transportable and positioning is less of a problem.
- Be realistic—will the patient comply with treatment over several visits? Will they tolerate prosthesis? Patients with advanced dementia may be less cooperative, and may refuse to wear dentures or lose them due to memory loss, contraindicating provision.
- Optimize the patient's oral health prior to extractions bearing in mind that ~25% of domiciliary patients have been found to be taking bisphosphonates.[1] Extract a single tooth and assess healing before proceeding with further extractions.

Mobile dental units (MDUs)

- These units are mobile vans with fully equipped dental surgeries. MDUs have their benefits for hard-to-reach groups who have limited

1 Shehabi Z (2014) *J Disabil Oral Health* 15, 5.

access to dental care, transportation problems, and poor appointment attendance.

- Often services that run MDUs liaise with other organizations that host local programmes to facilitate access (e.g. day centre projects for mental health patients).
- This can improve efficiency as the day centre team can prepare the patient beforehand by completing the medical history forms in advance and ensuring attendance.
- The MDUs should be designed to allow access for disabled people. All normal regulations that govern delivery of care and manage quality of care and risk should be adhered to (e.g. infection control, sterilization, COSHH).
- Other practical issues that need particular attention include records management and storage, and access to emergency appointments.
- At the end of each clinical session, the lead clinician must ensure that all equipment is fastened securely to prevent damage during transportation.
- Disadvantages of MDUs include cost of purchase and maintenance, insurance, overnight parking, and need for a competent driver. Lack of equipment and time restraints may limit surgical treatment and advanced restorative rehabilitation.

Prison dentistry

People in prisons are four times more likely to have caries and periodontal disease when compared to their peers in the general population.[2] This may be a result of poor lifestyle and lack of oral health education. They are also more likely to misuse illicit substances and suffer from mental health problems. Dental services are available in all prison categories (A (high security) to D (low security)), although they are often limited. Waiting lists are long, and the ongoing transfer of prisoners makes ongoing care almost impossible.

- Leave all mobile phones and sharp items at home as these will not pass through security. If you do accidently take them in, expect to get a formal warning.
- Always count instruments before and after every patient—dental instruments are ideal weapons for prisoners.
- Keep all instruments behind you so they are inaccessible to patients.
- Never leave a prisoner alone in the dental surgery.
- Always ensure a guard is present within the surgery especially in a high-security category A prison and identify all panic alarms.
- Use good behaviour management—prisoners too have dental anxiety.
- Prioritize treatment of symptomatic teeth especially if the prison waiting lists are long.
- Ask the patient if they are sentenced or on remand. Patients on remand are only entitled to emergency dental care.

2 Patel R (2014). A Survey of Dental Services in Adult Prisons in England and Wales. Public Health England.

Treatment under general anaesthesia

While the majority of patients are able to have treatment under LA or sedation, for those with challenging behaviour, treatment under GA may be the only option. The notes in this section are intended as a guide for DF trainees involved in GA procedures in SCD.

Preoperative work-up

* Formulate an accurate and realistic treatment plan. For many non-cooperative special care patients, this may simply be 'examine under anaesthesia and any necessary treatment'. Include all special investigations that need to be carried out.
* Obtain valid consent if the patient has capacity, or involve all parties for best interest decisions if the patient lacks capacity.
* Update current medical history and write to GMP for confirmation if necessary.
* Liaise with the anaesthetist for patients who are ASA III or IV or who have cardiorespiratory involvement—a full anaesthetic assessment and further testing may be required if the patient has some degree of cooperation (e.g. electrocardiogram, echocardiogram, lung function tests).
* Preoperative bloods (where possible): FBC, U&E, liver function tests, clotting, and haemoglobin electrophoresis (if sickle cell suspected).
* Give fasting instructions: usually NBM for 6 hours preoperatively for solids, 2 hours preoperatively for clear liquids. Most regular medications can be taken as normal with a sip of water.

Day of surgery

* Check availability of all dental and medical records.
* Update medical history.
* Check fasting instructions have been followed.
* Check appropriate postoperative care is available.
* Most special care patients are suitable for day case procedures, but you may need to book a bed if postoperative monitoring is required for medically complex patients.
* Admission nurses will usually carry out the following checks where possible: height, weight, blood pressure, pulse, SpO_2, blood glucose if diabetic.
* The anaesthetist and the dentist should reassess the patient and reconfirm consent in the admissions area.
* Premedication may be necessary if the patient has challenging behaviour. Usual premedication oral regimens include 20 mg midazolam, 20 mg temazepam but up to 80 mg if necessary; 3–5 mg/kg ketamine; clonidine.

Multidisciplinary input

For many patients with severe learning disabilities, the only way by which investigations and interventions are possible is under GA. It is therefore important that the special care team liaise with appropriate medical physicians to coordinate care under the same GA, thereby minimizing repeat anaesthetic procedures. Examples include liaising with the following:

- GMPs who may request routine blood tests and scans. Some genetic tests may be requested but require specific blood bottles and transport to specialized laboratories.
- Ophthalmology for eye assessments especially those who are diabetic.
- Gastroenterology for PEG insertions and changes.
- ENT for patients who are unable to communicate their pain but display behaviour which may indicate an ear problem (e.g. fingers in ears, discharge from ears).
- Theatre preparation and patient safety.

The WHO surgical safety checklist suggests a series of steps to be taken to minimize avoidable harm to patients (Table 8.2).

Table 8.2 Surgical safety checklist

Start of list	Equipment checked including anaesthetic machine and emergency equipment
Sign in Before anaesthetic induction	Anaesthetist & assistant & scrub team: Medication checked and labelled Patient airway assessed Patient temperature >36°C Verify patient details, allergy status, procedure, consent Surgical team checks all radiographs and equipment present
Time out Before draping	Team introduction Reconfirm patient name, DOB, hospital number, consent, procedure, and site VTE prophylaxis, pregnancy status checked, allergy status, infection risk, glycaemic control Anticipated problems discussed
Sign out Before wound closure	Full count of swabs, instruments, and sharps Surgeon confirms procedure performed Theatre team confirms throat pack and tourniquets removed Specimens labelled correctly Handover to recovery area

A comprehensive restorative treatment plan that takes into account long-term oral health is ideal. It is advisable to have the opinion of a second experienced clinician regarding the treatment plan for patients who lack capacity and who failed to cooperate with preoperative intraoral examination.

Conscious sedation

Definition

'A technique in which the use of a drug, or drugs, produces a state of depression of the CNS enabling treatment to be carried out, but during which communication is maintained' (Intercollegiate Advisory Committee for Sedation in Dentistry, 2015).[1]

Conscious sedation drugs

Midazolam

This is a benzodiazepine that exerts its effects on the CNS by enhancing the inhibitory actions of gamma-aminobutyric acid (GABA), thereby resulting in anxiolysis, sedation, muscle relaxation, and anterograde amnesia. Its wide safety margin and short duration of action (~30–40 minutes) has made it the most widely used drug of choice for chairside conscious sedation in dentistry. The elimination half-life is approximately 2–3 hours, a prime reason why an escort is essential until the following day. Midazolam is metabolized by the liver and excreted by the kidneys and any patients with advanced disease should be referred to secondary care. Remimazolam is a new drug that has a shorter half-life than midazolam and may offer benefits of a shorter recovery time. Its use in dentistry is in its infancy but current trials look promising, and its use may become more widespread in the near future.

Flumazenil

Competitive antagonist for the benzodiazepine receptor. The ring structure is absent on flumazenil which has a neutral effect on GABA. Has a decreased half-life than midazolam = 1–1.5 hours and reverses all the effects of midazolam except the amnesia. Although it has a shorter redistribution half-life than midazolam, re-sedation is unlikely to occur.

Opioids

Work via mu and kappa receptors to produce CNS depression. Have a synergistic effect when administered with a benzodiazepine, resulting in more profound respiratory depression, but can also improve the quality of the sedation especially in patients where midazolam alone has failed. A dose of 50 micrograms of fentanyl is the opioid of choice as a multidrug sedation technique.

Propofol

Has rapid onset of action, improved patient comfort, and rapid clearance (half-life = 2–4 minutes), as well as prompt recovery and hence earlier discharge. Patients should be NBM 6 hours preoperatively. It should be emphasized that adequate sedation can in the majority of patients be achieved with midazolam, and that propofol use should be limited to specific cases by trained clinicians (e.g. when midazolam sedation has failed, for extremely short/long procedures).

Ketamine

This derivative of phencyclidine is a dissociative anaesthetic with analgesic properties. It has been used as a sedative agent mainly in children and the

---

1 ♫ https://www.saad.org.uk/images/Linked-IACSD-2015.pdf

psychomimetic emergence disturbances that can result are of little concern to patients. As it is a stimulant, blood pressure and pulse rate may rise.

Nitrous oxide (N_2O)

Diffuses into blood down a gradient, concentrates in tissues of high blood flow but mechanism of action is unknown. It is a colourless, odourless, and non-irritant gas that has a low blood solubility. Titration is easy and recovery is rapid. Systemic effects include vasodilatation, reduction in rate and depth of breathing, gastrointestinal, and bone marrow suppression.

Respiratory physiology

Gas exchange of CO_2 for O_2 takes place in the capillary beds that line the alveoli. As the diaphragm and intercostal muscles contract, the thoracic cavity is enlarged as it is pulled outwards and downwards, creating negative pressure for air to be drawn in. Expiration is passive and relies on elastic lung recoil which reduces with age.

- Respiratory rate (RR) =12 18 breaths/minute.
- Tidal volume (TV) (air moved in one breath) = 500 mL.
- Minute volume = TV × RR= 12 L × 500 mL= 6 L.
- Dead space volume (DSV) (air not involved in gas exchange) = 150 mL.

For gas exchange to take place, TV should be > DSV. In the elderly, DSV is increased and breathing becomes more inefficient. In shallow breathing (which can happen during anxiety or sedation), the TV becomes insufficient to allow entry into the lungs, so encouraging patients to take slow, deep breaths would rectify this.

Inhalation sedation

A mixture of N_2O and O_2 is delivered via a nasal hood attached to a delivery system (e.g. Quantiflex). Gases are either stored centrally and are piped within the building or stored in the cylinders attached to the delivery units. Active scavenging is recommended.

- Indications: mild–moderate anxiety, where IV sedation is contraindicated, mild to moderate gagging.
- Absolute contraindications: nasal hood phobia, acute rhinitis.
- Relative contraindications: severe myasthenia gravis, severe chronic obstructive pulmonary disease, first trimester of pregnancy, severe psychological disease.
- Risks of complications: rare, but theoretically diffusion hypoxia may occur if O_2 is not administered at 100% on completion or the patient suddenly take off the nasal hood mid-sedation.

Preoperative checks

- Check consent—written consent is mandatory.
- Confirm medical history. An escort is not essential.
- Safety checks: check all in use and spare cylinders have enough gas (O_2 black cylinder with white shoulder, full = 2000 psi; N_2O blue cylinder, full 800 psi); check inflatable bag has no leaks; start flow at 6 L/minute (minute volume) then move mixer dial to 50% after which the gas flow should read 3 L/minute for each gas; switch off O_2 supply and ensure that the flow of N_2O falls to 0. This safety feature ensures that a hypoxic mixture of gas is never administered.

Method of administration
- 100% O_2 for 1 minute, relax the patient using semi-hypnotic suggestion throughout → 10% N_2O for 1 minute → a further 10% N_2O ($N_2O:O_2$ = 20:80) for 1 minute → increase N_2O by 5% increments until patient feels relaxed. Be wary of exceeding doses of >60% N_2O as you are in the third plane of anaesthesia which can potentially lead to a GA, but assess your patients clinically. Continue with psychological support throughout.
- Recovery = 100% O_2 for over 2 minutes.

The environmental impacts of N_2O are gaining widespread attention. N_2O cracking technologies are available but come at a cost. To minimize the contribution to greenhouse gases, the use of cylinders attached to the delivery heads eliminates the common issues of leakages from piped gases. Ensuring full use of the cylinders prior to returning back to gas suppliers avoids unused gas being expelled into the atmosphere.

Intravenous sedation

- Indications: moderate to severe anxiety, severe gagging, moderate to severe learning disability, involuntary movements, medical conditions exacerbated by stress (stable angina, asthma).
- Absolute contraindications: allergy to sedative drug, pregnancy.
- Relative contraindication: (may require additional monitoring, presence of an anaesthetist, or sedation in theatre) unstable cardiorespiratory disease, poorly controlled epilepsy, acute psychosis.

Preoperative checks
- Check consent—written consent is mandatory.
- Confirm medical history.
- Safety checks: O_2 present, drugs drawn up, labelled, and within expiry date, flumazenil present (for midazolam sedation), naloxone present (for opioid sedation), equipment checked and working, able and reliable escort present, suitable transport arranged.
- Record preoperative blood pressure, pulse, SpO_2.

Method of administration
1. Tie a disposable tourniquet around the arm and identify a suitable vein in the dorsum hand or antecubital fossa (for propofol, a large vein in the antecubital fossa is preferred as it reduces pain on injection).
2. Insert IV cannula (e.g. BD Venflon™, BD Nexiva™) using aseptic technique.
3. Monitor patient at baseline and throughout procedure:
   - SpO_2 using a pulse oximeter—set the audible alarm to 90%.
   - Respiratory rate (12–18 breaths/minute): also look at depth.
   - Pulse rate (60–80 bpm): often increases with anxiety and pain, so is often >100 bpm in anxious patients.
4. Administer drugs:
   - Midazolam: preferred concentration of midazolam is 5 mg/5 mL following the National Patient Safety Agency's rapid response report on midazolam overdose. Titrate 2 mg initial, wait 90 seconds, then 1 mg increments until patient appears more relaxed and is ready to accept treatment. In the elderly: 1 mg initial, wait 4 minutes, then 0.5 mg every minute.

- Fentanyl + midazolam: 50 micrograms fentanyl in 1 mL administered prior to midazolam.
- Propofol: requires separate operator and seditionist. Use target-controlled infusion or manual infusion pump. For manual infusion, administer 20–30 mg bolus depending on size and age, then place on a 200–300 mg/hour infusion rate. Adjust accordingly depending on level of sedation and observations.
5. Carry out necessary treatment then allow the patient to recover.

Postoperative checks
- Record postoperative blood pressure, pulse, SpO_2.
- Give postoperative instructions verbal and written: do not operate machinery, or sign legal binding documents, or drink alcohol until the following day, or drive.

Pre-cannulation sedation

- Indications: needle phobia, uncontrolled movements, severe learning disability, challenging behaviour.
- Advantages: facilitates cannulation.
- Disadvantages: risk of oversedation as not titrated—IV access is therefore mandatory for both oral and intranasal midazolam.
- Oral midazolam: 20 mg (formulations include 2.5 mg/mL syrup, draw up 8 mL; 5 mg/mL, draw up 4 mL) mixed with patient's preferred drink. As it can be quite bitter, use small quantities of a strong-flavoured drink. Wait at least 20 minutes then attempt cannulation.
- Intranasal midazolam: available as 40 mg/mL solution mixed with 20 mg lidocaine. Draw up 0.25–0.3 mL in a 1 mL syringe and attach a mucosal atomizer device to allow a quick spray up one nostril. Warn the patient of bleeding. Wait 7–10 minutes, then attempt cannulation.

Complications

- Conscious sedation using midazolam alone has an excellent safety profile in dentistry and serious complications are rare.[2]
- When CO_2 levels increase, H^+ ions are released into the cerebrospinal fluid and are detected by the brain's central chemoreceptors.
- An increase in tidal volume and respiratory rate results (the patient breathes deeper and faster) to blow off excess CO_2. Sedative drugs like midazolam reduce the sensitivity of central chemoreceptors to detect changes in H^+, and so the patient needs to be reminded to take deep breaths in.
- Respiratory depression occurs in all patients and rarely requires intervention more than simple tactile stimulation, airway manoeuvres, and O_2 via a nasal cannula.
- If SpO_2 continues to fall below 90%, then positive pressure O_2 and flumazenil should be administered.
- Other complications include paradoxical effects, disorientation, nausea, failed sedation, failed cannulation, hiccups (if midazolam given too quickly at high dose).

2 Shehabi Z (2018). *Br Dent J* 224, 98.

Training

Dentists wishing to carry out single-drug conscious sedation independently are encouraged to complete a training course that follows the curriculum set out by the Intercollegiate Advisory Committee for Sedation in Dentistry, which includes both theoretical and practical components, and competency assessments. For those wishing to carry out advanced multidrug techniques or propofol sedation, further training is required with a minimum pre-requisite of 100 cases in basic sedation over a 2-year period.

Substance misuse

Drug and alcohol abuse is common in patients seen within special care services. Dental implications of substance misuse include erratic behaviour, poor attendance, vague/unexplained symptoms, managing associated dental phobia, and interactions with anaesthetic drugs.

Stimulants

- Examples include amphetamine, caffeine, nicotine, cocaine, and ecstasy.
- Stimulants block the re-uptake of norepinephrine and dopamine, which cause exhilaration, increased alertness, increased heart rate, increased weight loss and metabolism, and increased respiration rate.
- *Cocaine*: coca bush leaf extract. Two main forms: (1) *powdered 'blow'*—dissolves in water then snorted/injected; (2) *hard 'crack'*—freebase form that is smoked. Oral use can numb lips and tongue and can cause soft tissue and dental erosion. It is advisable to defer dental treatment for 6 hours after last dose as the risk of cardiac arrhythmias is higher especially with LA. Sedation may be complicated by difficulty with venepuncture, and failure of adequate sedation to allow treatment.
- *Amphetamines* (speed, whiz, meth): smoked, sniffed, injected, or taken orally. No physical dependence, but associated problems with withdrawal. Dental affects include xerostomia, erratic attendance, bruxism, and interaction with midazolam and anaesthetics.

Depressants

- Examples include alcohol, benzodiazepines, inhalants, cannabis, and heroin.
- *Cannabis* (pot, grass, ganga, spliff, reef, dope, draw, herb): is derived from the Indian hemp plant that is grown in tropical countries. It uniquely has some medicinal uses and is now considered a class C drug. It may be smoked, eaten as 'cake', drunk. or injected IV. Cannabis causes euphoria, distorted and heightened images, colours, and sounds, altered tactile sensations, tachycardia, visual and auditory hallucinations, as well as extreme hunger. Complications include memory impairment, acute psychosis, schizophrenia, and bronchitis. Dental implications include abnormal behaviour, increased risk of oral cancer and caries, and difficulty achieving cooperation under sedation.
- *Heroin* (H, smack, junk, gear, horse): is an opioid derived from the opium poppy and is smoked or injected. The euphoric 'high' that it produces makes it highly addictive with severe withdrawal effects. Cardiorespiratory complications can ensue and may lead to death. Addiction programmes provide psychological and pharmacological support. Methadone is often prescribed and although it too can be addictive, withdrawal symptoms are far less. Due to its bitter taste, non-sugar formulations are preferred by addicts who tend to hold the syrup in the mouth for as long as possible for maximum euphoric effects, thereby increasing the risk of rampant caries.

Alcohol

- Alcohol misuse in UK is increasing.
- Maximum of 14 units a week spread over three days or more.
- Signs and symptoms of alcohol abuse are shown in Table 8.3.

Table 8.3 Signs and symptoms of alcohol abuse

System affected	Signs/symptoms
CVS	Blood pressure: 2× risk if drinking >6 units/day
	Arrhythmias: binge drinking affects heart conduction—palpitation and death (holiday heart syndrome)
	Cardiomyopathy → heart failure
CNS	Confabulation, Wernicke–Korsakoff disease
Vitamin deficiencies	A: night blindness
	B₁: Wernicke's encephalopathy
	B₁₂ and folate: macrocytic anaemia
	C: scurvy
	D: osteomalacia
	K: clotting deficiency
Gastrointestinal tract	Liver: hepatitis and cirrhosis
	Oesophagitis, Mallory–Weiss syndrome, cancer
	Reflux, gastritis, gastric carcinoma
	Pancreatitis: death if acute, diabetes if chronic

The dental implications of alcoholism include:
- Poor oral hygiene
- Tooth surface loss, attrition, and erosion
- Xerostomia, risk of caries, candidiasis
- Impaired wound healing (liver damage)
- Orofacial trauma
- Bleeding tendency and impaired wound healing.

Practical tips
- Enquire about the time of day the patient is likely to start drinking and arrange appointments accordingly.
- Avoid IV sedation if a patient is a heavy drinker as they may be difficult to sedate and may drink after the sedation.
- Take preoperative blood and test the FBC, U&E, liver function tests, and clotting screen.
- If alcohol is interfering with the patient's ability to consent to treatment, defer all elective procedures until the patient becomes more stable.
- Use local haemostatic measures post extraction—pressure, suture, use of haemostatic agents (e.g. surgical), and topical tranexamic acid.

Mental health disorders

Dementia

Dementia is an organic neurodegenerative disease that results in a lack of awareness of space and time. Its aetiology includes multi-infarct dementia, HIV, and trauma, but by far the most common cause is Alzheimer's disease. It is thought that Alzheimer's disease is caused by neurofibrillary tangles which can only be confirmed on autopsy.

Prevalence = 2–3% in >65-year-olds, 20% in >85-year-olds.

Stages and signs of dementia are listed in Table 8.4.

Completion of high-quality, low-maintenance treatment is critical in the early stages since the inability to cooperate increases as the disease progresses. Full mouth radiographs which may be impossible with progression of diagnosis should be taken for future reference. In the moderate–late stages of dementia, treatment under sedation/GA may be the only option. The use of clinical holding should be discussed with the patient/carers (➔ Consent), taking extreme care in the frail patient who is more prone to osteoporotic fractures.

Extractions should be carried out singly to assess healing if the patient is on oral bisphosphonates.

Table 8.4 The various stages of dementia

Stage	Signs	Dental implications
Early	Can function independently	May forget to brush teeth
	Some memory loss especially with new things, decreased concentration	Can cooperate with dental treatment with some behaviour mx
	Increasing trouble with planning or organizing	
Moderate	Confusing words, getting frustrated/angry	Poor oral hygiene
	Forgetfulness of past events	High caries rate
	Incontinence	Likely to require sedation
	Changes in sleep patterns delusions/repetitive behaviour	
Late	Decreased response to environment	As above
	Decreased ability to control movement	Treat under GA or in domiciliary care
	Decreased self-care	May decide to treat symptomatically
	Difficulty communicating	
	Vulnerable to infections, e.g. pneumonia	
	Vegetative state and death	

Schizophrenia

- Schizophrenia is characterized by thought disturbances including persecutory delusions (being spied on), thought broadcast and control, and hallucinations with a typical onset between late teens and mid-30s. It affects 1–2% of the UK population and men and women are affected equally.

- Specific causes are unknown but contributing factors include genetic predisposition, trauma, and abuse.
- Life expectancy is reduced in this group and may be due to a combination of poor diet, sedentary lifestyle, smoking (70%), obesity, coronary heart disease, and emotional problems.

Medications

- First generation: haloperidol, chlorpromazine.
- Second generation: newer, clozapine or risperidone. Less side effects.
- Side effects = tardative dyskinesia (reduced by anticholinergics).

Dental signs and symptoms

Patients with schizophrenia may exhibit the following orofacial signs and symptoms:

- Excessive drooling with clozapine which can be problematic. Patients often prescribed anticholinergics which cause xerostomia.
- Poor oral health due to lack of motivation.
- Advanced generalized periodontal disease.
- Involuntary movements of tongue, lips, jaw (tardative dyskinesias), female > male.
- Removable prostheses may be difficult to wear.
- Medication-related xerostomia, *Candida*, dysphagia, caries.

Dental management

- Reconfirm consent at every appointment as capacity may fluctuate.
- If patient is on clozapine, ask for a copy of recent bloods as it can cause neutropenia.
- Avoid inhalation sedation in patients with severe unstable psychiatric disease as hallucinations may occur.
- Do not feel pressurized to extract/treat sound teeth in patients who have false beliefs that their teeth may be a source of monitoring by external agencies.
- Ensure comprehensive records are kept, detailing conversations and incidents.

Bipolar disorders

This is a mood disorder that features manic–depressive alterations in mood and affects 1% of the population. There is a strong familial predisposition. Episodes (lasting ~3 months) of mania are characterized by feelings of elation, impulsiveness, sexual activity, excessive and theatrical speech, grandiose delusions, and little sleep. This rapidly shifts to anger then depression where there is detachment from daily life and these episodes are of a longer duration. Bipolar disorder has major impacts on social and working life as individuals find it difficult to focus on jobs and maintain relationships. Complications include substance misuse and suicide.

Medications

Manic phase = lithium (effective within 3 weeks in 70%) and neuroleptics (e.g. phenothiazine); depressive phase: antidepressants but relapses occur every 3–9 years.

Dental signs and symptoms
- Cervical abrasion due to vigorous brushing in mania.
- Drug-related xerostomia (lithium, first- and second-generation antipsychotics, anticholinergics) and its sequel.

Dental management
- Treatment in the manic phase may be difficult—avoid conscious sedation and defer elective treatment.
- Reinforce prevention, especially in the depressive phase. Prescribe 1.1% sodium fluoride toothpaste, reinforce oral hygiene, and give diet advice.
- Lithium toxicity has been reported with the use of metronidazole and prolonged use of non-steroidal anti-inflammatory drugs.[1]

1 Becker D (2008). *Anaesth Prog* 55, 89.

Movement disorders

Cerebral palsy

Aetiology

- *Prenatal*: prematurity, maternal rubella, syphilis, herpes, drugs (e.g. alcohol) diabetes, hypertension.
- *Neonatal*: hypoxia, birth injury, prolonged/difficult labour.
- *Postnatal*: trauma, brain tumours, infections (e.g. meningitis), toxins (e.g. lead).

Signs and symptoms

- Uncontrolled movements, learning disability, speech difficulties, visual and hearing impairments, epilepsy (30% of patients).
- Cerebral palsy may be classified as:
  - *Spastic* (50–60%): cortical motor area, exaggerated movements, increase in muscle tone hyperreflexia, tendency towards contractures/positioning/movement, increased spasticity, loud noises can precipitate flexion/extension.
  - *Athetoid* (20–35%): lesions of the basal ganglia (extra-pyramidal system). Writhing, wormlike movements.
  - *Ataxic* (7–15%): lesion of the cerebellum. Lack of coordination (hand to eye) and balance problems (gait).
- Dental signs include class II division 1 malocclusion, high palatal vault, drooling, caries—xerostomia, periodontal disease, bruxism.

Parkinson's disease

Aetiology

Caused by degeneration of dopamine-releasing cells in the substantia nigra. Can be genetic or idiopathic secondary to neuroleptic drugs (e.g. phenothiazines), viruses (encephalitis), and Alzheimer's disease.

Incidence of 1% in those >60 years of age (1:100) and 2% for people >85 years (1:50).

Signs and symptoms

- Symptoms occurs when 80% of dopamine producing cells are destroyed and usually appear >50 years of age.
- Resting tremor, limb rigidity, bradykinesia (slowness in the initiation and execution of movement), shuffling gait (with slow, short steps), mask-like face due to facial rigidity, and decreased spontaneous blinking.

Gold standard treatment is levodopa which is a precursor of dopamine given to help replenish the depleted dopamine in the basal ganglia. Due to its side effects (confusion, hallucinations, dystonia, xerostomia), prescription of an inhibitor of the degradation enzyme dopa decarboxylase decreases dosage and increases concentration of dopamine centrally.

Dental implications

Excessively rigid episodes may limit access and domiciliary care may be more appropriate. Insertion and removal of dentures may be facilitated with the addition of clasps. Tremors may be severe enough to warrant treatment under sedation.

Multiple sclerosis (MS)

Aetiology

With an incidence of 1:1000, MS is caused by damage to the myelin sheath of brain and spinal cord therefore → decreased conduction of impulses. Precise aetiology is unknown, but it is thought that genetic and environmental factors play a role.

Diagnosis of MS is usually made between the ages of 20 and 40 years and the male:female ratio = 3:2.

Signs and symptoms

Includes fatigue, muscle weakness, loss of sensation, speech and visual impairment, and as diagnosis progresses → urinary incontinence, breathing problems requiring tracheostomy, dysphagia requiring gastrostomy insertion, and aspiration pneumonia. Demyelination may show up as plaques on MRI but a clinical history of two or more episodes affecting two different parts of the CNS. Types of MS include:

- *Benign* (20%): few mild attacks then complete recovery.
- *Primary progressive* (15%): symptoms worsen over time.
- *Relapsing–remitting* (25%): symptomatic and symptom free periods—develops to secondary progressive after 15 years.
- *Secondary progressive* (40%): follows relapsing–remitting MS, where symptoms become continuous later in life.

Treatment

Disease-modifying drugs (e.g. interferon beta) decrease the number of relapses and slow progression. Physiotherapy and steroids during episodes speed up recovery. A range of drugs can be prescribed to treat associated fatigue, incontinence, neuropathic pain, tremors, spasticity, and depression.

Dental implications

- There has been some suggestion that MS may be associated with the presence of amalgam restorations, but the evidence is weak. Trigeminal neuralgia can be a presenting sign of MS and should be managed accordingly.
- The combination of drugs such antidepressants, anticholinergics, and corticosteroids can result in xerostomia and its sequelae. Cannabis use in patients with MS is not uncommon (➔ Cannabis).
- Consent may prove to be challenging in the later stages of MS where the patient has retained their cognitive function but is unable to speak. Use of non-verbal communication becomes important and the patient may be able to give their consent using facial gestures such as blinking.
- Treat patient when most relaxed and keep appointments short. A semi-upright position can decrease aspiration pneumonia risk if dysphagia is evident.
- Provide low-maintenance, high-quality dentistry, taking a more aggressive approach (e.g. extractions of carious molars) in those who are likely to deteriorate soon.

Stroke

Aetiology

- 80% ischaemic thromboembolic (locally or from a distant clot), 20% haemorrhagic (secondary to intracerebral or subarachnoid haemorrhage).

- Risk factors include atrial fibrillation, hypertension, diabetes, renal disease, obesity, alcohol, age (>65 years), polycythaemia.

Signs and symptoms
- Facial palsy on the affected side impacting swallowing and eating.[1]
- Dysphagia may increase risk of aspiration pneumonia, reduce oral clearance, and increase risk of caries; patient may be PEG fed.
- Mortality rate is 20–30% within 1 month.
- Aphasia (disorder of speech processing):
  - *Broca's (expressive) aphasia*: damage to frontal lobe—patients can understand most things but have limited words to respond (e.g. may reply with 'yes' to everything).
  - *Wernicke's (receptive) aphasia*: damage to temporal lobe—patient cannot understand information but will articulate a response that is unrelated to the question asked. Patients may create own words.
  - *Global aphasia*: affects large areas of the brain—patients are unable to understand or communicate.

Management of stroke
- Investigations include video fluoroscopy for swallowing, and cerebral scans to locate emboli.
- Surgical stenting to relieve carotid stenosis.
- Anticoagulant therapy: heparin initially, then warfarin (international normalized ratio (INR) 2–3).
- Multidisciplinary input is required early on and normally involves general medical team, SALT, physiotherapy, and neurosurgery.
- Communication aids such as text to speech devices may be beneficial.

Dental implications
- Dentists should be aware of the warning signs of a stroke (FAST = **F**ace weakness, **A**rm weakness, **S**peech difficulty, **T**ime to call 999).
- Reduced dexterity can make compliance with oral hygiene difficult, and patients may require toothbrush modification to improve grip or rely on assistance of carers.
- Fixed prosthesis may be better tolerated than removable prosthesis.
- INR should be checked if the patient is on warfarin (<4 for simple extractions, <3 for advanced surgical work).
- Consider shortened dental arch.

Huntington's disease

Aetiology
- Neurodegenerative disease.
- 12.3:100,000.
- Autosomal dominant.
- Faulty gene on chromosome 4 leads to cerebral atrophy results and mutated huntingtin protein.

---

1 British Society of Gerodontology (2010). Guidelines for the oral healthcare of stroke survivors. www.gerodontology.com/content/uploads/2014/10/stroke_guidelines.pdf

Signs and symptoms

Symptoms may vary from the age of 32 to 50 years, but will gradually worsen with time, and include:
- Lack of coordination, jerky movements
- Unsteady gait
- Speech difficulties
- Swallowing difficulties, eventually resulting in gastrostomy insertion for feeding and an increased risk of aspiration pneumonia.

Suicide risk is high as patients have often cared for a parent or relative with Huntingdon's disease, and are aware of the degenerative course of the disease.

Management of Huntington's disease

Diagnosis is made through a physical and psychological examination.

If symptoms are abrupt and have random timing and distribution, they suggest a diagnosis of Huntington's disease. The *unified Huntington's disease rating scale* is used and involves motor, behavioural, cognitive, and functional assessments, MRI, and positron emission tomography scans.

Dental implications
- Reliance on carers and transport may make access difficult.
- Communication may become more problematic as speech deteriorates.
- The patient may lack capacity in the later stages. Dentists should enquire about advanced directives regarding treatment (e.g. do not resuscitate directive in the event of a cardiac arrest).
- Consider conscious sedation or GA for those with advanced disease.
- Dental disease: xerostomia, diet supplements, dexterity.

Further reading

British Dental Association. Case mix tool. ℘ https://bda.org/dentists/governance-and-representation/craft-committees/salaried-primary-care-dentists/Pages/Case-mix.aspx

British Society for Disability and Oral Health (2009). The provision of oral health care under general anaesthesia in special card dentistry (2009). ℘ http://www.bsdh.org/documents/BSDH_GA_in_SCD_2009.pdf

Equality Act 2010. ℘ https://www.legislation.gov.uk/ukpga/2010/15/contents

Intercollegiate Advisory Committee for Sedation in Dentistry (2015). Standards for conscious sedation in the provision of dental care. ℘ https://www.saad.org.uk/images/Linked-IACSD-2015.pdf

Mental Capacity Act 2005. ℘ https://www.legislation.gov.uk/ukpga/2005/9/contents

National Patient Safety Agency (2008). Reducing risk of overdose with midazolam injection in adults. ℘ https://www.sps.nhs.uk/wp-content/uploads/2018/02/2008-NRLS-1074A-midazolam-RRR-mation-2008-12-09-v1.pdf

Oral and maxillofacial pathology

Introduction to oral and maxillofacial pathology

Oral and maxillofacial pathology (OMFP) is a dental specialty concerned with the diagnosis, assessments, and pathogenesis of disease affecting the head and neck region. As such, biopsies may come from many different tissues including the oral cavity, salivary glands, sinuses, jaw bones, pharynx, larynx, and thyroid. As well as providing a diagnostic service, a large portion of the workload involves examining tumour resection specimens. This is important to allow tumour staging and grading and for the adequacy of the surgical margins to be assessed. This can influence whether any further postoperative therapy or surgery is indicated for the patient.

Some consultants are closely affiliated with dental and medical schools which creates opportunities to teach dental and medical undergraduates about the disease processes which can affect the oral and maxillofacial apparatus. Many consultants also undertake research or supervise students undertaking higher degrees.

Training in OMFP

- Specialist training in OMFP normally takes 5 years. Some positions include the opportunity to complete a PhD, which means training can take longer.
- You will usually be based at a teaching hospital, either in a separate OMFP department or as part of a general pathology service.
- The first few years are spent working closely with OMFP consultants and other trainees; this allows time for your knowledge of the basic disease processes and tumour types to develop.
- Following this, 1 year is spent in a general pathology department. Here, the specialist trainee (ST) rotates through the various branches of pathology which may include:
  - breast
  - cardiothoracic
  - cytology
  - dermatopathology
  - endocrine
  - gastrointestinal (upper and lower)
  - gynaecology
  - lymphoreticular
  - neuropathology
  - renal
  - soft tissue
  - urology.
- This allows the ST to gain an appreciation of the anatomy, physiology, and histology of different organs. This knowledge also ensures that the ST is able to recognize metastases from these organs if they were to present in the head and neck region.
- As many pathological processes and mechanisms are similar throughout the body, this year of training develops the ST's general pathology knowledge base and diagnostic skills.

- After approximately 3 years of training, the ST will sit their first professional exam called the Fellowship of the Royal College of Pathologists (FRCPath) Part 1. This is a written exam which takes the format of short answer questions.
- After a further 2 years, the ST will sit FRCPath Part 2 which is more practical and composed of numerous unseen cases to assess diagnostic accuracy. There are also practical and viva elements to this exam.
- On satisfactory completion of these exams and other requirements of training, the ST is eligible to apply for a consultant post.

The oral and maxillofacial pathology team

- Consultants/professors in OMFP.
- STs/academic clinical fellows or lecturers.
- DCTs.
- Research staff (readers/senior lecturers/lecturers/postdoctoral staff/ PhD students)—that is, non-clinical staff. They may be able to assist if you are interested in becoming involved with laboratory-based work.
- Technicians/biomedical scientists—responsible for the day-to-day running of the laboratory, including cut-up, embedding and staining specimens, and quality control within the laboratory.
- Administrators/managers—responsible for the day-to-day running of the department.
- Secretaries—typing of reports and letters.

How do I secure a DCT post?

- Applicants will be expected to have completed DFT, including experience in general dental practice and hospital environments.
- Applicants should have a broad range of experience and ideally in specialties linked to OMFP e.g. OMFS and oral medicine. Experience in pathology either by work shadowing or previous DCT experience is also desirable. Satisfactory completion of the Diploma of Membership of the Faculty of Dental Surgery (MFDS)/Membership of the Joint Dental Faculties (MJDF) is also expected and is usually listed as 'desirable' in the person specification for jobs. Posts in OMFP at DCT level are advertised as part of a central recruitment process.

How do I secure an ST post?

- Applicants will have completed placements as described for DCT posts. When applying for ST posts, applicants will have normally completed DCT posts in OMFP or be able to demonstrate they have had considerable experience of the specialty.
- As with other dental specialties, applicants who have completed audits, presentations, publications, and who have evidence of teaching will be scored highly. The most important thing is to have enthusiasm for the specialty.

What is expected of the trainee in DCT?

- Cut-up of small and medium-sized specimens according to experience.
- Reporting of the pathology (apart from major cancer cases).
- Preparing cases for the head and neck cancer MDT (➜ The Multidisciplinary team meeting).
- Help organize material for referral cases (e.g. requesting radiographs).
- Help with teaching of undergraduate students.
- Perform departmental audits and service evaluations.

Receiving specimens in the laboratory

- Specimens are received by the laboratory and assigned an identifier. Patient details on the specimen pot should be cross-referenced with the request form to make sure they match. Specimens may be received from the local dental hospital, general hospital, and all around the region; referral cases from further afield may also arrive, for the attention of the OMFP consultant(s).
- Specimens usually arrive in plastic pots containing formal saline (10%). This fixes the tissue so that it can be processed adequately. Specimens can remain preserved in formalin for many years. Most small biopsies need 24 hours to fix; larger resections may take several days. Remember, tissue shrinks when placed in formalin.
- Formal saline is harmful if inhaled or swallowed.
- It is irritating to the eyes, respiratory system, and skin and there is limited evidence of a carcinogenic effect.
- Your workspace should be sufficiently ventilated—ideally, a fume cupboard or similar.
- This material and/or its container must be disposed of as hazardous waste according to the Special Waste Regulations 1996 or according to local regulations, in compliance with Duty of Care Regulations and Special Waste Regulations.
- Sometimes 'fresh' tissue is needed for diagnosing diseases such as pemphigus and pemphigoid, so that direct immunofluorescence can be carried out. It should be sent in Michel's solution as a transport medium. Care should be taken as this medium is also irritant to the eyes, respiratory system, skin, and the gastrointestinal system, if swallowed. The tissue is frozen on arrival at the laboratory, using liquid nitrogen.
- Urgent cases should be brought to the attention of the ST or consultant to allow for timely processing and reporting.

The cut-up process

- The 'cut-up' or 'macroscopic description' involves looking at, describing, and measuring the specimen. The specimen is then cut to allow embedding into wax blocks. The laboratory staff will then prepare the blocks and slides (➔ Embedding).
- One should be mindful of:
  - cross-infection control: personal protective equipment must be worn at all times in the laboratory (laboratory coat, protective eye wear, and gloves)
  - ensuring the screen on the fume cupboard is down (if present) and the extractor fan is on.
- For each case:
  - Confirm that the patient's name and laboratory number are the same on the request form, pot, and cassette. Read it out loud. Mistakes at this stage are easily made; if there is any confusion, the requesting clinician should be contacted. Read the request form.
  - Take the specimen from the pot and place it on the board, using forceps. Describe the specimen (➔ Describing specimens).

- Measure the specimen in three dimensions in millimetres (mm).
- Trim the specimen as necessary.
- Clean equipment to prevent cross-contamination of specimens.
- Each laboratory is different so always take advice from colleagues working in your department.

Describing specimens

- Macroscopic description of specimens forms the first part of the pathology report.
- Describe:
  - the shape (e.g. ellipse, triangular, circular, fragment)
  - the nature of the tissue (hard, soft)
  - if there is any overlying mucosa
  - the colour and consistency
  - any noticeable feature (e.g. a central fissure, ulcer, cyst)
  - the size (measure length × width × depth in millimetres)
  - any distinguishing features on sectioning (e.g. presence of cyst cavity/tumour)
  - the way it has been cut (e.g. bisected, trisected)
- For example: 'an ellipse of pale brown soft tissue, with overlying white mucosa, with a central fissure, measuring 8 ×5 × 3 mm. Bisected'.
- If a tooth is present, describe it (➔ Tooth specimens).

Embedding

- Most biopsies are bisected along their long axis and embedded on their cut surfaces. Larger mucosal biopsies may be trisected.
- If the biopsy is very small (<3 mm in diameter), the specimen should be embedded 'on edge'.
- Always state how you want the specimen to be embedded during the cut-up; the chosen surface can be marked with a dot of special ink.
- Each separate representative part of a specimen, once it has been embedded in wax, is referred to as a 'block'.
- Usually, specimens are stained with haematoxylin and eosin (H&E). Other commonly used stains are described later (➔ Routine histological stains). If it is clear that other stains will be required, they can be requested during cut-up.
- A ST will monitor the DCT for the first few weeks until he/she is happy that the DCT is competent at doing cut-up. It is only by watching and doing that you learn.

Large specimens and resections

- The ST will usually be in charge of these.
- Larger specimens and specimens containing a lesion which the surgeons hope to have completely excised need more careful sampling; the consultant pathologist is always informed of their arrival.
- Excision specimens should have been orientated by the clinician either by way of a diagram on the request form or, more accurately, by placing at least one marker suture in the tissue itself.

- The site of the suture should be indicated on the request form. If orientation is impossible, the clinician is contacted and asked to supply the required information.
- Photography may be necessary (completed by the laboratory staff) as sampling will probably involve taking a number of representative slices through the tissue at different sites.
- For cancer resections, the tissue must be sampled appropriately to allow reporting of margin involvement and to report prognostic information (e.g. maximum depth of invasion).
- Margins should be inked in different colours to aid orientation when performing histological examination.
- Jaw resections and specimens containing hard tissue can be radiographed in two planes at right angles to each other so that the extent of bone involvement can be assessed.
- Slices of bone must first be decalcified before being processed; this process can take several days to weeks.

Tooth specimens

- Teeth may be submitted for diagnosis of either enamel, dentine, or cementum defects or attached hard or soft tissue lesions. Usually, soft tissue lesions can be detached from the tooth and cut up in the usual way as for a small biopsy.
- The anatomical relationship between the tooth and soft tissue must be accurately recorded in the macroscopic description (e.g. tissue attached at amelocemental junction).
- If a tooth is to be examined for caries or a dental/enamel defect, then either decalcified or ground sections can be examined.
- Enamel can only be examined microscopically in ground sections. If examination of enamel is essential, half the tooth is initially prepared for ground section, and the other half is then decalcified for paraffin embedding.
- The tooth itself should also be described: describe the crown, shape, colour, presence of pitting, caries, and so on. Also look at the roots and describe whether they are completely formed and of normal morphology and number.

Laboratory stages following cut-up

The following information is included to give you a flavour of what happens in the laboratory after the cut-up:

Tissue processing

After cut-up, all specimens (apart from frozen and occasional special cases) are processed and embedded into paraffin blocks for sectioning. To do this, the tissue is dehydrated by passing it sequentially through graded alcohol solutions, followed by xylene, before it is then impregnated with hot wax. This is usually completed on an automated machine in the laboratory.

Embedding

Unless otherwise requested, all specimens are routinely embedded in paraffin wax. Resin embedding is requested when it is required to study fine cellular detail and is particularly useful for diagnosing lymphoid lesions such as lymphomas. Resin is a plastic which is harder than paraffin and enables thinner sections to be cut. Resin may also be used to embed hard tissues when it provides support for either decalcified or ground sections.

Sections

Unless otherwise requested, one or two stained 5 μm sections from the cut surface of the tissue block are provided and are mounted onto a single slide. During the reporting of the specimen, it may be felt necessary to look at further sections to establish the diagnosis: levels are requested when the suspected lesion is not present in the first section, or if the clinical history arouses suspicion of possible malignancy. They may also be requested if the section is poorly oriented or too superficial.

'Deepers' may sometimes be requested if the section appears to be completely unrepresentative (e.g. epithelium is missing). In this case, the laboratory will discard the initial microtome sections (ribbons) and provide you with a section taken from deeper within the specimen.

How to set up a microscope

- Turn the microscope on (the power switch is usually present on the side of the microscope).
- Position your chair so that your back is straight, and the eyepieces are level with your eyes.
- Place the slide with the details face-up and on the right of the stage. Use the clip to secure the slide.
- Adjust the interpupillary distance on the eyepiece so that you see one image through the microscope.
- Look at the slide on low power and work your way up to high power, by rotating through the lenses.
- When using high power, the upper part of the condenser needs to be rotated into place using the small lever next to it.
- You can look at different parts of the slide by using the stage controls on the right of the microscope.
- The level of light can be adjusted using the brightness control.

Routine histological stains

- All specimens are stained with H&E. Other 'special' stains you might see include the following:
  - Periodic–acid Schiff (PAS): stains carbohydrate molecules bright pink (e.g. glycogen, mucins, glycoproteins, and proteoglycans); can also be used for detecting fungal hyphae.
  - PAS/D: the 'D' stands for diastase, which will lyse any glycogen (e.g. to differentiate glycogen from mucins).
  - Congo red: stains amyloid red and should show apple-green birefringence under polarized light.
  - Perls: stains iron deposits/haemosiderin blue.
  - Fontana–Masson: stains melanin black.
  - Martius Scarlet Blue (MSB): muscle and fibrin stain red, erythrocytes are yellow, and connective tissue blue.
  - Ziehl–Neelsen (ZN): stains mycobacteria red on a blue/green background.

- Gram stain: stains Gram-positive bacteria blue and Gram-negative bacteria pink.
- Grocott: stains fungal organisms black.
- Sometimes, further investigations are required, such as:
  - immunohistochemistry
  - immunofluorescence

Writing a report

- A report may be drafted by the trainee in DCT which will subsequently be checked by the responsible consultant, which allows for excellent teaching opportunities.
- At first, report writing is difficult. All of your reports will be checked by the consultant and amended (if necessary) before being typed, so it is a worthwhile learning exercise. Use the textbooks to help you but develop your own style of writing.
- View the slide in a methodical way rather than moving around the slide too quickly. Trainees often choose to look through the high-power lenses, but a lot can be learnt from viewing the biopsy under low power first.
- Develop a methodical approach to reporting specimens. If you are reporting a mucosal biopsy, first give a general description of the tissues present and then focus on the specifics, that is, the features that support your diagnosis.

Examples of excellent reports

Example 1

Histopathological examination shows hyperplastic hyperparakeratinized stratified squamous epithelium overlying fibrovascular connective tissue with muscle at the deep aspect. The epithelium shows basal cell loss, apoptotic bodies, and lymphocyte-epithelial tropism. No dysplasia or malignancy is seen.

The features are those of a *lichenoid tissue reaction* consistent with the clinical suspicion of lichen planus.

Example 2

Hyperparakeratinized stratified squamous epithelium, overlying a nodule of relatively uninflamed and variably dense fibrovascular connective tissue. Towards the deep aspect, collections of skeletal muscle fibres and small neurovascular bundles are identified. In addition, a lobule of minor salivary gland tissue, showing acinar atrophy and ductal ectasia, is also identified.

The features are those of a *fibroepithelial polyp*.

Example of a moderately good report

Histological examination reveals a nodule of uninflamed connective tissue covered with hyperkeratinized stratified squamous epithelium.

The features are those of a *fibroepithelial polyp*.

Learning points

- The report mentions all salient features of the pathology but does not give a detailed description of the specimen.
- Hyperkeratinized is used, rather than hyperparakeratinized or hyperorthokeratinized.

Example of an unacceptable report

The basal cells in this biopsy are destroyed by lymphocytes and there is muscle at the deep aspect of the biopsy. The epithelium is atrophic. No dysplasia is seen. The epithelium also contains apoptotic bodies associated with lymphocytes. Lymphocytes are also seen in the lamina propria and extend into the epithelium.

The features are of *lichen planus*.

Learning points
- The report has poor structure.
- It begins by mentioning a very specific feature rather than giving a general description of the specimen.
- Three separate sentences regarding lymphocytes could have been grouped together.
- Important negatives such as whether dysplasia is present or not, should be mentioned in the last line of the report so it can be clearly seen by the clinician reading the report.
- The conclusion is too specific as the histological diagnosis is a lichenoid tissue reaction. Lichen planus can only be diagnosed after clinic-pathological correlation.

Sometimes a diagnosis is not straightforward. This may be because the biopsy is not representative of the lesion, too small, or because the lesion is obscured by inflammation or artefact.

In these cases, it is important to review the clinical notes and radiology to see if they may offer any more information. However, sometimes it may be necessary to ask for a further biopsy or suggest a less-specific diagnosis. For example:
- 'The biopsy is insufficient for diagnostic purposes and a repeat biopsy is recommended', or
- 'The appearances are of granulomatous inflammation. The differential diagnosis includes Crohn's disease, orofacial granulomatosis, tuberculosis, and sarcoid. Clinicopathological correlation is advised.'

It is important to realize that what you write will affect the patient's management. Incorrect diagnosis may lead to unnecessary surgery and medico-legal intervention

Pathological features of oral and maxillofacial lesions

Common lesions

Fibroepithelial polyp

A nodule of dense fibrous tissue covered by normal or hyperplastic/hyperkeratotic epithelium. The connective tissue may contain a few inflammatory cells and some metaplastic bone, especially when they occur on the gingiva.

Frictional keratosis

This is characterized by a thick layer of para- or orthokeratosis and usually a prominent granular cell layer. The epithelium may be hyperplastic or atrophic but is cytologically bland. It often occurs in sites of trauma such as the retromolar pad or along the occlusal lines on the buccal mucosa.

Pyogenic granuloma

The epithelium is ulcerated beneath which there is an exuberant mass of granulation tissue containing numerous blood vessels and plump fibroblasts. As they mature, they usually become more fibrous in nature, resembling fibroepithelial polyps.

Squamous cell papilloma

This lesion is characterized by hyperkeratotic and hyperplastic epithelium with a papillary surface pattern overlying cores of vascular connective tissue. The epithelium is often mitotically active. Koilocytes may be visible in the epithelium.

Chronic hyperplastic candidosis

Varying degrees of epithelial hyperplasia and atrophy with broad-based rete processes and neutrophils within the superficial epithelial layers, forming microabscesses. Fungal hyphae will be present and can be highlighted with PAS staining. There may be cytological atypia in reaction to the fungal hyphae.

Lichen planus/lichenoid reaction

Hyperkeratosis, basal cell liquefaction, and a band-like infiltrate of lymphocytes in the lamina propria. You may also see apoptotic bodies, hyalinization of the basement membrane, and lymphocytes extending into the epithelium.

Haemangioma

Capillary, cavernous, and mixed variants are seen. Cavernous haemangiomas consist of dilated vessels within the connective tissue, often with thrombus formation and calcification. Capillary haemangiomas contain many tiny vessels with an endothelial lining; connective tissue is often scant.

Epithelial dysplasia

Various grades are seen (mild, moderate, and severe) according to whether the dysplasia affects the lower, middle, or upper 1/3 of the epithelium. Features of dysplasia include cellular and nuclear pleomorphism, increased nuclear:cytoplasmic ratio, increased mitoses, loss of normal stratification, low-level keratinization, acantholysis of epithelial cells, and bulbous rete processes.

Squamous cell carcinoma

Infiltrative islands of malignant epithelium within the connective tissue. There is usually overlying epithelial dysplasia and you may be able to see where the tumour has 'budded-off' from the surface. Tumour islands will show the features of dysplasia. Tumours are graded according to how well differentiated they are (e.g. well, moderate, or poorly differentiated). A well-differentiated squamous cell carcinoma will show keratin pearl formation whereas a poorly differentiated one will show little or no keratinization and may not resemble squamous epithelium at all. Look for perineural or lymphovascular invasion, if the advancing front is cohesive or not, and the presence of a host response to the tumour.

Radicular cyst

Macroscopically, the cyst should be attached to the root of a tooth, although the tooth is not always sent to the laboratory. Microscopically, a mature fibrous tissue wall is lined by non-keratinizing stratified squamous epithelium, which is usually heavily inflamed with acute and chronic inflammatory cells. The cyst lumen often contains further inflammatory cells and necrotic material.

Mucous retention cyst

This cyst is lined by ductal type epithelium and the lumen is filled with mucin, foamy macrophages, and a few neutrophils.

Mucous extravasation cyst

This cyst does not have an epithelial lining but instead is lined by compressed granulation tissue. The lumen is filled with mucin, foamy macrophages, and a few neutrophils.

Dentigerous cyst

Macroscopically, the cyst should be attached to the crown of a tooth, with attachment at the amelocemental junction. Microscopically, the cyst lining may show a varying appearance of non-keratinizing stratified squamous epithelium, respiratory-type epithelium, or cuboidal-type epithelium. The cyst wall is often composed of fibromyxoid connective tissue. These cysts are developmental and are typically uninflamed.

Less common lesions

Pleomorphic adenoma

Usually, an encapsulated tumour composed of epithelial and myoepithelial components. Bilayered ducts are often present, with spindle-shaped myoepithelial cells 'melting' into the surrounding stroma. The stroma can vary, including myxoid and chondroid appearances.

Ameloblastoma

An odontogenic tumour characterized by islands of odontogenic epithelium in a fibrous stroma. The peripheral cells of these islands are columnar in shape and palisaded, resembling ameloblasts. The central portions resemble the stellate reticulum. Follicular and plexiform patterns exist but have no bearing on management.

Odontogenic keratocyst

A fibrous cyst wall lined by parakeratinized stratified squamous epithelium. The lining epithelium often has a corrugated surface pattern and flat basement membrane. Basal cells are normally palisaded against the basement membrane.

Pemphigus

This is an autoimmune vesiculobullous condition characterized histologically by intraepithelial separation. This means the prickle cell layer of the epithelium breaks apart and lifts away from the rest of the epithelium, creating a bulla. The diagnosis is confirmed by direct immunofluorescence whereby IgG antibodies can be detected in a typical 'fish scale' pattern within the epithelium.

Pemphigoid

Histologically, pemphigoid forms subepithelial bullae, such that the full thickness of the epithelium separates from the underlying connective tissue. Again, direct immunofluorescence needs to be used to substantiate the histological appearance and will show a band of IgG antibodies along the basement membrane.

Necrotizing sialometaplasia

This lesion is often mistaken for malignancy as it frequently presents with a large area of ulceration and swelling, commonly on the palate. Histologically, beneath an area of ulceration, there are rounded islands of squamous epithelium and areas of necrosis which may mimic infiltrative squamous cell carcinoma. Characteristically, however, these squamous islands are arranged in lobules and represent salivary ducts which have undergone squamous metaplasia.

Granulomatous inflammation (e.g. oral Crohn's)

Granulomas often form deep within the tissue and may be absent in superficial biopsies. They are usually round in shape and composed of collections of epithelioid histiocytes. Multinucleate giant cell may be present, as well as plasma cells and lymphocytes. Further clinical tests are needed to confirm the exact diagnosis.

Common words used in pathology reports

- Acanthosis: increased thickness of the prickle cell layer of the epithelium.
- Acantholysis: separation of the prickle cells.
- Basal cell liquefaction: destruction of basal cells.
- Capsule: a dense connective tissue structure enclosing a tumour or organ.
- Epithelial atrophy: decreased thickness of the epithelium.
- Epithelial dysplasia: disordered growth of the epithelium.
- Epithelial hyperplasia: increased thickness of the epithelium.
- Hyperkeratosis: increased thickness of keratin.
- Lamina propria: the connective tissue immediately below the epithelium.
- Lumen: a hollow cavity, often used when describing cysts.
- Mucosa: a mucous membrane composed of several layers including the epithelium and lamina propria.
- Stroma: the connective tissue of an organ or tissue but often used to describe connective tissue around a tumour.

The multidisciplinary team meeting

Standard format for MDT meeting

The multidisciplinary team meeting

- All new cases of head and neck cancer are discussed at the MDT meeting, which may be held weekly or bi-weekly. Cases are also discussed following surgery, to assess the adequacy of the surgery and in the event of recurrences or if the patient dies. Clinicians may list cases for discussion at any time during a patient's care if a management decision would benefit from multidisciplinary input.
- Participants may include oral and maxillofacial surgeons, oncologists, radiologists, pathologists, restorative dentists, SALTs, dieticians, and clinical nurse specialists.

Standard format for MDT meeting

- Clinical presentation: the patient's general health and the clinical features of the disease will be discussed.
- A radiologist may then present the findings of any radiological investigations (e.g. MRI/CT scans).
- The pathologist will then be asked to present the histopathology; For cancer resections, this will involve describing the completeness of the excision and any prognostic factors likely to influence management decisions e.g. bone invasion. The number of lymph nodes found within a neck dissection specimen and the number of nodes containing cancer will also be presented if applicable; a pathological TNM stage can then be presented.
- A list of cases being discussed at the next MDT meeting will be published prior to the meeting. Any cases requiring a discussion of relevant pathology will need to be compiled, so that the consultant pathologist can review the cases prior to the MDT meeting.
- For each patient being discussed, ensure the following are available:
  - The most recent report and slides.
  - Relevant previous reports and slides for the same patient.
  - Photographs if available.

Common audits in oral and maxillofacial pathology

Turnaround time (TAT) audit

Local or national guidance often dictates how long it should take a biopsy or resection to be reported by a pathologist. This is known as the TAT and is measured from the time the specimen arrives at the laboratory to when a histological report arrives back with the requesting clinician. TAT audits are commonly completed in pathology departments and are important for highlighting ways in which the unit may become more efficient in its processing or reporting of specimens.

Minimum dataset for head and neck cancer reporting

When cancer resections are reported by pathologists, certain details must always be present within the body of the report. For squamous cell carcinoma of the head and neck, examples include the size of the tumour, its depth of invasion, its degree of differentiation, and whether there is lymphovascular of perineural invasion. The RCP publishes 'Minimum datasets' which stipulate the key things which must be included in the report. A simple departmental audit would involve measuring how many reports meet this gold standard.

Audit of request forms

When specimens are sent to the pathology laboratory, they must be accompanied by a request form. This gives details of patient demographics, the surgeon involved, and a clinical description of the lesion biopsied. It may also include a relevant medical history and any previous reports for the patient. A common audit completed in OMFP assesses whether minimum data on the request form has been completed. Again, minimum data is given on the RCP website. This is a very useful audit because data on request forms can help enormously when making a diagnosis. Providing details of previous diagnoses may help to prevent unnecessary tests, saving time and money.

Top tips

- Read about the basic anatomy of the head and neck as it will help enormously when trying to orientate specimens. It will also help you to appreciate where tumours have derived from and their spread through different structures.
- Read reports written by consultant and STs—this is useful when trying to decide on the correct language and phrasing to use in reports.
- Join the British Society of Oral and Maxillofacial Pathology and attend their meetings; you will meet other trainees to share your experiences with. It is a great opportunity to network with like-minded individuals and ask your seniors questions. You can also present posters or oral presentations which will help build your personal portfolio.
- Speak to the consultants about trying to get an article published. You are likely to see rare and unusual tumours, which may be interesting enough to write up as a case report.
- Don't get demoralized in the first few weeks of training when everything under the microscope looks like another series of pink dots! You are not expected to be an expert but only to have enthusiasm and a willingness to learn. You'll be surprised what you can diagnose after a year.

Further reading

British Society of Oral and Maxillofacial Pathology (BSOMP): ℞ www.bsomp.org.uk

Odell EW (2017). *Cawson's Essentials of Oral Pathology and Oral Medicine* (9th ed). Churchill Livingstone.

Robinson M, Hunter K, Pemberton M, Sloan P (2018). Soames' and Southam's Oral Pathology (5th ed). Oxford University Press.

El-Naggar AK, Chan JKC, Grandis JR, Takata T, Slootweg PJ (Eds) (2017). WHO Classification of Head and Neck Tumours (4th edition). IARC: Lyon

General Dental Council (2015). Specialty training curriculum for oral & maxillofacial pathology. ℞ www.gdc-uk.org

Dental trauma

Dental traumatology definitions

Injuries to dental hard tissues

- *Enamel infraction*: incomplete fracture of enamel without loss of tooth structure.
- *Enamel fracture (E#)*: fracture resulting in loss of enamel.
- *Enamel–dentine fracture (ED#)*: fracture resulting in loss of enamel and dentine but not involving the pulp.
- *Enamel–dentine–pulp fracture (EDP#)*: fracture resulting in loss of enamel and dentine involving the pulp.
- *Root fracture*: fracture involving dentine, cementum, and the pulp.
- *Crown–root fracture*: fracture of enamel, dentine, and cementum. Can be uncomplicated (not involving the pulp) or complicated (involves the pulp).

Injuries to periodontium

- *Concussion*: no mobility or displacement of tooth (i.e. no rupture of PDL fibres), but marked reaction to percussion.
- *Subluxation*: increased tooth mobility (i.e. rupture of some PDL fibres), but no displacement. Bleeding from the gingival sulcus. Often tender to percussion.
- *Extrusion*: partial displacement of the tooth out of the socket (i.e. rupture of PDL and damage to the pulp). Bleeding from the gingival sulcus. Excessive mobility. Often tender to percussion. Radiographic examination will show a widening of the PDL space at apical foramen.
- *Lateral luxation*: displacement of the tooth other than axially (i.e. rupture of PDL and pulp with damage to alveolar plates). Usually gives a high metallic sound upon percussion. Tooth usually immobile. Radiographic examination may reveal a widened PDL space.
- *Intrusion*: displacement of the tooth into alveolar bone (i.e. extensive damage to PDL, pulp, and alveolar plates). Usually gives a high metallic sound upon percussion. Tooth usually immobile. Radiographic examination reveals an absent PDL space from all or part of the root.
- *Avulsion*: loss of tooth from the socket (i.e. extensive damage to PDL, pulp, and alveolar plates).

Injuries to alveolar bone

- *Fracture of socket wall*: fracture confined to socket wall.
- *Fracture of alveolar process*: fracture of alveolar process that may involve the tooth sockets.
- *Fracture of maxilla or mandible*: may or may not involve the sockets.

Dental trauma in the primary dentition

- Common: by the age of 5 years, 1/3 of children will have experienced dental trauma.
- Luxation injuries occur more frequently than fractures in the primary dentition due to the more elastic nature of alveolar bone in young patients.
- Factors that influence the management of trauma in the primary dentition:
  - Relatively short period of time the teeth are present.
  - Close proximity of root of primary teeth to developing permanent successors.
  - Patient's cooperative ability.
- Aims of management:
  - Support the family.
  - Avoid inducing dental anxiety.
  - Minimize risk of further damage to permanent successor (e.g. chronic infection associated with non-vital primary tooth).

> A torn labial frenum is no longer believed to be pathognomonic of child abuse. However, a torn labial frenulum in a non-ambulant child where there are concerns regarding the history given should be regarded as a suspicious injury.

Management of injuries to dental hard tissues

- *Enamel infraction*: often just requires monitoring for signs and symptoms of loss of vitality.
- *Enamel fracture (E#)*: smooth sharp edges. Ongoing monitoring for signs and symptoms of loss of vitality.
- *Enamel–dentine fracture (ED#)*: cover exposed dentine with GI cement or place composite restoration if patient deemed cooperative. Ongoing monitoring for signs and symptoms of loss of vitality.
- *Enamel–dentine–pulp fracture (EDP#)*: often extraction is the only viable option due to the cooperative ability of young patients. For cooperative patients, it may be possible to perform a partial pulpotomy under LA prior to coronal composite restoration as for permanent teeth (➔ Pulpotomy for traumatized permanent tooth). Clinical examination at 1 week, 6–8 weeks, and 12 months with radiographic review at 12 months or as indicated by clinical examination.
  - Missing tooth fragments should be accounted for.
- *Root fracture*:
  - No/minimal displacement of the coronal fragment: monitor tooth for signs and symptoms of loss of vitality at 1 week, 6–8 weeks, and 12 months. If loss of vitality occurs, extraction is indicated.
  - If coronal fragment is displaced, consider repositioning and splinting under LA. Review at 1 week, 4 weeks (remove splint), 8 weeks, and 12 months.
  - Mobility of coronal fragment: extraction of coronal fragment. Apical fragment should be left *in situ* to undergo physiological resorption. Review at 12 months.

- *Crown–root fracture*: rare in the primary dentition. Extraction often indicated.

Management of injuries to periodontium

- *Concussion*: review at 1 week and 6–8 weeks (Box 10.1).
- *Subluxation*: review at 1 week and 6–8 weeks (Box 10.1).

Box 10.1 Advice following luxation injuries

- Soft diet for 10–14 days and good oral hygiene should be encouraged following luxation injuries.
- Consider use of 0.1% chlorhexidine gel on gauze swabs or a soft toothbrush twice daily for 7 days.
- Regular analgesia: paracetamol sugar-free (SF) oral suspension + ibuprofen SF oral suspension as needed.

- *Extrusion*: management depends on the degree of displacement, mobility of the tooth, and the child's cooperative ability.
  - In cases where there is no occlusal interference, monitor for signs and symptoms of loss of vitality.
  - Where there is occlusal interference repositioning and splinting, or extraction is indicated.
  - Review at 1 week, 6–8 weeks, and 12 months.
- *Lateral luxation*:
  - Where there is no occlusal interference, the tooth should be allowed to reposition spontaneously.
  - In cases with mild occlusal interference, grind down the traumatized primary tooth to remove the interfering contact.
  - In cases with more significant occlusal interference, reposition tooth under LA and splint for 4 weeks.
  - In cases with severe displacement, consider the need for extraction.
  - Monitor for signs and symptoms of loss of vitality—if these occur, extraction is indicated.
  - Review at 1 week, 4 weeks (for splint removal, if required), 8 weeks, 6 months, and 12 months.
- *Intrusion*:
  - Record the degree of displacement (between incisal edge of intruded tooth and incisal edge of non-traumatized adjacent tooth/teeth).
  - Classification:
    - Mild: partial intrusion, >50% crown visible.
    - Moderate: <50% crown visible.
    - Severe: crown not visible.
  - Radiograph to confirm diagnosis and determine proximity to permanent successor.
  - Inform parents of risk of damage to permanent tooth: greatest risk is for children <3 years of age.
  - Management options:
    - Leave to spontaneous erupt: spontaneous re-eruption occurs in the majority of cases and usually occurs within 6 months.

○ If spontaneous eruption does not occur, there is a risk of acute inflammation—extraction indicated. In rare cases, ankylosis may occur.
- Review at 1 week, 6–8 weeks, 6 months, and 12 months.
- Monitor eruption of permanent incisors, especially in severe cases.
- *Avulsion*:
  - If possible, take an intraoral radiograph to confirm primary tooth has been avulsed as opposed to severely intruded.
  - Where tooth has not been accounted for, consider the need for a chest radiograph in cases where consciousness was impaired at the time of trauma.
  - Replantation of avulsed primary teeth is not indicated due to the risk of damage to the permanent successor.
  - Review at 6–8 weeks.
  - Monitor eruption of permanent incisors as the tooth may have been displaced towards the developing successor during the avulsion injury.

Management of injuries to alveolar bone

- *Fracture of alveolar process*: manual repositioning and splinting of displacement segment for 4 weeks. Often requires GA. Monitor for signs and symptoms of loss of vitality at 1 week, 4 weeks (splint removal), 8 weeks, and 12 months. Review eruption of permanent teeth in the line of the fracture.
- *Fracture of maxilla or mandible*: urgent referral to OMFS.

Potential sequelae

Colour changes
- Grey discoloration can be transient or permanent; 50% of cases of permanent discoloration are associated with pulp necrosis.
- Common following luxation injuries.
- Majority of discoloured primary teeth do not develop clinical/radiographic signs of infection and exfoliate naturally.

Pulp canal obliteration (PCO)
- Frequent finding following luxation injuries.
- Often associated with yellow discoloration of crown.
- Pulp necrosis occurs in <13% of cases and is often related to a new trauma as an obliterated pulp has less healing potential.

Pulp necrosis
- Confirmed by signs and symptoms and radiographic examination.
- Extraction indicated as the presence of chronic infection is associated with enamel defects in the permanent successor.

Damage to permanent dentition
- Depends upon type and severity of injury to primary tooth and stage of tooth development of permanent successor.
- Enamel hypomineralization and hypoplasia: injury to primary tooth between the ages of 2 and 7 years.
- Dilaceration of permanent tooth: injury around 2 years of age.

Trauma in the permanent dentition: injuries to dental hard tissues

- Most commonly involves upper permanent central incisors.
- Fractures are more common than luxation injuries in the permanent dentition.
- Missing tooth fragments should be accounted for.

Enamel infraction

- Monitor for signs and symptoms of loss of vitality.
- Extensive infractions may need to be sealed with resin (after etching) to prevent discoloration of the infraction lines.

Enamel fractures

- Smooth sharp edges or restore with composite.
- Clinical (including sensibility testing) and radiographic examination after 6–8 weeks and 12 months.

Enamel–dentine fractures

- Commonest injury in the permanent dentition.

Aim of management

- Cover exposed dentine as soon as possible to prevent loss of vitality.

Management options

- Ideally a definitive restoration should be placed at presentation but where this is not possible, the exposed dentine should be covered with a provisional GI restoration.
- Definitive restorations:
  - Composite restoration under LA.
  - If tooth fragment is available, this can be reattached using flowable composite resin.
- Where pulp tissue is showing through the dentine, consideration should be given to performing a direct pulp cap or a partial pulpotomy (➔ Pulpotomy for traumatized permanent tooth).

Follow-up

- Clinical and radiographic review after 6–8 weeks and 12 months or as guided by clinical and radiographic findings.

Enamel–dentine–pulp fractures

Aim of management

- In immature teeth, the rationale for management is to preserve pulp vitality to enable continued root development.

Key considerations

- Time since fracture.
- Degree of contamination of fracture site.
- Stage of root development.
- Size of exposure.

Management options

Pulp capping

- Indications: pinpoint exposures <1 hour old; open/closed apices.

- Procedure: under LA and dry dam, wash exposure with saline, cover exposure with NSCH + GIC/MTA/other biocompatible material prior to definitive restoration. NB: risk of discolouration with use of MTA.
- Success: 88% (NSCH).[1]

Partial (Cvek's) pulpotomy

- Indications: exposure larger than pinpoint up to 24–48 hours old often in teeth with incomplete root development. Can also be performed in teeth with closed apices.
- Procedure under LA and dry dam:
  - Removal of 1–2 mm of pulp around the exposure site with tungsten carbide bur (jet 330).
  - Achieve haemostasis with a small cotton pledget soaked in saline placed in the pulpotomy site for 5 minutes.
  - If haemostasis is not achieved after this time period, remove another 1 mm of pulp tissue and repeat the application of a saline-soaked cotton pledget. Repeat this until healthy pulp tissue is reached.
  - Once haemostasis is achieved, place Biodentine™ or MTA over the pulp stumps prior to the definitive restoration. An alternative option is NSCH in the pulpotomy site then interim layer of GI liner before definitive composite restoration. NB: risk of discolouration with use of MTA.
- Success: 96%.[2]

Coronoradicular pulpotomy

- Indications: exposure larger than pinpoint that is 3–6 days old or a grossly contaminated exposure in teeth with open apices.
- Procedure under LA and dry dam:
  - Removal of entire coronal pulp.
  - Achieve haemostasis and restoration as for partial pulpotomy.
- Success: 79%.[3]

Pulpectomy and root canal treatment

- Indications: necrotic pulp.
- Procedure: complete chemomechanical cleansing of the root canal prior to root canal treatment. For management of the immature non-vital permanent incisor, see ➔ Management of the immature non-vital central incisor.

Most advocate the partial pulpotomy technique as the treatment of choice for enamel–dentine–pulp fractures in teeth with open and closed apices where the pulp is deemed to be vital. It has a higher success rate than direct pulp capping. Even in teeth with closed apices with delayed presentation, every effort should be made to maintain pulp vitality to allow continued apical root development and dentine deposition on the root canal walls.

---

1 Ravn J (1981). *Scand J Dent Res* 89, 213.
2 Cvek M (1978). *J Endodont* 4, 232.
3 Gelbier M (1988). *Dent J* 164, 319.

Follow-up
- Clinical and radiographic review after 6–8 weeks.
- Further follow-up guided by clinical and radiographic findings, usually after 3 months, 6 months, and 12 months.

Root fractures

- Prevalence: 0.5–7% of traumatic injuries affecting the permanent dentition.
- Classification:
  - Single/multiple.
  - Horizontal/vertical.
  - Apical, middle, or apical 1/3.
- Diagnosis: clinical examination may reveal mobility and/or displacement of the coronal fragment:
  - Radiographs should be taken from two different angles in order to locate the fracture line by applying principles of parallax.
  - Establish the stage of root development, site of the fracture, degree of displacement, and presence of multiple fractures.
- Immediate management:
  - Where there is no mobility or displacement of the coronal fragment, advise analgesia, encourage good oral hygiene, and advise a soft diet for 10 days.
  - Where there is mobility or displacement of the coronal fragment, administer LA and reposition the coronal fragment prior to placing a physiological splint. Optimal repositioning favours hard tissue healing and reduces the risk of pulp necrosis.
  - Where the coronal fragment is avulsed, immediate management should be as for avulsion injuries (→ Trauma in the permanent dentition: avulsion).
  - Where a splint has been placed, this should remain *in situ* for 4 weeks. In cases where the fracture involves the cervical 1/3 of the root, prolonged splinting for up to 4 months may be required.
- Referral to a specialist following immediate management, if required.
- Follow-up: clinical and radiographic examination at 4 weeks, 6–8 weeks, 4 months, 6 months, 12 months, and annually for at least 5 years.
- Prognosis:
  - Dependent upon the stage of root development, location of the fracture, presence of a concomitant crown fracture, and degree of displacement of coronal fragment (chance of hard tissue union reduces with displacement >0.5 mm; chance of necrosis increases with displacement >1 mm).[4]
  - Pulp necrosis may be indicated by a persistent lack of response to sensibility testing and a radiolucency at the fracture site upon radiographic examination. The apical fragment remains vital in the majority of cases and therefore, root canal treatment should only be performed to the fracture site after placement of an MTA or Biodentine™ barrier.
- Healing can occur by the following methods:
  - Hard tissue union:

4 Andreasen J (2004). *Dent Traumatol* 20, 192.

- o Affected by pulp vitality, tooth maturity, and degree of displacement.
- o Fragments are in close contact and the fracture line may only just be visible on radiographs.
- Repair with connective tissue:
  - o Healing with interposition of soft tissue.
  - o Radiographs show that fragments are close but separated by a radiolucent line.
- Interposition of bone and connective tissue:
  - o Fragments become separated by bone.
  - o Due to a displaced root fracture occurring during growth of the alveolar process.
- Interposition of granulation tissue:
  - o Indicates no healing and coronal pulp necrosis.
  - o Radiographs reveal a persistent/widened space between the fragments and a radiolucency in the alveolar bone adjacent to the fracture line.

Crown–root fractures

- Prevalence: 5% of injuries affecting permanent dentition.
- Classified as uncomplicated (not involving the pulp) or complicated (fracture involving the pulp).
- Diagnosis: based on clinical and radiographic findings.
- Immediate management:
  - The coronal fragment can be stabilized with a physiological splint until definitive treatment can be provided.
- Definitive management may involve:
  - removal of coronal fragment under LA and composite restoration (electrosurgery or orthodontic extrusion of the apical fragment may be needed to expose fracture margins)
  - in cases of complicated fractures, a partial pulpotomy or pulp extirpation to the fracture line may be required prior to the placement of a composite restoration (as for uncomplicated fractures)
  - alternative management options include root submergence or extraction.
- Follow-up: clinical and radiographic review at 1 week, 6–8 weeks, 3 months, 6 months, 12 months, and annually for at least 5 years.

Trauma in the permanent dentition: injuries to periodontium

Concussion

- Usually, no treatment indicated (➲ Box 10.1).
- Keep under clinical review (including sensibility testing) to monitor pulpal status for at least 12 months.
- Follow-up radiographic examination should be guided by clinical findings and is often indicated at 4 weeks and 12 months.

Subluxation

- Clean area with saline if needed.
- Occlusal adjustment may be needed if there is occlusal interference (➲ Box 10.1).
- Keep under clinical review (including sensibility testing) to monitor pulpal status for at least 12 months.
- Follow-up radiographic examination guided by clinical findings and is usually indicated at 2 weeks, 12 weeks, 6 months and 12 months.

Extrusion

- Clean area with saline if needed.
- Give LA and reposition tooth gently.
- Place physiological splint for 2 weeks.
- Clinical and radiographic review at 2 weeks, 4 weeks, 8 weeks, 3 months, 6 months, and 12 months, then annually for at least 5 years.

Lateral luxation

- Give LA (buccal and intrapapillary infiltrations and consider need for further palatal analgesia).
- Clean area with saline.
- Reposition tooth with digital finger pressure supporting the tooth from the buccal and palatal aspect. Gentle use of forceps may be needed to disengage the tooth from bone.
- Reposition displaced bone with finger pressure from palatal and labial aspects simultaneously.
- Stabilize tooth with physiological splint for 4 weeks (Box 10.2).

> ### Box 10.2 Splinting traumatized teeth
>
> - Physiological splints should be extended to one tooth either side of the traumatized tooth/teeth and should allow physiological mobility in order to reduce the risk of ankylosis.
> - Favourable splints: titanium trauma splint (TTS), composite and wire splint (e.g. a passive 0.018 twist-flex wire or stainless steel wire up to 0.4 mm diameter).
> - Unfavourable splints: vacuum-formed splints, suture splints, rigid splints, such as composite resin splint (without the wire).
> - Splinting duration:
>   - 2 weeks: extrusion, avulsion.
>   - 2–4 weeks: intrusion.
>   - 4 weeks: lateral luxation, root fracture*, alveolar bone fracture.
>
> * Where the fracture is in the cervical third of the root, prolonged splinting for up to 4 months may be required.

- Remove splint at 4 weeks.
- Clinical and radiographic examination at 2 weeks, 4 weeks, 8 weeks, 12 weeks, 6 months, and 12 months, then annually for at least 5 years.

Intrusion

- Comprises ~0.3–1.9% of injuries to permanent teeth.[1]
- Often associated with severe damage to the tooth, periodontium, and pulp.
- Lacerations should be cleaned and sutured as needed.
- Consider the need for systemic antibiotics if wounds appear contaminated.
- Management dependent upon stage of root development and degree of intrusion.[2]
- Incomplete root development:
  - Allow re-eruption without intervention.
  - If no movement after 4 weeks, commence orthodontic repositioning.
- Complete root development:
  - Mild intrusion <3 mm: passive repositioning initially. If no movement within 8 weeks, orthodontic repositioning or surgical repositioning and place physiological splint for 4 weeks.
  - Moderate intrusion 3–7 mm: orthodontic repositioning or surgical repositioning (preferable) under LA and placement of physiological splint for 2 weeks.
  - Severe intrusion >7 mm: surgical repositioning under LA.
- Remove splint (if placed) at 4 weeks.
- Clinical and radiographic examination at 2 weeks, 4 weeks, 8 weeks, 3 months, 6 months, and 12 months, then annually for at least 5 years.

Following initial trauma management, consider the need for an urgent specialist referral to consider medium- and long-term management.

1 Andreasen J (2006). *Dent Traumatol* 22, 83.
2 Bourguignon C (2020). *Dent Traumatol* 36, 314.

Trauma in the permanent dentition: avulsion

- Comprises ~0.5–3% of dentoalveolar trauma to permanent teeth.[1]
- Upper central incisor most frequently involved.
- Injury represents damage to pulp, PDL, and alveolar bone.
- Prognosis dependent upon initial emergency management.
- Avoid unnecessary delays prior to replantation.
- The patient and person with parental responsibility need to be made aware of the likely outcome from the outset and the potential sequelae.

Immediate management

At the scene of the accident

- If possible, the tooth should be replanted prior to urgent definitive repositioning and placement of a splint by a dentist.[2]
- If tooth is dirty, briefly wash it (<10 seconds) in milk or saline (or the patient's saliva) prior to replantation.
- After replantation, the tooth should be stabilized by biting on gauze or a handkerchief until the patient attends an emergency dental appointment as soon as possible.
- If immediate replantation is not possible, the tooth should be placed in suitable storage media (in order of preference: milk > saliva > physiological saline > water (in preference to leaving the tooth dry)) and the patient should attend an emergency dental appointment as soon as possible.

In the dental surgery

- Place tooth/teeth in milk or saline as soon as possible if the tooth has not already been replanted.
- Take clear history and examination to exclude presence of a head injury of other injuries requiring urgent medical management.
- Determine the extra-alveolar dry time and total extra-alveolar time along with any storage medium used.
- Be aware that some dental injuries are the result of non-accidental injury. Follow local safeguarding policy if there are any safeguarding concerns.
- Check tetanus status.
- If tooth has already been replanted:
  - Leave the tooth *in situ* and encourage patient to bite on gauze to stabilize tooth.
  - Clean area with saline/chlorhexidine gluconate.
  - Check correct position of the tooth clinically and radiographically.
  - Give LA, if needed.
  - Place a physiological splint for 2 weeks.
  - Consider the need for endodontics. Pulp extirpation within 2 weeks for teeth with closed apices. NSCH dressing for up to 1 month

---

1 Andreasen J (2007). *Textbook and Color Atlas of Traumatic Injuries to the Teeth* (4th ed), pp. 444–488. Blackwell Munksgaard.

2 Fouad A (2020). *Dent Traumatol* 36, 331.

followed by obturation. If a corticosteroid/antibiotic paste is used as an intracanal medicament, place as soon as possible after replantation and leave for at least 6 weeks (NB: potential risk of coronal discolouration). For teeth with open apices stored in physiological medium or stored in non-physiological medium with extra-alveolar time <60 minutes, consider the likelihood of revascularization of the pulp against the risk of infection-related resorption to determine whether pulp extirpation within 2 weeks is needed.

- Prescribe systemic antibiotics.
- Give postoperative instructions and arrange follow-up.
- If the tooth/teeth were replanted incorrectly, consider repositioning up to 48 hours after avulsion.
- If tooth has not already been replanted:

For teeth with closed apices

Cases where tooth kept in physiological storage medium or stored in non-physiological conditions, with extraoral time <60 minutes:

1. Place tooth in milk or physiological saline.
2. Remove any contamination on root surface by gently agitating it within the storage medium/briefly rinse in saline.
3. Administer LA (preferably without vasoconstrictor) to achieve buccal and palatal analgesia.
4. Irrigate the socket with sterile saline.
5. Handle the tooth by the *crown only*.
6. Replant the tooth with firm digital pressure. Where resistance is felt, remove the tooth and place back into storage medium. Gently introduce a blunt instrument into the socket to reposition and bony fragments that may be preventing the tooth from being fully replanted.
7. Replant the tooth slowly with digital pressure.
8. Once replanted, encourage patient to bite on gauze swab.
9. Check position of tooth clinically and radiographically.
10. Place physiological splint for 2 weeks.
11. Suture any lacerations.
12. Prescribe systemic antibiotics.
13. Pulp extirpation within 2 weeks.
14. Give postoperative instructions and arrange follow-up appointment.

Teeth with extraoral time >60 minutes:

- PDL will become necrotic and ankylosis is inevitable. Ankylosis-related (replacement) root resorption is likely to occur.
- In all cases of avulsion, the patient and person with parental responsibility need to be aware of the treatment required and the likely outcome.
- In most cases, even though prognosis is poor, the tooth will be replanted after gaining appropriate informed consent.
- Follow steps 1–14.

For teeth with open apices

Cases where tooth kept in physiological storage medium or stored in non-physiological conditions, with extraoral time <60 minutes:

- Follow steps 1–12.

- Revascularization of the pulp space is a possibility which would lead to continued root development. This possibility should be considered against the risk of infection-related resorption which occurs rapidly in children. Pulp extirpation and endodontic management is indicated as soon as pulp necrosis is diagnosed.
- Provide postoperative instructions and arrange appropriate follow-up.

Teeth with extraoral time >60 minutes:
- As described for extraoral time <60 minutes, but note that revascularization is much less likely to occur.

Postoperative care

- Prescribe systemic antibiotics (amoxicillin or penicillin unless allergic in which case prescribe a suitable alternative) for 5 days and encourage use of 0.12% chlorhexidine gluconate mouth rinse twice daily for 2 weeks.
- Advise continued toothbrushing, with a soft toothbrush, if necessary, after each meal.
- Advise/prescribe appropriate analgesia and soft diet for up to 2 weeks.
- The patient should avoid contact sports for at least 2 weeks.
- Consider the need for a tetanus booster (if tooth has been contaminated) and refer the patient to their GMP if needed.
- The family should be informed of the tooth's prognosis as soon as possible. The online dental trauma guide[3] can be referred to.
- Follow-up care should be coordinated between the initial provider and specialist services as a multidisciplinary approach to medium- and long-term management may be required.

Replantation is usually always indicated, even in cases with poor prognosis as this will allow for the eventual loss of the tooth to be planned appropriately by a MDT.

Contraindications to replantation:
- Primary teeth.
- Injuries requiring urgent medical attention.
- Patient could be at risk if tooth is replanted (e.g. active chemotherapy, immunosuppressed patients). For children with complicated medical histories (e.g. congenital heart disease), liaison with the child's medical specialist is advised.

Follow-up

- For teeth with closed apices: clinical and radiographic review at 2 weeks (+ splint removal), 4 weeks, 3 months, 6 months, 12 months, and annually for at least 5 years.
- For teeth with open apices: 2 weeks (+ splint removal), 1 month, 2 months, 3 months, 6 months, 12 months, and annually for at least 5 years.

---

3 ☞ www.dentaltraumaguide.org

4 Fouad A (2020). *Dent Traumatol* 36, 331.

- Immature teeth will require frequent review due to the risk of infection-related resorption which leads to rapid loss of the tooth.
- Immediate pulp extirpation is indicated if pulp necrosis is diagnosed (➔ Management of non-vital immature permanent incisor).

Prompt referral for specialist interdisciplinary planning and management is often indicated in cases of avulsion.

Prognosis

PDL

- Factors that influence PDL healing[5]:
  - Extra-alveolar time.
  - Dry time.
  - Storage media.
  - Contamination of root surface.
  - Splinting.
- Chance (>10%) of PDL healing with extra-alveolar dry time <30 minutes and total extra-alveolar time <90 minutes when stored in appropriate storage medium (e.g. milk, saline, or saliva).[5]
- Ankylosis likely with extra-alveolar dry time >30 minutes or total extra-alveolar time >90 minutes.

Pulp

- Factors that influence pulpal healing[5]:
  - Root length.
  - Stage of root development.
  - Extra-alveolar time.

5 Day PF, Gregg TA (2012). UK National clinical guidelines in paediatric dentistry. Treatment of avulsed permanent teeth in children. ✍ https://www.bspd.co.uk/Portals/0/Public/Files/Guidelines/avulsion_guidelines_v7_final_.pdf

Trauma in the permanent dentition: injuries to alveolar bone

Fracture involving alveolar bone

- Diagnosis:
  - Clinical and radiographic findings.
  - Displacement of alveolar segment.
  - Segmental mobility (i.e. when one tooth is moved, several teeth move together).
  - Occlusal interference.
  - Radiographs at different angles may reveal fracture lines.
- Management:
  - Reposition displacement segment under LA and place physiological splint for 4 weeks.
  - For extensive fractures, urgent referral to OMFS to consider the need for ORIF.
  - Advise soft diet and analgesia for 7 days.
  - Encourage good oral hygiene and use of 0.2% chlorhexidine gluconate.
  - Consider the need for systemic antibiotics (e.g. contaminated injuries).
- Follow-up:
  - Splint removal at 4 weeks.
  - Clinical and radiographic review at 4 weeks, 6–8 weeks, 4 months, 6 months, 12 months, and annually for at least 5 years.

Fracture of maxilla or mandible

- Urgent referral to OMFS on-call team.

Trauma in the permanent dentition: potential sequelae

There are various sequelae that could occur and therefore regular clinical and radiographic reviews are indicated. At each review appointment, as a minimum, the following should be recorded:

- Any patient concerns.
- Pain history.
- Discoloration of traumatized tooth/teeth and adjacent teeth.
- Tenderness to percussion of traumatized tooth/teeth and adjacent teeth.
- Mobility of traumatized tooth/teeth and adjacent teeth.
- Sensibility testing of traumatized tooth/teeth and adjacent teeth.
- Radiographic changes in PDL space and apical region (or at fracture line for root fractures) when radiographs are indicated.

Use of a trauma proforma helps to ensure all the information is clearly recorded.

Potential sequelae following all injuries

Pulp necrosis

- Can occur following injuries involving the dental hard tissues, periodontium, and alveolar bone.
- Clinical and radiographic signs of pulp necrosis: dark discoloration of crown, no response to sensibility, acute/chronic signs of infection, periapical radiolucency, arrested root development.
- Prognosis of luxation injuries is affected by the type of luxation injury and the stage of root formation.[1]
- Prevalence of pulp necrosis for luxation[1]:
  - Intrusion (85%) > lateral luxation (58%) > extrusion (26%) > subluxation (6%) > concussion (3%).
  - Complete root development (38%) > incomplete root development (8%).
- There is an increased risk of pulp necrosis where there has been a combination of injuries.
- When a diagnosis of pulp necrosis is made, pulp extirpation and root canal treatment is indicated.

PCO

- Related to pulp revascularization and therefore PCO is a healing response.
- Often accompanied by yellow discoloration of the crown.
- Seen most frequently following luxation injuries, particularly in teeth with open apices.
- Occurs in ~15% of luxation injuries.
- A late complication of PCO is pulp necrosis (seen in ~7–12% of cases of PCO) if further trauma is experienced.

1 Andreasen F (1985). *Endod Dent Traumatol* 1, 207.

Potential sequelae specific to luxation injuries

Ankylosis

- Occurs when an area of PDL between 4 and 9 mm^2 has been damaged—this area has been described as the critical defect.[2]
- Almost always followed by infraocclusion and replacement resorption in children.
- Clinically detected by a high metallic note on percussion once 20% of the root surface is affected by root resorption.
- An ankylosed, infraoccluded permanent incisor should be decoronated in patients <15 years old when the incisor is infraoccluded by >1 mm. Decoronation is performed to maintain the bone level at the correct height.

Ankylosis-related replacement root resorption (replacement resorption)

- In the absence of PDL (as in cases of ankylosis), osteoclasts resorb cementum and then the root which gets replaced by bone.
- Tooth root becomes incorporated into the remodelling cycle of bone.
- Speed of replacement resorption is governed by the age of the child and rate of bone turnover.

Infection-related inflammatory root resorption

- Related to the presence of infected, necrotic pulp in the root canal and damage to the cementum secondary to luxation injuries.
- Due to the loss of the protective cemental layer, inflammatory cells and toxins from the root canal can enter the surrounding bone resulting in infection-related resorption.
- Radiographic appearance of root resorption with an adjacent radiolucency within the bone.
- Histological findings are of bowl-shaped areas of resorption of both cementum and dentine with inflammation of the adjacent periodontal tissue.
- Requires immediate extirpation and dressing with NSCH for 3 weeks. This should be replaced every 3 months until the resorptive defects disappear. Obturation should be delayed until bone repair is visible radiographically.

Repair-related resorption

- Often not detected clinically or radiographically.
- Root surface shows superficial resorption lacunae repaired with new cementum visible upon histological examination.
- No intervention needed as is self-limiting and shows spontaneous repair.

Internal root resorption

- Unusual finding.
- Reported in 2% of luxated permanent teeth.
- Consider the possibility that external root resorption affecting the labial or palatal root surface may mimic internal root resorption on radiographs. Therefore, take PA radiographs at different angles and

apply the principles of parallax (if the radiolucency representing the resorption defect doesn't move, it is located centrally within the root indicating internal resorption).

Transient apical breakdown

- Temporary resorption of bone surrounding root apex and dentine within the apical foramen of mature extruded and laterally luxated permanent incisors.

Loss of marginal bone support

- 5% of laterally luxated and 31% of intruded permanent incisors demonstrated changes in the marginal periodontium.[1]

Internal bone formation

- In severe luxation injuries, invasion of bone and PDL into the pulp canal can occur.

Gingival recession

- Can be seen following the more severe injuries.

Further reading

Bourguignon C (2020). International Association of Dental Traumatology guidelines for the management of traumatic dental injuries: 1. Fractures and luxations. *Dent Traumatol* 36, 314–330.

Day P (2008). Dental trauma: managing poor prognosis anterior teeth. Part 2. *J Orthod* 35, 143–55.

Day P (2020). International Association of Dental Traumatology guidelines for the management of traumatic dental injuries: 3. Injuries in the primary dentition. *Dent Traumatol* 36, 343–359.

Day P, Gregg TA (2012). UK National Clinical Guidelines in Paediatric Dentistry. Treatment of avulsed permanent teeth in children. 🔖 https://www.bspd.co.uk/Portals/0/Public/Files/Guidelines/avulsion_guidelines_v7_final_.pdf

DiAngelis A (2012). International Association of dental traumatology guidelines for the management of traumatic dental injuries: 1. Fractures and luxations of permanent teeth. *Dent Traumatol* 28, 2–12.

Fouad A (2020). International Association of Dental Traumatology guidelines for the management of traumatic dental injuries: 2. Avulsion of permanent teeth. *Dent Traumatol* 36, 331–342.

International Association of Dental Traumatology. The dental trauma guide. 🔖 www.dentaltraumaguide.org

Kindelan S (2008). Dental trauma: an overview of its influence on the management of orthodontic treatment. Part 1. *J Orthod* 35, 68–78.

Malmgren B (2000). Decoronation: how, why and when? *J California Dent Ass* 28, 846–854.

Sandler C (2021). Guidelines for the orthodontic management of the traumatised tooth. *J Orthod* 48, 74–81.

Trope M (2002). Root resorption due to trauma. *Endodontic Topics* 1, 79–100.

Chapter 11

Monitoring progress

Introduction to monitoring progress

- Work-based assessments (WBAs) and supervised learning events (SLEs) have become increasingly important methods of assessing trainees both in medical and dental areas. They comprise several different tools used to assess the progress and development through the training programme, evidencing the progress to clinical competence.
- Monitoring the progress of dental trainees can have its challenges. The aim of DFT and DCT is to develop competency within a range of procedures and this needs to be evidenced. It therefore requires the trainee to be proactive to provide the evidence of developing competency.
- Each individual patient encounter has to be seen as an opportunity to develop skills and knowledge but also as a way of providing evidence of progress in trainee development and skill, ultimately evidencing competency in a certain procedure.
- At the start, it may seem rather tedious to complete these WBAs or SLEs, but these form the evidence of competence and ultimately enable your educational supervisor and training programme director to confirm satisfactory completion of training.
- The onus is on the trainee to lead and ensure completion of such assessments; however, guidance can usually be sought.
- WBAs or SLEs need to be seen as opportunities for development rather than solely proving competence. There is a great deal of learning possible from undertaking a procedure and gaining feedback on this throughout training. As highly trained professionals, we have the inherent need to perform procedures to a high level. The aim of SLEs and WBAs is not to 'prove' competence, but to show development in your abilities.
- Assessments can be formative, and the assessment comprises feedback and reflection or there may be an associated point score for different assessment items.
- Regardless of the score achieved, it is always worth gaining feedback from the assessor.
- It is important to check your programme requirements about how many assessments are required. There will be a minimum requirement, which is often seen as the number required. The authors' advice is to use every opportunity possible to gain feedback on your abilities and methods to improve your skills (clinical and communication), to develop your abilities. Do not wait until you feel competent at a certain procedure before undertaking a SLE or WBA, there may be more benefit in the feedback when you are less competent rather than when you feel competence has been gained.

Work-based assessments

Case-based discussion

- The main purpose of this tool is to evaluate clinical judgement, decision-making, and management.
- Areas that are assessed include:
  - clinical note keeping
  - patient assessment
  - appropriate radiographs, study casts, tests and investigations, and justification
  - diagnosis
  - treatment options and plan
  - patient management including delivery of treatment and further management and follow-up
  - making judgements
  - overall performance in presenting the case
  - trainee's reflection into own performance.
- The assessment is based on the discussion between the trainee and the assessor.
- Although a patient may not be present, having all available items such as study models, clinical photos, and records should help form part of the discussion.
- One aspect of the assessment is case presentation skills. It may be beneficial to do this as a multimedia presentation.
- Clinical judgement is being assessed; therefore, it can be useful to investigate any relevant research or evidence to support any particular decision made prior to the discussion.
- A case-based discussion can also be completed mid-way through a treatment plan. A current problem list can be useful along with proposed follow-up plans.
- In a hospital setting, a diagnosis and treatment plan may have already been formulated from the consultant's clinic. Try not to simply recite information from the consultant's notes. Instead, try to understand how the diagnosis was formulated, identify the patient's current symptoms, and make a contemporary diagnosis—this actually shows thought in the process rather than simply reading notes!

Direct observation of procedural skills (DOPS)

- The assessor directly watches the trainee perform a clinical procedure and the entire patient encounter is assessed.
- Areas that are assessed include:
  - understanding of the theory behind the procedure including indications and contraindications; can talk through the procedure; anatomy; and instrument and material use
  - can obtain valid and informed consent
  - carries out all preoperative procedures
  - provides all necessary analgesia
  - demonstration of technical ability
  - shows respect for infection control
  - gains help and assistance if necessary
  - carries out all postoperative procedures

- professionalism and communication skills
- overall performance.
- Before undertaking a DOPS, ensure the following:
  - an assessor is available and fully free for entire time slot for that assessment to take place—this may require forward planning of several weeks
  - the planned procedure fits in with the rest of the patient's management plan
  - additional time may be required to enable feedback
  - any special or unusual instruments are ordered in advance or check there are adequate numbers beforehand
  - the patient is aware of the assessment, as an additional person will be present throughout the procedure
  - Ensure that any pre-procedure reading has been performed and that you have researched the options available and any alternatives.
- Practise on models or simulators where you have the opportunity, as this will assist in your confidence in providing the procedure.

Mini clinical evaluation exercise (mini-CEX)

- The assessor directly observes the trainee in a patient encounter which mainly looks at information gathering and clinical judgement.
- Areas that are assessed include:
  - history taking
  - performing a clinical examination
  - verbal and non-verbal communication skills
  - making clinical judgements based on the information gained
  - organization skills and professionalism
  - overall management.
- Try to work to a logical format. Make sure you are familiar with the system of clinical note keeping, whether that involves history sheets, proformas, or computerized systems as well as any forms for requesting investigations or radiographs.
- Practise a good number of cases and become familiar with the important parts of history taking and examination for the area you are working in.
- In general practice, these cases may be selected from a standard day; however, in hospital settings it may be undertaken from a new patient clinic, which may limit the opportunity to carry out this assessment.
- Before starting, make sure you have a systematic way of carrying out your history and examination.
- Make sure any necessary equipment, such as periodontal probes and electric pulp testers, are readily available if necessary and be familiar with using the specific model of equipment.

'A Dental Evaluation of Performance' (ADEPT)

- ADEPT is another type of assessment involving a patient encounter which is observed by the assessor who then completes the assessment and provides feedback.
- This type of assessment may be used instead of a mini-CEX and DOPS.
- It assesses an entire patient episode which may involve clerking a patient in, taking a history and examination, a technical procedure, or a review.

- Areas that are assessed include:
  - history taking
  - performing a clinical examination
  - treatment planning
  - knowledge of performing a procedure
  - technical performance
  - verbal, written, and non-verbal communication
  - keeping professional standards
  - time management
  - reflection.
- There is great flexibility in this type of assessment as it allows for a range of clinical encounters to be assessed.
- The best opportunity to complete these would be during supervised sessions that may be available.
- In general practice this could be virtually any case, however any cases used during tutorial sessions could be particularly useful. In a hospital setting, any consultant-led new patient clinics can be useful as can any other sessions that are supervised.
- Try to follow the same preparation as you would for a mini-CEX or DOPS assessment.

Early-stage peer review (ESPR)

- This assessment is generally unique to DFT.
- It occurs in the first few weeks of the programme.
- The outcome of an ESPR is based on the standard of a newly qualified dentist. All other assessment outcomes are based on the standard expected at the end of the training year.
- The assessment is carried out in the following way:
  - A series of cases or procedures is proposed by the trainer to discuss.
  - A series of cases or procedures is proposed by the trainee to discuss.
  - The trainer provides general feedback.
  - A judgement of either satisfactory or unsatisfactory is made.
- If an unsatisfactory judgement is made, then remedial work may be required as decided between the DFT trainer and trainee.
- The procedures themselves need not be complete treatment plans or even treatment items. They could include specific elements of treatment such as:
  - giving LA
  - writing a prescription
  - placing a rubber dam
  - gaining appropriate valid consent
  - writing a referral letter.
- This assessment identifies a trainee's strengths and weaknesses early on the in the programme.

Multi-source feedback

- A form is given to several (usually a minimum of five) assessors who have worked directly with the trainee over a substantive period of time sufficient to be able to make judgements on the trainee.
- There are two different assessments: team assessment of behaviour and peer assessment tool.

- Each assessor is given a standard form to complete to assess the trainee ensuring that any comments cannot identify the assessor.
- The feedback should focus on an overall impression rather than one-off occurrences.
- This assessment gives a general holistic view from the people the trainee works with, whereas the other assessments focus more on individual encounters or single cases.
- A deadline is issued for the complete collection of the forms to the educational supervisor, who then collects all the responses together.
- A discussion then occurs with the trainee.

Team assessment of behaviour

The following areas are assessed:
- Constructing a professional relationship and building trust with patients.
- Verbal communication skills.
- Working with colleagues and teamwork.
- Being accessible.
- Areas of positive performance.
- Areas that need improvement.

Peer assessment tool

The following areas are assessed:
- Diagnosis and treatment planning skills.
- Ability to use own initiative and use resources appropriately.
- Understanding the psychological and social aspects of illness.
- Time management and set priorities.
- General technical ability.
- Communication skills with patients and their family.
- Respecting confidentiality.
- Written and verbal communication skills with colleagues.
- Recognizing the contributions of other colleagues.
- Being accessible and reliable.
- Trainees' probity and health.
- Areas of positive performance.
- Areas that need improvement.

Patient assessment questionnaire

- This gains patient feedback on the trainee concerned.
- Questions that are asked would normally focus on the professional manner and behaviour of the dentist rather than seeking opinions on the technical quality of treatment.
- Each practice or institution would design its own questionnaire based on the service they provide.
- Things that could be asked include questions around:
  - how the patient was greeted by the trainee
  - enquiring about the patient's visit
  - explaining procedures and examinations prior to doing them
  - informing the patient of any findings without any undue delay
  - discussing the options with the patient and helping them decide
  - inform the patient of the estimated costs in advance of treatment and not waiting until the end
  - showing sensitivity and empathy

- indicating if there is likely to be any pain or unpleasant sensation prior to it occurring and offering appropriate analgesia
  - using language that the patient understands and avoiding jargon
  - inspiring confidence
  - providing preventative advice
  - taking questions.
- Patients would also be asked about the likelihood of them:
  - recommending the dentist to a friend
  - wanting to see the same dentist again.
- This provides a proactive method of assessing patient views. The views of many patients go unheard and when a patient is not happy most do not do anything about it.
- A patient questionnaire allows dentists to identify concerns and comments from a patient perspective.

Other logs required

Other logs required

- Buddy assessments:
  - Occur throughout the year, but not with the same frequency as the other assessments.
  - These mainly consist of ADEPT and case-based discussion where an educational supervisor of a different practice attends and carries out the assessment with the trainee.
  - The main purpose is that it can provide quality assurance and reduce bias between different educational supervisors.
- Other logs that need to be kept:
  - Clinical experience log: to ensure that a sufficient range of procedures are being carried out.
  - Complex treatment log.
  - Non-working day log (including annual leave and sick leave): this ensures that the training is not affected by excessive leave.
  - Learning needs.

Reflection exercises

- Reflective practice is an important part of any dentist's career.
- It is very easy to go through each working day, tackling problems and attending courses without actually learning from them and using the experiences to improve.
- By being a reflective practitioner, you evaluate each situation, whether good or bad, and use it to improve as a professional.
- Similarly, you can attend lots of courses which may seem very productive at the time; however, some months later you may question what the value of the course actually was and has anything actually changed—reflection is now essential for any CPD you declare to the GDC.
- After any patient encounter that went particularly well or not so well, ask yourself the following questions:
  - What was the whole patient encounter?
  - What went well?
  - What were the challenges?
  - What didn't go as well as expected?
  - Why didn't it go as well as expected?
  - What could you do differently?
  - What were the thoughts of others around you, such as the nurse or patient, and your own thoughts on the matter?
  - Try to identify the causes of these things in terms of both good and bad.
- When a situation has not gone as well as expected, try not to be overly critical as this can produce an overall negative outcome. Accept it for what it was, analyse the situation, and look for a way to improve.
- When something has gone particularly well, try to identify why it went well, as this will help identify how a similar result could be achieved again in the future.
- After attending a course or completing any CPD activity, it is worth reflecting on this.
- Ask yourself the following questions:
  - What was your current level of practice in this particular area?
  - What have you learned from this CPD activity?
  - What do you aim to change about your current practice?
  - How will you go about making this change?
  - How will you measure the improvement of your outcomes as a result?
- In these situations, it is worth documenting any reflections made, as it will enable you to think more carefully about each encounter and gain value from it.

Further reading

COPDEND: ℜ www.copdend.org
Health Education England: ℜ www.hee.nhs.uk

Chapter 12

Modern aspects of clinical practice

Evidence-based dentistry

Introduction to evidence-based dentistry

- Patients and the public expect their professional to be competent and contemporary in their approach. It is expected that a professional will be keeping abreast of any new developments and have an understanding of the evidence they are using to inform their decisions.
- Evidence-based practice consists of three aspects:
  - Clinical expertise and knowledge.
  - Patients' preferences and choices.
  - Use of the best available evidence.

Clinical expertise and knowledge

- Long-term experience of the practitioner makes a big difference in this area.
- Pre-existing knowledge.
- CPD.
- Skills of the practitioner.
- To some extent, the individual practitioner's own clinical expertise and knowledge is less important as this could be compensated for by referral to another practitioner who does have the skills and knowledge required—however, the availability of such practitioners can influence this.

Patients' preferences and choices

- Individual patient's views.
- Patient's capacity to make decisions concerning their health.
- Medical status of the patient.
- The patient's own cultural and religious beliefs.
- Social circumstances of the patient.
- Anxiety.
- Patient's perception of the risk/s and benefit/s.
- Patient's willingness to accept the risks.
- Consent.
- Financial circumstances.
- Patient's overall dental attitude.
- For children, the parental views and wishes as well as assent from the patient.

Use of best available evidence

Rank of evidence

In vitro studies

- These are studies undertaken on non-living organisms or tissue.
- Major drawbacks are that the study does not take into account the effects on the whole biological system and potential complications that can result.
- Useful aspects are that subjects can be tested in a standardized way. This is useful when testing for physical properties such as material strengths, or for tests which would not be possible on living subjects.

Animal studies
- Such studies use animals to test an intervention and observe an outcome as a substitute for a human trial.
- The main reason why they are regarded as low levels of evidence is due to the biological differences between animals and humans.
- Where there are close or similar biological situations, these can be used to demonstrate the use of an intervention prior to using it on humans as the studies can also show any gross significant biological incompatibilities of the technique.
- The other reasons include the lack of behavioural factors including patient-centred outcomes such as symptoms, compliance, and aesthetic factors, which are more difficult to assess.

Expert opinion
- This is generally classed as one of the lowest levels of evidence as it is potentially the opinion of one or a group of individuals.
- What constitutes being an expert is not defined.
- It may be one individual specialist, or it could be a committee compiling a consensus document.

Case series/case reports
- Case series and case reports are used to report on unusual conditions or demonstrate a novel technique.
- They are regarded as lower levels of evidence as they are usually one-off events. It may be difficult with rare or unusual conditions to have the number of subjects required be able to conduct large clinical trials or observational studies; however, there may be others (albeit a small number) suffering from similar conditions worldwide who may be able to benefit from a possible strategy used to manage their condition. As such, a case report is the best way of disseminating these ideas.
- There may be unusual/rare reactions to established treatment which may be of significance to report, such as aberrant anatomy—a case report would be best way to share these types of occurrences.
- With regard to case series, these are multiple cases managed with the same technique, although the numbers treated are often small.
- Case reports are often used to show how an established technique could be used in a different way or could be used to solve another problem.

Retrospective studies
- Retrospective studies are based on data that have already been collected.
- Retrospective studies are often chosen due to the ease by which data can be collected as the cases have already been treated, so data collection is much quicker and cheaper.
- There is an increased risk of bias with these studies, in particular that subjects could be selected to exaggerate a particular association and a lot of information gathering in terms of the causative or associated characteristic relies on the patient history, which can be unreliable.
- An example of a retrospective observational study would be a case–control study. This is where there are two groups of subjects: one with the disease (case) of interest and one without (control). With the

exception of the characteristic that is being investigated, all the cases and controls should be as similar as possible.

- There are many treatments that become obsolete after a few years as short-term studies show them to be ineffective. If every treatment option underwent an expensive prospective trial with a 20-year follow-up, then there would be a large number of trials that would either have to terminated early if the results showed them to be ineffective or there would be published studies showing long-term follow-up of a treatment that has long been discontinued. Selective retrospective studies of current established treatments to determine the long-term efficacy cost less, but are more subject to bias.

Prospective studies
- A prospective study is one where the data are collected after the study starts and therefore can be subject to strict inclusion criteria and has greater validity. This is because the terms of the study can be set depending on the area of interest to ensure all details are collected in a consistent and fair way.
- A type of prospective observational study would be a cohort study.
- A cohort study involves observing two groups of subjects—one with the characteristic of interest and one without—and following them both up over a period of time.
- An example would be a group of smokers and a group of non-smokers who do not have periodontitis. They can be followed up over a period of 10 years and the incidence of periodontitis can be measured and the two groups can be compared.
- While prospective observational studies are regarded as a lower level of evidence, they still have great importance. In a clinical trial, it is possible to make an intervention and measure the effect of such an intervention; however, this would have to undergo ethical approval. When a causative agent is being investigated, it would not be considered ethical to have a group of subjects given genuine cigarettes and another group placebo cigarettes as you would effectively be exposing the subjects to harm and measuring the harmful effect rather than measuring anything positive.
- In most cases aetiological agents are often harmful and therefore if a trial wishes to investigate the effect of such an agent on a particular disease, it may only be possible to do this on an observational basis.

Other non-randomized, non-controlled clinical trials
- The value of such trials needs to be questioned.
- Where such a clinical trial lacks randomization, there is a risk of allocation bias, lack of blinding can lead to operator bias, and lack of a control can lead to a lack of ability to make comparisons.

Randomized controlled trials
- These are considered to be the gold standard of clinical trials to test the effect of an intervention, controlling as many variables as possible to determine the true effect of a treatment/intervention.
- The trial will have a control group which may be untreated, treated with a conventional treatment, or receives a placebo treatment.

- The placebo treatment would be identical in every way to that received by the test group but contain no active component and is otherwise indistinguishable and would have no therapeutic effect. The use of a placebo is less common due to ethical considerations.
- The aim of a randomized controlled trial is to determine whether there is a difference between two or more groups. The groups should be matched so that each group is as similar as possible.
- In many cases, the control group cannot be allocated a placebo. The reason behind this would be that if there is already a known established treatment and a new drug or intervention was being tested, then it may be considered unethical to withhold a known effective treatment simply to find out how much better the test intervention is compared to no treatment. In this case, the control group would be allocated the established treatment rather than a placebo.
- When looking at such studies, where an established treatment is used for the control group, it is important to establish the effects of the treatment in the control group compared to the effects shown in the test group.
- You cannot assume that an established intervention has no effect like a placebo in the control group treated. For example, if a study was testing the effect of a sensitive toothpaste, it may be deemed unethical to use a placebo toothpaste. If, however, the control group used a whitening toothpaste than this may distort the conclusions as a whitening toothpaste may be abrasive and hence exacerbate sensitivity. Therefore, if the test group shows a significant difference than this may not be due to the effectiveness of the sensitive toothpaste, but rather the negative effect of the whitening toothpaste which generated the result.
- There is also a recognized placebo effect, which may occur. This is where there is a positive effect on the condition after receiving a treatment with no active component. This can occur due to a range of reasons including the following:
  - The condition is self-limiting and so would have resolved regardless of whether the placebo or treatment was given; however, the resolution of the condition may be attributed to the provision of the treatment even if this was a placebo.
  - Providing a subject with a treatment can give them recognition of their condition and any of the symptoms they are experiencing, enabling them to cope better with their situation and hence reduce the effect of the condition. The subject may then attribute the improvement to the treatment even if it was a placebo.
- The next part of the study is the randomization. The subjects need to be randomly allocated to the treatment groups. If there was no random allocation, this would lead to bias. Random allocation ensures that there are no particular characteristics of the subjects that have been intentionally placed into a specific group.
- Allocation concealment is also important as it ensures that the allocation of the next subject is not known until the moment of allocation.
- Blinding is another significant aspect in the reduction of bias within a trial. If either the operator or subject are aware of the group they have

been allocated, this may affect their compliance or behaviour which may alter the results. If either the subject or the operator/assessor is unaware of their allocation than it is termed a single blind study. If both the operator/assessor and subject are unaware, this is considered a double blinded study. It is not always possible to blind a trial, but every effort should be made to blind to reduce the risk of selection, performing, or detection bias.

- The CONSORT statement is a useful reference for the minimum dataset for randomized controlled trials.[1]
- Typically, in dentistry, these can be parallel studies, where each group gets one treatment only, or cross-over groups, where each group gets both treatments either in different parts of the mouth or at different times.

Systematic reviews

- Systematic reviews and meta-analyses of the literature are generally regarded as the highest standard of evidence.
- 'A systematic review aims to identify, appraise and synthesise all the empirical evidence that meets pre-specified eligibility criteria to answer a specific research question. Researchers conducting systematic reviews use explicit, systematic methods that are selected with a view aimed at minimizing bias, to produce more reliable findings to inform decision making.'[2]
- The authors of these type of articles systematically search through all the published literature on a particular subject, evaluating the quality of each study and presenting the results. Systematic reviews may limit their search to randomized controlled trials, thus increasing the level of evidence and therefore reducing the risk of bias.
- By mathematically combining the data (meta-analysis) from several studies, more subjects are included than in any one study alone, therefore increasing the reliability of the results.
- The method would have to have a clear and precise search strategy such that it could be repeated by anyone and they would get the same results.
- A systematic review is really only as good as the studies it includes.
- Not all systematic reviews would be regarded as being of uniform quality. The search strategy should clearly state the type of studies that are being included. Ideally, randomized controlled trials should be used when researching interventions; however, often other non-randomized trials are used.
- The PRISMA (Preferred Reporting Items for Systematic review and Meta-Analysis)[3] Statement consists of a 27-item checklist and four-phase flow diagram to improve the reporting of systematic reviews.
- The PRISMA statement can be used to critically appraise a systematic review but not quality assess it as there may be items missing, but this does not necessarily take away from the quality of the review.

---

1 www.consort-statement.org/consort-2010

2 www.cochranelibrary.com

3 Moher D (2009). *Br Med J* 21, 339.

- This should not be mistaken for a narrative review, which is a review of literature without any particular search strategy and is used by authors to illustrate a point by showing some literature in favour of the article contents. While a narrative review does not have a high standard of evidence, they are often useful in terms of generating ideas, sharing information, and are usually much easier to read and understand, particularly as they tend to have a lower use of statistics.
- Cochrane reviews are specific systematic reviews undertaken with prescriptive guidelines[4] to ensure standardization in the level of the reviews and therefore reduction of the risk of bias.

Guidelines

- Guidelines are evidence-based statements that are used to inform ideal or best practice.
- They differ from policies or protocols as these refer to practice or procedures that must occur, whereas it may be acceptable to deviate from a guideline.
- While it is generally acceptable to deviate from a guideline if there is a justified reason, it would not be considered acceptable to not follow a guideline because you were unaware of it.
- Often when guidelines are written, they will state the piece of evidence that it is based on as a way of justifying the statement.
- There may also be an indication to the level of evidence that it refers to. Not all statements will be based on the highest level of evidence—it may be the case that the guidelines are based on expert opinion alone.
- Guidelines are developed by many bodies including the NHS, usually via NICE. There are many professional societies and associations including specialist and general bodies that issue guidelines. See ⮞ Professional societies and associations for sources of information on guidelines.
- Locally, a hospital trust will issue a large number of guidelines to help with local decision-making and onward referral.
- The Royal Colleges are also sources of guidelines.
- Guidelines are also a good source for use in audits when looking for examples of best practice—these can often be used with audits to suggest changes to improve local standards.

basics of research design and statistics

Basics of research designs and statistics

This section aims to describe common terms used in studies and some statistical concepts.

Basic terms

- Variables: these are either qualitative, when used for a variable that cannot be assigned a numerical value such as a colour, or quantitative, such as length where a numerical value can be used. Variable are data that are collected or measured.
- Factor: usually used to describe the causative variable.
- Parameters: characteristics of the populations such as incidence or prevalence rate.
- Interaction: this is where the effect of an invention can differ for different groups—for example, the use of stickers as a reward for paediatric dental patients may have a different response in male compared to female patients if the same type of stickers are used.
- Confounders: this is where other factors contribute to the overall effect being measured and therefore may result in a distortion of the actual effect of the variable being measured. For example, smoking may cause stained teeth. Smoking may cause heart disease. It would be incorrect to state that an association exists with stained teeth and heart disease.
- Bias:
  - Allocation: subjects allocated to different groups may not be comparable because of the way they were allocated to each group. Randomization can help with this.
  - Assessment: the differences in the interpretation of the responses to the treatment. This can be reduced by blinding, so patients or observers do not know what treatment is being provided and so the interpretation is more accurate.
  - Observer: when the person carrying out the observation may not be reporting the findings or measuring them in a consistent way.
  - Selection: the sample selected is an inaccurate representation of the population concerned.
  - Publication: the choice of publishers as to whether or not to publish results or decline publication for what they may deem insignificant.
  - Recall: subjects' ability to give an accurate history.
- Confidence intervals: generally, 95% confidence intervals are used. This means that there is a probability of 95% that the true effect will fall within this interval. This is calculated using the standard error. The size of the standard error is determined in part by the sample size. A large sample size would give a small standard error which would in turn give a smaller confidence interval. Where a confidence interval includes the no-effect value (e.g. with relative risks where the no effect value is 1), then this means that the true value of the effect could include no effect, which can happen with large confidence intervals. For this reason, a large sample size would give a smaller confidence interval and give a more accurate estimate of the effect and better conclusions can be drawn.

- Intention to treat: often in many trials there may be patients who drop out as a result of change in address, side effects of treatment, and so on. Intention-to-treat analysis involves including all withdrawals in the analysis and acts as if they continued in the treatment group originally allocated. This goes against natural instinct about the scientific value of managing withdrawals; however, in real practice there also will be patients who withdraw from a treatment regimen and so this takes on a pragmatic approach.

Screening and diagnostic tests terms

- Variance: this is the degree of variability in the observations made.
- Sensitivity: the chance that someone with the condition will generate a positive result in the test.
- Specificity: the chance that someone without the condition will generate a negative result in the test.
- Positive predictive value: the percentage of individuals who have a positive result on the diagnostic test who actually have the condition.
- Negative predictive value: the percentage of individuals who have a negative result on the diagnostic test who are free of the condition.

Hypothesis, null hypothesis, and significance

- Hypothesis: this is the question being asked—for example, to see if there is a difference between two interventions.
- Null hypothesis: this is where there is no effect between the two interventions being questioned in the hypothesis and hence no difference in the two interventions being tested.
- P-value: this is the value used to determine statistical significance. The most common value used is 0.05. If the p-value is 0.05 or lower then it is likely to be statistically significant. 0.05 is used as this represents 5% probability which is the accepted arbitrary figure. In effect, it means that there is a very small chance that the results obtained were by chance alone. A p-value of 0.05 means there is a 95% probability that the result has not been achieved by chance alone. A p-value of 0.01 means that there is a 99% probability that the result has not been achieved by chance alone.
- Statistical significance: this is the ability to reject the null hypothesis of a no-effect situation. This is determined using the p-value. Being statistically significant does not mean that the result has clinical significance. Statistically significant simply means that the result is unlikely to have been made by sampling error alone. For example: if two restorative materials were being investigated for longevity, if restorations with material A survived 10 years and restorations with material B survived 10 years and 1 day, the result may be statistically significant based on a large sample size and other factors.
- Clinical significance: this is how important the actual difference is in clinical practice. A result may be statistically significant which indicates the result was not achieved by chance alone; however, using the same example of material A and B, a 1-day difference over a 10-year lifespan may not be very important particularly if:
  - there was a large cost of material B compared to A
  - other serious side effects.

- Important point for statistical significance: if a result has a p-value >0.05 then it means that the null hypothesis cannot be rejected. It does *not* mean, however, that the null hypothesis can be accepted either. Other reasons for having a result that is not statistically significant are:
  - that the sample size is too small to detect a difference
  - that there is a real difference, but the sample selected did not show it.
- Important point for clinical significance: the actual difference needs to be in the context of other factors. The example of two restorative materials shows something of small clinical significance; however, having a small difference does not mean that it is not clinically significant. An example is the WHO surgical checklist[1] which results in a 2% reduction in potentially serious errors. While 2% seems like a small difference, the checklist is a relatively easy thing to implement and has virtually no cost implications, therefore, to get a 2% reduction in serious errors is considered to be clinically significant.
- Type I error: this is the probability of the null hypothesis being true and being rejected. This otherwise known as alpha (α). Generally, α should not be >0.05. This is because p ≤0.05 as this would be the accepted value for statistical significance.
- Type II error: this is the probability of the null hypothesis being false and not being rejected. This is otherwise known as the beta (β).
- Power: this is $(1 - \beta)$. In effect, it is the probability that the null hypothesis is false and is rejected. This should be at least 80%.

1 WHO (2009). Implementation manual: WHO surgical safety checklist 2009: safe surgery saves lives. ℛhttps://apps.who.int/iris/handle/10665/44186

Sample size

- The sample size of studies is important:
  - Very small sample sizes may not be able to detect a difference or it may be concluded that any difference that has been detected would be by chance alone and so have little relevance.
  - Very large sample sizes may add undue expense to the study, any additional difference may not be significant and may be unethical as there may be too many individuals subjected to experimentation for no real benefit.
- It is therefore vital that the sample size is correct when looking at studies to see if it actually makes a difference.
- Most studies would document in the methods section the way the sample size was calculated and from this information it should be possible to determine if it was appropriate.
- Some published pilot studies may not state the sample size calculation as the purpose of the pilot study may be to generate the information needed to determine an estimate of the actual difference and this can then be used to determine a sample size for a larger study.
- The type of information needed will vary depending on the type of study; however, the following is a list of information that is useful in seeing if the study is of an appropriate size:
  - The expected variance of the data: data that have a high variance are likely to need more subjects as it will be difficult to determine a real difference with a smaller number of data.
  - The expected clinically important differences in the areas being studied: if there is only a subtle difference between treatments, then a greater sample will be required to detect this subtle difference, whereas if a large difference is being expected, then this can be more easily detected with a smaller sample.
- The statistical significance level: this is usually set at 0.05 or less.
- The power: this is usually 80% or higher.

Example of how sample size and significance are linked

Example of how to assess for clinical and statistical significance using three fictional studies. Each study compares the survival of composite A compared to composite B for restoring a class I cavity after 4 years. Each subject has only one restoration. Assume all other factors are similar between each group.

- Study 1: composite A has five patients of which all five restorations have survived after 4 years and composite B has five patients of which four restorations have survived after 4 years. This implies that composite A has a 20% difference in survival compared to composite B. This could therefore be regarded as being clinically significant. The sample size is very small. The p-value for this result is likely to be $p > 0.05$, and therefore is not statistically significant. This means that the null hypothesis cannot be rejected as there is not a large enough sample size and the result could have occurred simply by chance alone.
- Study 2: composite A has 200 patients of which 190 restorations have survived after 4 years. Composite B has 150 patients of which 120 restorations have survived after 4 years. For the results it could be

concluded that composite A has a 15% difference survival compared to composite B. The sample size is large and so the p <0.05 which indicates this is statically significant.

- Study 3: composite A has 10,000 patients of which 9504 restorations have survived after 4 years. Composite B has 20,000 patients of which 16,000 restorations survived after 4 years. The sample size is large and so p <0.01. Composite A has a survival difference of 15.04% compared to composite B which is clinically significant. The sample size is extremely large. The cost of the study would have been high. There would also be doubt that such a study would get ethics approval as it is subjecting a large number of people to experimentation when a smaller number could have shown a similarly meaningful result.

Critically appraising literature

- Being able to critically appraise literature is a really useful skill to have to correctly apply study results to practice.[1]
- There is a huge amount of literature available and not everything is useful—it is important to be able to look at the study and see what use, if any, it has rather than simply take on the conclusions and assume they are universally applicable.

Overall assessment of a paper

- Is there a clearly defined question that is being investigated?
- For review articles, were the correct type of studies searched for? Is there a clear method which is reproducible to carry out the search? How have the results been combined?
- For trials: think about the allocation of patients to treatment groups, randomization, blinding, similarities between the treatment groups, and follow-up.
- For studies looking at cause and effect: think about the type of study used and if it was appropriate, how the subjects were selected and defined, the time frame for the study, were the controls appropriate with a sufficient number and good response rate, the exposure and if it was appropriate, measurements taken, confounders, and were the groups representative of the population.
- Think about the power of the study, sample size, and bias.

Results

- What were the overall results?
- How precise were the results, were there confidence intervals?
- Are they statistically significant? What were the p-values?
- What adjustments have been made for confounders?

Local application

- Do the results apply to the local population?
- Is the setting of the study similar and does this make a difference (hospital/practice)?
- Consider the cost versus the benefit.
- Are the results significant enough to be worthwhile?

---

1 Critical Appraisal Skills Programme (CASP UK): ⅋ www.casp-uk.net

Clinical governance

Introduction to clinical governance

- 'Clinical governance is a system through which NHS organizations are accountable for continuously improving the quality of their services and safeguarding high standards of care by creating an environment in which excellence in clinical care will flourish.'[1]
- The main aspects of clinical governance are:
  - research and development
  - education and training
  - clinical and cost-effectiveness
  - clinical audit
  - information governance
  - risk management
  - openness and accountability.

Education and training

- This has in part already been covered in aspects of postgraduate training.
- The main focus of this would be CPD.
- As a dentist, CPD is a compulsory part of remaining on the dentist register—this is not necessarily the case for other healthcare professionals, but it is part of QI of clinical governance.

Clinical effectiveness

- Clinical effectiveness is concerned with measuring, monitoring, and improving clinical care.
- While this may seem obvious, it is a constantly changing area which has its foundations in evidence-based practice.
- It is also about the appropriateness of treatment and patient safety.
- It emphasizes the need to discontinue outdated and unsafe practices.
- Within a state-funded system such as the NHS, other factors also need to be considered including cost-effectiveness.

Clinical audit

- Clinical audit is a cycle (Fig. 12.1) composed of the following elements:
  - Identify a problem: the very purpose of clinical audit is to identify a clinical problem and look to improve on it. In all areas of our practice, it will be possible to identify things we feel are not going right or could be done better. An audit is a way of making things better.
  - Identify the gold standard: this is important for it to be regarded as an audit. Without a gold standard, the project may be considered as research and as such would have to be considered differently with ethic committee approval, although audit may lead to research. Such standards can be from established guidelines (e.g. NICE guidelines), predefined targets (e.g. 18-week referral to treatment target), published literature, or locally set standards.
  - Collect data that are relevant to the standards being measured: this includes data collection methods such as tables or forms. Aspects

1 Scally G (1998), *Br Med J* 317, 61.

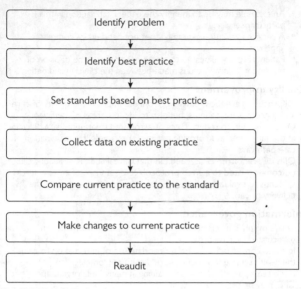

Fig. 12.1 The audit cycle.

of information governance need to be considered if asking patients questions. The data should be collected strictly to identify the current standard and not to generate new information.
- Compare against the set standard: process the data and identify if the standards are being achieved. Where there is a deficiency in the standards being met then identify the cause of such a shortfall.
- Implement change: after identifying what needs to be changed, take the steps to implement such change. In certain institutions this may not be the choice of the individual clinician, but of the department or practice.
- Repeat the audit cycle: in doing so, it may be important to review any changes to published literature or guidelines to identify change or other issues—identify if there is still a shortfall and, if so, then implement further change and repeat.
- Service evaluations are similar to audits; however, there may not be a gold standard:
  - This should not be confused for research. Research aims to identify new knowledge; a service evaluation aims to evaluate the effectiveness of existing evidence-based practice or service with the aim to gain information on that particular service to assist with local decision-making.
  - It is otherwise known as a baseline audit.
  - The results cannot be generalized to other departments or units—this is the role of research.

- An example may be to identify the patient satisfaction with a particular service.
- A service evaluation generally does not need ethics committee approval.
- Patients are not allocated to treatment groups—the decision of treatment is known and is made between the clinician and patient.

Quality improvement

- QI processes are those aiming not only to improve the quality of care and outcomes for patients, but also to identify areas of inefficiency.
- QI can also aim to reduce costs of associated treatment/care delivery at the same time as improving quality, for example, by examination of care pathways.
- QI is different from clinical audit in that clinical audit is evaluating clinical outcomes related to a given protocol/gold standard of care, whereas QI tends to evaluate the patient experience or the process of the delivery of care.[2]

Information governance

- This is mainly concerned with the use of patient information in particular clinical records.
- It is also concerned with the appropriate use of information to guide the health service to produce good health outcomes.
- It is often a part of mandatory training in many NHS organizations and CPD may be required in this area.

Caldicott

- A senior person in each NHS organization is required to act as the Caldicott guardian,[3] whose duty it is to oversee any aspect of patient-identifiable data. This includes the flow of information between individuals.
- There are seven Caldicott principles that need to be adhered to:
  - The purpose of using patient-identifiable data must be clearly justified for each use.
  - Patient-identifiable data must not be used unless necessary and essential. The continuing need for this type of data must assessed.
  - Only the minimum amount of patient-identifiable data required must be used.
  - There must be a need-to-know basis for the use of patient-identifiable data. That essentially means if someone is not contributing positively with the use of the data then they do not need to know it.
  - Those who do have access to patient-identifiable information must be aware of their individual responsibility towards it including confidentiality. This includes all staff, not just healthcare professionals.
  - All those involved must comply with the law.

2 Limb C (2017). *Int J Surg Oncol* 2, e24.

3 Lea W (2013). Information: to share or not to share? The information governance review. ℬ https://assets.publishing.service.gov.uk/government/uploads/system/uploads/attachment_d ata/file/192572/2900774_InfoGovernance_accv2.pdf

- All those with access to patient-identifiable data must be aware when it is appropriate to share such information and the policies surrounding this and do so when necessary.
- Understanding of the Caldicott principles is essential and may even come up in an interview question.
- In secondary care settings, there are often several healthcare professionals managing a single case and therefore it is essential to know who should have what information.
- The purpose of this policy would be to ensure that information is readily available and accurate when required and that it is adequately protected from undesirable disclosure.
- There are several policies that are often included within this including:
  - confidentiality and security policy
  - mobile computing policy
  - records management policy
  - corporate records management policy
  - freedom of information policy
  - social networking policy.
- The General Data Protection Regulation 2018:
  - There are rights for individuals including the right to be informed, access to data, correcting or rectifying the data, erasing data, place restrictions on processing, to data portability, to object, not to be involved with automated processing.
  - Subject access requests must be made within 1 month and should be without charge.
  - If a request is refused, the individual can complain to the Information Commissioners Office.
  - There has to be a lawful basis for holding information: consent, contract, legal obligation, vital interest, public interest, or legitimate interest.
  - Consent is required for marketing.
  - Where there is a data breach then this may have to be reported to the Information Commissioners Office and possibly the Individuals concerned.
  - For public bodies (including those dental practices providing NHS care) a data protection officer would need to be appointed to take responsibility for compliance.
- The Freedom of Information Act 2000 also applies which concerns public bodies holding information and giving public access to such information. The act is also covered by the Information Commissioners Office.
- Individuals or organizations that process personal information would be required to register with the Information Commissioners Office as data controllers.
- The Information Commissioners Office has the power to take action including issue fines or prosecute those who fail to comply with the Data Protection Act or Freedom of Information Act.

Research and development

- This is the development of guidelines, strategies, and changes in policy depending on newly available research.

- This can also include the development of other protocols, local policies, and pathways which would be based on research.
- Examples include the WHO surgical checklist[4] implementation.

Risk management

- Risk management is mainly concerned with the risk to the:
  - patients
  - professionals
  - organization.

Risk to patients

- Many risks to patients are reduced by the use of clinical guidelines, statutory regulation, and local policies and protocols. All of these help to reduce or even prevent risks occurring to patients.
- Examples include the use of NICE guidelines for wisdom tooth extraction, local prophylactic regimens for management of patients with a history of bisphosphonate use, and completion of VTE risk assessments.
- Undergoing safeguarding training for both children and vulnerable adults and being aware of local safeguarding policies as well how to escalate matters.
- Being able to complete critical incident forms and be able to honestly report untoward actions.

Risk to professionals

- Immunization of blood-borne viruses such as hepatitis B virus.
- Regular training in risk management topics such as:
  - manual handling
  - slips, trips, and falls
  - fire safety
  - compliance with working hours directive on rest periods
  - ensuring indemnity cover is adequate and up to date.

Risk to organization

- Ensuring staff are compliant with equality and diversity training.
- Quality assurance procedures.
- Ensuring good recruitment procedures including for those being recruited as locums.
- Ensuring that the building and facilities conform to health and safety regulations.
- Registration and continued compliance with CQC requirements.

Openness, honesty, and accountability

- It is generally accepted that any sort of medical or dental treatment is not free from risk and mistakes can occur, whether this is as a result of human error or as a result of a system problems within an organization.
- The duty of candour[5] is about being honest with patients when things go wrong and giving a frank explanation of what happened, what is

---

4 WHO (2009). Implementation manual: WHO surgical safety checklist 2009: safe surgery saves lives. ⅁ https://apps.who.int/iris/handle/10665/44186

5 RCS England (2015). Duty of candour: guidance for surgeons and employers. ⅁ https://www.rcseng.ac.uk/-/media/files/rcs/standards-and-research/standards-and-policy/good-practice-guides/new-docs-may-2019/rcs-_duty-of-candour.pdf

going to be done to manage the situation, and what steps are going to be undertaken to prevent the situation from happening again.
- This is about ensuring that mistakes and errors are not covered up.
- This can be associated with risk management by reporting the incident following the practice's or organization's procedures.
- Following an incident, it is worth reflecting on the situation and most portfolios for both DFT and DCT would normally have a section to document a reflection on the issue concerned and what steps are to be taken. This is worth doing after discussion with any colleagues.
- The duty of candour and being open and honest is not focused on attributing blame on an individual but should be more focused on the needs of the patient, including the need to be honest about what happened and how this can be managed better in the future.
- A key aspect of clinical governance is about 'creating an environment where excellence in clinical care can flourish', therefore care must be taken not use this as an opportunity to put blame on individuals or use it as a disciplinary process, which can often be counterproductive. This could create a hostile environment and as such may discourage other staff from reporting incidents in the fear that it may work against them—which can have far-reaching consequences.
- Following the situation and after the patient has been managed safely, it is therefore important to ensure that the colleagues involved with the situation are properly supported. This is to ensure that the colleagues can understand the actions with a focus on improvement rather than punishment and so that they can be encouraged to continue to be open and honest in the future.

Management

All workplace environments (general dental practices, community dental services, and hospital departments) have a management framework to work within. Part of the management process includes implementation of guidelines, protocols, policies, and procedures.

Infection control policy

- Should include details on training requirements for all staff.
- Immunization requirements and testing for immunity and consequences for not being having sufficient levels of immunity.
- Personal protective equipment that is required for clinical work.
- Hand hygiene details and requirements.
- Decontamination of reusable instruments including disinfection, inspection, sterilization, and storage, with details either within the same policy or another on how different instruments would be decontaminated such as the difference between solid instruments and those with hollow tubes and hand pieces (HTM 01-05).[1]
- Disposing of single-use instruments and sharps.
- Cleaning of the water lines in each dental unit.
- Decontamination of laboratory work.
- Management of inoculation injuries.
- Management of spillages including body fluids and mercury.
- Management of aerosol-generating procedures and standard operating procedures.

Complaints policy

- Every dental workplace environment must have a complaints policy or procedure.
- This must comply with the GDC standards principle 5.[2]
- The policy should be clearly visible and include time scales for dealing with complaints, regular updates should this not be possible, and how the patient can escalate the complaint should they feel that there is not a satisfactory response.
- Any complaint needs to be acknowledged within 3 days of receiving the complaint, apologizing for the patient's dissatisfaction whether the complaint is justified or not. An apology is not an admission of guilt but is empathetic to the patient's concerns.
- A constructive manner should be adopted rather than a defensive one when dealing with a complaint and lessons learnt wherever possible, which should be shared with the rest of the team.
- Where appropriate and possible, a solution should be offered.
- Local resolution is preferred, but if this is not possible, it may be necessary to escalate the complaint. If this is an NHS patient, this may be to the local area team or may require you to inform the patient of their right to take the complaint to the ombudsman.[3]

---

1 ℘ www.gov.uk/government/publications/decontamination-in-primary-care-dental-practices

2 GDC (2013). Standards for the dental team. ℘ https://standards.gdc-uk.org/

3 ℘ www.ombudsman.org.uk

Radiography standards

- Every exposure must be recorded with a clinical justification and report.[4,5]
- Justification must bear in mind the following:
  - Risk of harm through ionizing radiation versus the diagnostic benefit of the radiograph.
  - The clinical justification of the exposure compared to other means such as non-ionizing imaging.
  - Any other image that the patient may already have.
- The quality of each exposure must be recorded:
  - A: acceptable.
  - N: not acceptable.

Local radiography rules

- The location to which these rules apply must be recorded. This will usually be the practice or department address.[5]
- The local radiation protection advisor must be recorded. This may be a person but could also be another external agency who fulfils this role.
- The radiation protection supervisor must be recorded. This could also be an external agent commissioned to fulfil this role.
- The designated controlled and supervised area must be recorded.
- Details of the radiography equipment must be recorded.
- The use of the radiography equipment must be explained including articles such as films or sensors.
- Contingency planning needs to be made clear if for example:
  - there is a failure of the ionization to stop
  - there is a defect to the lead shielding around the tube.
- Means of processing the radiographs to be explained.
- Test objects to ensure consistency in quality.
- Record the roles of classified people.
- The need for dosimeters needs to be recorded.
- Operator position needs to be recorded along with estimated hourly dose.
- Any direction that the beam cannot be directed towards—for example, a window.
- Number of exposures per week to be carried out.

Child safeguarding policy

- There should be a clear protocol to state that should a child be in immediate danger than the police may have to be informed.[6]
- In many other cases a telephone referral will be needed to the local child protection unit and followed up with a written referral within 24 hours.

4 Faculty of General Dental Practitioners (2018). Selection criteria for dental radiography. ℘ https://cgdent.uk/selection-criteria-for-dental-radiography/

5 Public Health England (2020). Guidance notes for dental practitioners on the safe use of X-ray equipment (2nd ed). ℘ https://www.rqia.org.uk/RQIA/files/44/449bdd1c-ccb0-4322-b0df-616a0de88fe4.pdf

6 Public Health England (2019). Safeguarding in general dental practice: a toolkit for dental teams. ℘ https://www.gov.uk/government/publications/safeguarding-in-general-dental-practice

- Things to consider when assessing patients for possible child safeguarding issues:
  - The interaction between the child, parent, and/or carers seems inappropriate.
  - Unduly inappropriate delay in presentation of injury.
  - An immobile child with bruising.
  - There is inconsistency in the history, reason for attendance, or reasons relating to the injury.
  - Multiple attendances.
  - Drug/alcohol/domestic abuse.
  - Mental health issues that may affect parental capacity.
- Examples of abuse and how to possibly recognize it:
  - Physical: particularly on immobile children, bruising on areas where there is a lack of bony prominences, disclosure made by child, torn labial frenum, fracture to the skull, bleeding within skull.
  - Emotional: this is the persistent ill treatment of a child so as to cause adverse effects on the child's development. There can be persistent inappropriate adult interaction, and feeling in the child of worthlessness or being unloved. There can also be overprotection of the child or preventing the child from participation.
  - Sexual: from a dental perspective, recognition of this can include disclosures by the child, pregnancy, and reporting of sexually transmitted disease.
  - Neglect: inappropriate clothing for the child and includes the persistent failure to meet physical and psychological needs, which can start from pregnancy. There may be a failure to provide food, shelter, or clothing as well as failure to protect the child from physical and emotional harm. This includes a parent's failure to bring the child to appointments.
  - Fabrication: when symptoms or illness has been deliberately caused or exacerbated in a child or vulnerable adult by someone else such as the parent or carer.
  - Extremism: opposition to British values such as liberty, democracy, rule of law, and tolerance of various beliefs and faiths.
  - Discrimination: unequal treatment on the basis of a protected characteristic.
  - Female genital mutilation: all procedures relating to injury or removal of the external female genitalia (either partial or total), for cultural or non-therapeutic reasons.
  - Forced marriage: when one or both parties are married without either or both of their consent.
  - Modern slavery: holding an individual in forced or compulsory labour or slavery.
- Risk indicators which may increase a child's susceptibility to neglect or abuse include:
  - parents with mental illness, previous history of domestic or substance abuse
  - parents with poor experience or ability to parent
  - parents who were abused themselves
  - disability.

- For the purpose of safeguarding, a child means one of the following:
  - Any person up until their 18th birthday.
  - An unborn baby.
- The only individuals that have parental responsibility are the following:
  - Mother unless parental responsibility is removed by a court or child arrangement order.
  - In the case of surrogacy, the host mother retains parental responsibility not the commissioning parents.
  - Father, if married to the mother at the time of conception or shortly after or currently married to the mother or named on the birth certificate.
  - The local authority if the patient is being fostered; however, the mother still can also retain her parental responsibility.
- Only someone with parental responsibility can give consent for a child under the age of 16 years, unless they are deemed to be Gillick competent. A child (usually aged 14–15 years) who has not reached their 16th birthday, is perceived to have the maturity to be able to understand and recall the information given, weigh up the risks and benefits, and come to a rational decision. If this is the case, then the patient may give consent for a procedure.
- In any case where consent has been obtained, then the child's assent should also be sought to show respect for their growing autonomy.
- A patient from the age of 16 years until just before their 18th birthday can give consent to treatment but cannot refuse treatment if a parent has given consent to it.
- From the age of 18 years, only the patient can give consent.

Safeguarding of vulnerable adults

- This includes individuals who are above the age of 18 years who may lack the ability to self-care or the lack of ability to protect themselves from harm or exploitation [6]
- A culture of abuse can form when long-standing poor practices become the accepted norm.
- They can be subject to abuse similar to children but may present differently.
- Examples include the following:
  - Physical: force feeding an adult; rough handling including causing pain (with or without visible injury). Adults may disguise injuries possibly by covering them up with extra clothing and there may be weight loss. This can be caused by a person or people who are more powerful physically, in terms of hierarchical position, or by taking advantage of someone with a lower degree of mental capacity. Injuries that are inconsistent with a history can indicate physical abuse as can an unusual reaction to physical contact.
  - Sexual: occurs if the adult lacks capacity, or without consent, or under pressure. Signs include depression, stress, change in sexual behaviour, and incontinence.
  - Emotional: this can include the threat or perception of violence, bullying, humiliation, and using language to disrespect the individual. Indicators include being emotionally withdrawn, passivity, negativity towards others, and need for reassurance.

- Neglect: can be due to general omission causing the needs of the individual to be neglected including failure to follow guidelines or protocols. Indicators include poor dress, not in a physically well position, regularly misses appointments, or failure to take medication. Although these may be signs of neglect, they can also be lifestyle choices made by an individual with capacity.
- Discriminatory: this is where there is unfair segregation based on protected characteristics including age, disability, gender reassignment, marriage and civil partnership, pregnancy and maternity, race, religion or belief, sex, and sexual orientation.
- Financial abuse: control or restriction of the individual's right to free movement, stealing, preventing the individual from seeking advice, or using the identity of the victim for other gains. This can be shown by an individual's lack of ability to make choices or pay for things that they would otherwise be able to do.
- Institutional/organizational: where staff concerns or convenience is put ahead of that of the patient and possibly using punitive means to achieve control.

Documentation, reporting, and escalating in safeguarding

- If a disclosure is made or safeguarding issues are identified, then it is important to document this.[6]
- If possible, ask the individual to document this; if not, try to use the victim's own words.
- Avoid extensive questioning, particularly if the alleged abuser is present. Take the individual elsewhere, make sure you are chaperoned, and ensure others are involved including senior colleagues.
- Do not approach the alleged abuser.
- Ensure details are recorded as best as possible including times and locations.
- Follow local policy which should be made available and decide how to escalate according to local protocol. Never handle these situations on you own—always ensure it is escalated appropriately.
- Where incidents occur, this must also be appropriately documented through critical incident reporting.
- Ensure any advice that is received is also documented.

Confidentiality

- All members of the dental team, including dental nurses (both registered and trainees) and clerical and domestic staff need to be aware of the confidentiality policy.
- As a dentist, other members of staff may request advice when being asked to disclose information to third parties.
- With the exception of when a patient gives consent, there are a limited number of cases when a patient's confidentiality may have to be breached and professional judgement should be used in such cases.
- When patients call asking about their own information such as appointment time or treatment details then measures should be taken to verify the patient's identity such as the date of birth, address, postcode, telephone number, or next of kin details.

- Ensure that patients' names or details are not announced in the waiting area, for example, avoid stating the patient's name when telling another colleague in the waiting room of a cancellation—instead, state the appointment time slot and the clinician they were due to see.
- Outside of work do not discuss patient details.
- Outside the surgery do not discuss treatment as this could be overheard by other patients.

Data security

- Reference to the confidentiality policy is essential.
- Any physical hard copies of data must be stored within lockable fireproof containers with restricted access.
- The premises must have good security.
- Original hard copies of the data should not leave the practice.
- Where data are stored on computer then there should be the means of backing up the data on a regular basis as well as a full audit trail to prevent overwriting the original data as well as tracking of the individuals who made such amendments.
- Staff training should include the use of such systems.

Consent

- All treatment and interventions as well as examinations and investigations should have informed consent.
- There are exceptions where the treatment is being completed in the patients' best interests, in which case this may need to be done with the use of a best interests meeting when the patient does not have capacity to consent.
- In the case of examinations, consent may be implied by the patient sitting back; however, it is usually customary to advise the patient of what you are doing as you are doing it.
- It is important that the consent process conforms to GDC standards for the dental team principle 3.[2]
- The important aspects of consent are that it is informed and valid. For this to happen, it is important that a full discussion happens with the patient, informing them of the risks and benefits in a way they can understand and checking that it has been understood. Ensure that the patient is able to ask questions and is able to weigh up the information to come to a decision and for them to communicate that.
- Patients should be allowed time to go away and think about the options.
- It may also be beneficial to provide patient information leaflets as this can help the patient recall any necessary information.
- The use of written consent can also be helpful, although a signature on a form does not substitute for a discussion with the patient. Where consciousness is impaired, such as treatment under conscious sedation or GA, then written consent is required.
- In many cases the consent process may be delegated to other members of staff; however, every member of staff involved in the patient's treatment should ensure consent has been obtained and not simply rely on others to do it.
- Costs also need to be mentioned in any consent policy as well as the explanation if the treatment is being done on a private or NHS basis.

Harassment, grievances, and bullying in the workplace policy

- There should be a policy surrounding grievances, harassment, and bullying, particularly in hospital units.
- It should state who to approach in the first instance to get resolution.
- Often resolution is considered preferable at a local level within the department; however, there are stages where this may need to be escalated and the policy should detail how to do this.
- There are some who believe in 'training through intimidation' which has no place in work-based training and therefore anyone subject to this should consider consulting the policy. Like most policies, this should be on the workplace intranet.

Referral to treatment time (RTT) policy

- This generally applies to those who are in hospital departments where RTTs apply and there are financial penalties for the trust for failing to meet those targets.
- RTT is the time period from referral to receiving the first definitive treatment.
- The RTT is usually 18 weeks and 90% of inpatients must meet this target while 95% of outpatient-only treatment will need to meet this target.
- There are different rules for cancer cases.
- There are often policies or procedures to help meet the target.
- Examples include how to manage a patient who fails to attend an appointment and those patients who cancel appointments.
- The aim is to reduce wasted appointments so that other patients can be seen and the RTT is kept to a minimum.
- Often the financial implication of failing to meet the target is proportional to the income.
- Nonetheless, it is usually customary to check with the consultant prior to discharging patients.
- A good working knowledge of outcome coding within hospitals is required to ensure appropriate 'stopping of the 18-week RTT clock'.

Risk assessment

This includes assessment of the significant hazard, those at risk, measures taken to reduce the risk, and any particular actions that may be required with respect to the following:
- Autoclave.
- Blood and body fluids such as saliva.
- Disposal of hazardous and infectious waste.
- Display screen equipment such as visual display units.
- Eye injury from aerosol and splash.
- Electrical particularly from equipment.
- Fire.
- Hazardous substances.
- Ionizing radiation.
- Manual handling.

- Sharps and inoculation injuries.
- Slips, trips, or falls.

Health and safety

- There should be a practice policy relating to health and safety.
- The regulations concerned should address at least those mentioned in the health and safety section of ➲ Key skills portfolio.

Professional societies and associations

Introduction to professional societies and associations

- Within dentistry there are a huge number of bodies that you can join.
- Joining such bodies can be beneficial to your overall career as they can provide advice and updates within their particular area of interest, and identify training and professional development.

Requirements to become a member

- In order to become a member, most if not all will require a membership fee which would normally be renewed annually and may have other conditions such as:
  - passing a stipulated examination
  - being recommended by an existing member for membership
  - being within a certain GDC registrant group or eligible for such a group such as a dentist or specific dental care professional, so may not be available to undergraduate students
  - there may be a requirement to be working in a specific environment or be in a specific job role such as a registrar or practice manager.

Benefits of becoming a member

- Benefits commonly offered by many dental societies and bodies include the following:
  - Attendance at their conference or events or discounted entry into such events.
  - Subscription to journals or periodicals.
  - To be able to enter prize competitions such as case or audit prizes.
  - Access to research funding.
  - Access to their own publications such as guidelines or policy documents.
  - Advice or support either via published fact sheets or phone lines.
  - Opportunities to influence the profession by participating in committees.
  - There may also be some additional non-dental-related benefits such as discounts on travel or financial services.
  - Professional advice.
- There are many job descriptions which may have membership of certain bodies as being a desirable or essential requirement, such as membership with a Royal College.
- By being a member there is a possibility of tax benefits with some membership subscriptions being tax deductible. Consult an accountant if necessary or check with HMRC.
- Many bodies (both within and outside of the dental sector) provide the use of post nominals if you are a member of that body. When using such post nominals, care must be taken to ensure that it does not mislead the public or patients.

Levels of membership

- Many bodies that are either colleges or academies may have a staged approach to their membership such as:
  - member

- accreditation
- fellow.
- Progression within such academies or colleges would usually be by the completion of cases, oral viva or written examinations, completion of CPD in specific fields, teaching, or other academic requirements.
- To retain membership at that level there may be further activities required on an annual or other periodic basis, with the risk of demotion otherwise.
- There may also be different annual fees required at each stage with a fee for being considered for promotion of membership.
- For many other bodies that are not academies or colleges there may be different levels of membership with each progressive level corresponding to further enhanced benefits—effectively more benefits for more premium membership levels and upgrades can occur by simply paying more money.

Tips for choosing a society or association to join

- Take a look at the website of the society and see what benefits they offer.
- Look through your PDP and identify areas that the society could help with.
- When considering the level of membership, aim to bear in mind the long-term commitment that may be required in terms of:
  - time commitment (e.g. the time taken to complete any extra CPD or produce cases or be available for teaching)
  - financial implications
  - patients (is there a sufficient patient base in your current situation to be able to produce the necessary cases required to maintain or achieve a higher level of membership?)
  - practice resources: for example, if you need to produce sedation cases, are nurses trained to assist with sedated patients?
  - is the level of benefits actually being used or is there a plan to use them?
- Is this something you need to join for career progression? If not, is this something that can benefit you in other ways (e.g. a reduced rate for journal subscription)?
- Review any memberships that you have and do not be afraid to stop being a member of one if you find that there is no longer a benefit to you. For memberships that provide post nominals, these will no longer be able to be used if membership subscriptions cease.

List of relevant professional organizations/societies

- Several bodies have been listed under different categories which should be used as a reference. Some of these bodies may have cross links with other categories so it is important to look them up for yourself to see how they may be applicable.
- None of these bodies are endorsed or recommended and there are likely to be many more available including many local or regional bodies which can also have a great benefit.
- Some of these bodies may be international and there may be different rules that may apply to them.

General
- British Association of Private Dentistry.
- British Dental Association.
- British Society for General Dental Surgery.
- College of General Dentistry.

Royal Colleges (surgical)
- Faculty of Dental Surgery within one of the royal colleges.
- Royal College of Physicians and Surgeons of Glasgow.
- Royal College of Surgeons Edinburgh.
- Royal College of Surgeons England.
- Royal College of Surgeons in Ireland.

Colleges (other)
- Faculty of Medical Leadership and Management.
- Royal College of Physicians London.
- Royal College of Radiologists.

Child oral health, orthodontics, and craniofacial
- British Orthodontic Society.
- British Society for the Study of Cranio-Mandibular Disorders.
- British Society of Paediatric Dentistry.
- European Academy of Paediatric Dentistry.
- European Cleft and Craniofacial Association.
- European Orthodontic Society.
- International Association of Paediatric Dentistry.
- International Confederation of Cleft Lip & Palate and Related Craniofacial Anomalies.
- World Federation of Orthodontists.

Dental public health
- British Association for the Study of Community Dentistry.
- Faculty of Public Health.
- Royal Institute of Public Health.
- Royal Society for Public Health.

Special care dentistry
- British Society for Disability and Oral Health.
- British Society of Gerodontology.
- International Society for Disability and Oral Health.
- Special Care Dentistry Association.

Research
- British Society for Oral and Dental Research.
- International Association for Dental Research.

Restorative dentistry
- British Academy for Cosmetic Dentistry.
- British Academy of Aesthetic Dentistry.
- British Academy of Restorative Dentistry.
- British Endodontic Society.
- British Society for Restorative Dentistry.
- British Society of Periodontology.
- British Society of Prosthodontics.

- European Federation of Periodontology.
- European Prosthodontic Association.
- European Society of Endodontology.
- International Academy of Periodontology.
- International College of Prosthodontists.
- International Federation of Endodontic Association.
- Restorative Dentistry UK including the Specialty Registrars in Restorative Dentistry Group.

Implant dentistry
- Association of Dental Implantology.
- European Association of Osseointegration.

Oral and maxillofacial surgery
- British Association of Oral and Maxillofacial Surgeons.
- British Association of Oral Surgery.
- European Association of Cranio-Oral and Maxillofacial Surgery.
- International Association of Oral and Maxillofacial Surgery.

Oral medicine, pathology, and radiology
- British and Irish Society for Oral Medicine.
- British Society for Oral and Maxillofacial Pathology.
- British Society of Dental and Maxillofacial Radiology.
- European Academy of Dento-Maxillofacial Radiology.
- European Association of Oral Medicine.

Examinations and qualifications

Introduction to examinations and qualifications

- Many dentists following graduation will undertake further examinations or qualifications.
- See the postgraduate training section (➔ Postgraduate education) for details on undertaking various types of postgraduate training or education which can lead to a qualification.
- One of the most common qualifications gained would be a membership diploma of one of the Royal Colleges (e.g. MFDS).
- Membership diplomas of one of the Royal Colleges are popular postgraduate qualifications as they assess knowledge appropriate for 1–2 years after a primary dental degree, thus the content of the examination would have been covered during DFT or DCT. They are also desirable qualifications for further development such as applying for specialist training.
- Unlike memberships or specific CPD courses there are often post nominals associated with qualifications.
- The regulations of each qualification must be read, particularly with membership examinations as there are often clauses which stipulate membership fees must be paid to retain the qualification.
- Awarding bodies are generally universities and colleges, with some academies.

How qualifications can benefit career paths

- In many careers, individual workers may have an annual appraisal as part of their employment and having a qualification may result in an increase in income—this is not often the case as a dentist.
- Having a qualification from any particular body shows that you have met the standard they expect and adds credibility to your knowledge and skills which may add 'value' in other ways—for example, meeting parts of person specifications for jobs or training posts or being more valuable for specific practices.
- Like everything else in this handbook, care needs to be taken when choosing qualifications to undertake. Obtaining multiple membership diplomas based on the same curriculum or content may come across as very authoritative to many patients looking at a practice website; however, many others in the profession may not see it in the same light. This may be a way of attracting patients but may not be a good way to gain referral from other colleagues if this was the objective.
- Similarly, if you are trying to build a referral practice, having a smaller number of qualifications that represent more in-depth study and training and are well known for this among colleagues may have higher value.

Credit scheme for qualifications

- Many university postgraduate courses run a credit scheme whereby qualifications produce a number of postgraduate credits. Generally, it is as follows:
  - Postgraduate certificate = 60 credits.

- Postgraduate diploma = 120 credits.
- Postgraduate master's degree = 180 credits.
- One credit would equate to ~10 hours of study time. This study time may not necessarily mean didactic teaching as it could include self-directed learning.

Courses, examinations, and qualifications

- As mentioned in the postgraduate training section (➲ Postgraduate education), there is a compulsory CPD scheme expected for all dental professionals to maintain their registration, which is measured in terms of hours dedicated to the activity.
- Dedicating a certain amount of time in terms of CPD hours to a particular subject does not in itself provide external evidence of competency in a particular area.
- There are many courses that also have examinations or assessments attached. This may sound somewhat daunting, but one of the major benefits of such assessments is that it introduces quality assurance.
- The courses that have assessments attached to them may often take a variable number of hours to achieve as it may take different people a different amount of time to complete the study required to pass the assessment. Such courses may not then have a stipulated verifiable CPD associated with it and, as such, may not be eligible for verifiable CPD hours.
- However, while the courses with assessments may not have CPD hours that can be used, by having the assessment it allows the quality assurance for the stated outcome. In other words, it is more likely to provide rigorous evidence of skills and achievements made. Many courses that have assessments attached to them may state that completion of the course renders it a qualification from that body—this should still be regarded as valuable due to the quality assurance it brings.
- Further courses attended even by non-dental or even non-clinical-based providers can also provide a good portfolio. For example, a course developed by business industries in communication skills, customer services, and leadership can still have great value within dentistry.

Chapter 13

Career development

Introduction to career development

- The opportunities within dentistry are almost limitless, with development of a career following further training or experience.
- As a dentist, the majority of employed positions are found within the NHS and universities, with few employed options outside of this, although there are more employed options emerging within primary dental care, particularly within the corporate bodies.
- The NHS hospital system or community dental service has pay progression with experience, although advancing to a higher banding will most likely involve further training.
- Outside NHS institutions (NHS trusts), the majority of dental positions are self-employed posts either as an associate, principal or partner of a practice, either in general or specialist practice, which may be private, NHS, or mixed.
- There are opportunities within these settings to be able to develop your career, taking into account your strengths, interests, and local dental health needs.
- Within a local network of practices, it may be possible to offer additional dental services based on enhanced skills developed through training. In doing so, you will not only be able to provide care and treatment to a high level, but also have a career that is much more fulfilling.
- At DF/Dental Core trainee level, there are ways to enhance your portfolio in order to be more successful in developing your future career, including delivering presentations, webinars, publications, and additional postgraduate training and education.
- Participating in such activities is a marker of commitment to a particular pathway or specialty; however, it also allows you to develop skills and knowledge and develop into a more proficient practitioner.
- Career development in one of the dental specialties can be undertaken within primary care (e.g. restorative mono-specialties), but the majority of specialist training is through NHS specialty training programmes through HEE/NES/HEIW/NIMDTA. These training posts may be located within primary (general/specialist/community) or secondary care (teaching hospitals or district general hospitals), training to specialist or consultant level.

Presentations

How to find a project

- Presentations are a good way to develop your portfolio, showing initiative, communication skills, and resilience and will develop your confidence in speaking to other professionals for your future career development.
- When looking to present, many think that this only includes conferences or nationally publicized events; however, opportunities to present locally are some of the best ways to start.
- If this is something that you are interested in doing, take every opportunity available to present. Presenting to a large group of individuals may be a very daunting prospect to many, but taking every opportunity will enable you to thrive and develop your skills in this area. Start presenting to small groups and develop this further in time. Feedback from close colleagues is a very useful tool to enable you to improve your performance.
- During DFT there will usually be some opportunities where you can present to your group or practice, including presentation of a case that you have treated.
- Find a topic to present on, such as:
  - clinical audit/governance/quality improvement (QI) project
  - case presentation
  - update on clinical skill/knowledge
  - update on clinical guidelines.
- The easiest way to find a topic which others will be able to benefit from or find useful is by looking at your own practice. Identify something you find difficult, or where there is a problem, or where you think things can be done better.
- Investigate solutions. If it is a clinical problem, then carry out a PubMed search of the literature and look for a solution. If it is a practice management problem, investigate information available from the BDA, and look up advice sheets and practice management manuals. Present these findings to a peer group.

Clinical audits/QI

- This is an ideal opportunity to present clinically relevant information to a group of peers and to gain feedback on your presentation performance. Within primary and secondary care, clinical governance projects need to be undertaken and there are often good opportunities to present your project locally or regionally.
- Show how you identified a problem, compared the current standard to the accepted best practice or gold standard, implemented changes, and improved your own clinical standards and patient care via the audit cycle.
- Not all QI projects will fit into clinical audit. Service evaluations are also good areas to present relevant information to your department/practice to enable improvements in the service you deliver.

Case reports

- This can be a good presentation of a treated case or a case to discuss relevant treatment options.
- Showing an unusual technique or method of solving a clinical problem can often be very interesting; however, it is important that the idea you are showing is not considered inappropriate and that patients are properly consented for such techniques.
- Similarly, the risks must be carefully discussed as well as accepted practice and any ethical considerations.
- A safe area that could be considered would be a new approved material licensed for a particular use and indicated in a specific situation—a case report could be presented to demonstrate favour for its use.

Research

- Involvement in research can be rewarding both personally and professionally but is also a useful addition to your CV/portfolio to enable career development.
- Being involved in research as part of DFT or DCT can be challenging due to the time constraints of the post and realistic timeframes need to be applied.
- Interest in being part of a research project needs to be identified early within your training due to the time required to conduct the project, particularly if ethical approval is required, and it is easy to underestimate the time required for patient recruitment and so on. You may be able to continue participation in the project beyond your post, but this may not be feasible.
- At DFT or DCT level, it is useful to identify research supervisors or identify a project that is already ongoing that you can assist with, such as data collection.
- See ➔ Publications for further details of types of research and producing a publication.

Local presentations

- Giving a presentation locally can be very beneficial; as a developing clinician as you will be able to gain feedback and it is often in a more informal environment.
- There may be compulsory presentations, such as a case report as mentioned previously as part of the DFT. Other areas could include the development of dental nurses in practice.
- Volunteer to present, even if this is something that you find challenging. These presentations can be added to your portfolio of evidence of teaching. You can also gain formal feedback on your skills as part of a SLE.
- Journal clubs are another area where there are good opportunities to present. Journal clubs usually occur within the department, group or local study circle. A relevant paper is chosen and circulated for critical appraisal. One person (usually a trainee) would take the lead in presenting the paper and their critical appraisal, followed by a group discussion.

Regional meetings

- There may be regional events organized by a local division of a national society, a group of hospital departments, or regional boards.
- Ask local committee members of societies, audit leads in hospitals, or check correspondence from other societies. They may be able to direct and advise of areas that you can get involved in.
- There are often opportunities to join specialist societies as a training grade, at a reduced fee, which will highlight any local meetings, which you may be able to be involved with. Speak with your trainers/ consultants for advice.

National and international conferences

- Most conferences provide the opportunity to submit abstracts for presentation as posters or oral presentations. It is worthwhile investigating these opportunities at conferences for a particular society that is of interest to your clinical practice or future career aspiration. There are often prizes available for presentations at conferences, which again will add weight to your portfolio.
- Conference fees can be quite high, and you may be required to join the respective society to be able to present. Some societies have reduced fees for those in training. Some conference fees may be covered as part of your training (DFT or DCT), depending on whether this is included in your curriculum delivery matrix and the agreed local funding. Generally, financial support is considered to enable trainees to attend a conference where you are presenting, as this is seen as career development.

Producing the presentation

Posters

- There will be specific guidance on any poster presentation. Read the set guidelines. This will dictate the size of the poster, orientation, font size and format, word count, and any specific content that must be included.
- Check if it will be presented as a hard copy or electronic display. Ensure you allow sufficient time and a budget for quality printing.
- Focus the presentation on making a few succinct points, with clear illustrations. A poster is not appropriate to display a full written dissertation. A successful poster is designed to draw the reader in, to spend time reading the information presented.
- Avoid copious text wherever possible. Many posters will be looked at between main presentations and so there may not be time to carefully read every word.
- Use diagrams, illustrations, and graphs to make the point where possible.
- Choose colour schemes carefully; clarity and first impressions are important—a poster is more likely to be read if it stands out. Ensure there are contrasting colours or background and text, and that images do not appear to be distorted or blend into the background.
- Printing services are readily available. Within hospitals, there is likely to be clinical photography, which can often print for you, or within universities, printing services. Many conferences are moving towards arranging their own printing of posters and display.

- Print an A4 version and ask other colleagues to read it through prior to making the final print—this gives a good opportunity to make changes.
- Make sure it is printed in good time as this gives the opportunity to inspect printing quality and reprint if necessary.
- Ensure you have a good medium of transport to the event to reduce damage to the poster prior to the event.

Oral presentations

- As with a poster—read the set guidelines.
- Check if any adjuncts such as slides, images, or other multimedia facilities are available.
- If there is a template, then you are advised to use it.
- Where no template exists, use good contrasting colours but consider some viewers may have more difficulty in seeing certain colours.
- Avoid more than four lines of text per slide. Any more than this is unlikely to be read.
- Use the slides and multimedia as an adjunct to your presentation rather than the other way around otherwise you will find yourself simply reading the text off the slide.
- Ensure the presentation keeps to time, out of respect to other presenters, to avoid running into their slot. The chairperson of the session may very well force closure to your presentation at the end of your allocated time and much of your hard work may not be presented.
- Rehearse the presentation and record it if possible—this gives you the chance to see how you are heard in front of others and if you are coming across the way you would like.
- Know your material. There may be questions after your presentation and therefore you need to be prepared for these and potential answers.

Publications

- In addition to papers on scientific studies and novel case reports, publications include letters in journals, book reviews, narrative reviews, and abstracts which can all feature in peer-reviewed journals.
- Other publications include patient information leaflets and conference abstracts.

Peer-reviewed journal publications

Book reviews

- While these commonly feature in peer-reviewed journals, book reviews are not peer-reviewed publications.
- The author is allocated a book and a deadline to write a review that is published in the journal.
- There is often a given word limit (usually ~500 words).
- The author of the book review is usually allowed to keep the book as a reward for producing the review and their name is stated as the reviewer of the book.
- Undertaking such an activity shows commitment to reviewing the current literature and providing objective thoughts to members of the profession regarding new information/resources, which can show dedication to the chosen pathway/specialty.
- Opportunities to be involved in reviewing new titles can be achieved by contacting the editor of the journal concerned.

Abstracts

- Abstract publication usually relates to a larger publication or presentation (oral or poster).
- These are often published in journals that are associated with a conference where posters or other presentations occur and the submitted abstract is often published as conference proceedings.

Letters

- These are not peer-reviewed publications even though they may be in a peer-reviewed journal. The purpose of such letters is often on the basis of an opinion, idea, or thought which a practitioner may wish to share with others.
- They often have word limits of ~500 words.
- They are usually on any topic—clinical, managerial, or political.
- There are often rules which prohibit anything inflammatory; however, letters promoting intelligent or stimulating debate may be accepted.
- Look up guidelines to suggest what is accepted in journals in terms of letters.

Papers

- Publishing a paper is often a desirable criterion for entry into specialty training.
- Publishing a paper can be seen as a difficult task to deliver as a trainee in DFT or DCT.
- It is important to identify a possible area in which you can deliver a publication within a relatively short timeframe. As a trainee in DFT/ DCT, you will be looking to gain a publication within your current training post to enable you to move to the next level of training. It

is therefore often not feasible to undertake clinical research due to the time involved in setting up a project, obtaining ethical approval, undertaking the research, and ultimately publishing the results.

- Publications may be divided into several areas:
  - Research.
  - Case report/case series.
  - Opinion.
  - QI.
- One of the more likely areas in which you will be able to publish a paper is by submitting a case report or case series.
- It is beneficial to identify a project and then identify a relevant journal that may be likely to accept your publication.
- Many journals restrict the type of work they are willing to consider for publication both in terms of subject area and the grade of evidence. There are others that are more willing to accept work of a wider variety and may have a greater audience.
- The 'impact factor' is a measure used to assess the quality of the research contained within a journal. Essentially, it is the number of times that the articles in the journal have been cited over 2 years divided by the number of articles published within that period. If the journal publishes very few articles, but those articles are cited on many occasions then it stands to have a high impact factor. Impact factors within dental journals tend to be relatively low in comparison to medical journals (e.g. The Lancet).
- Look up the guidelines of the journal—these will state how the journal want the manuscript to be written. These are often very specific and are worth reading even before starting to write the manuscript.
- The majority of journals will require submissions to be sent electronically via a portal on their website.
- If your project is less conventional or through your research of that specific journal, your manuscript may not be what they would currently accept, but you feel that it would be well suited to that journal's audience, it may be beneficial to contact the editor with a brief summary of your idea to see if this is something they will consider for publication. This may save a lot of time, particularly if other journals you may be considering have very different guidelines.
- Be aware that some journals charge a fee for submission, even if the paper is not accepted.
- Where patients are involved, a specific consent form may be required.
- Ensure all authors are aware of the submission and are happy with the content prior to submission.
- Author order convention. It is customary that the lead author responsible for the project/manuscript is the first author. The last author is generally the overall supervisor of the project or head of department involved.
- The journal will give a decision, which would usually be:
  - accepted
  - accepted, but requires amendments
  - declined.
- Any amendments should be made quickly and the paper resubmitted.

- Any unsuccessful submissions would usually be returned with some feedback from the editorial team. It is worth considering this carefully before resubmitting to another journal.
- It is considered unethical to submit the same manuscript to several journals at the same time. You must choose your preferred journal first and if rejected, only then can you consider an alternative journal.
- Once accepted, proofs are sent for all authors to check prior to final publication.

Non-peer-reviewed publications

Patient information leaflets

- These may not seem particularly high profile, but they can demonstrate non-verbal communication skills by being able to translate complex procedures to lay people.
- This should not be considered an easy, quick option to build a CV. Often, particularly in hospitals, the leaflet has to undergo approval from a panel to ensure it is produced in clear English and can be understood by lay people. This process can take up to a year to complete—sometimes longer depending on the trust concerned.
- Find a topic you are interested in and which has not already been covered.
- Look at what information leaflets have already been produced.
- Take note of the amount of text, diagrams, and level of information provided.
- Be careful when it comes to the use of images—most photos and illustrations are protected by copyright and cannot be reproduced without permission.
- It may be the case that you would have to approach a medical illustrator to produce images or consent may need to be obtained from patients to take photos for the purpose of publication.
- Ask someone who is not involved in healthcare to read the leaflet. A good way of checking if it is properly understood is to then ask them to explain it to another lay person with you observing the conversation to ensure that it is properly understood—this can save lots of time later as it is more likely to be accepted by the patient information panels.
- Providing information in writing such as on leaflets can increase patient understanding and retention of information compared to just explaining a situation verbally and so this can make a significant difference to a patient's overall experience.

Manuals

- Often when starting a new job there can be a lot of things that are unfamiliar and different systems and procedures to get to grips with, which can be very overwhelming.
- Once you have found your way, you can usually follow procedures and pathways that are currently in place easily.
- Many trainees create manuals for future cohorts to go over any particular problems or situations or how to approach a particular procedure or process, such as admitting patients.
- This can be a useful exercise as it will demonstrate your ability to understand procedures to keep patients safe and show effective

communication to colleagues, particularly at a time when new members of staff come into a department/practice and there may be lots of omissions due to lack of familiarity. Such a manual can therefore increase patient safety.

Postgraduate education

Introduction to postgraduate training

- While adherence to the GDC CPD scheme is compulsory, there are ways that postgraduate training can significantly contribute to career development.[1]
- Completion of undergraduate training is only the beginning of your dental education. Through your career there will be continued and significant changes and developments in the pattern of disease, clinical techniques, materials, and professional and patient attitudes to oral healthcare. You will need to be proactive, identifying areas in which you wish to develop your skills and knowledge, and undertaking the necessary training to ensure that you are contemporary in your approach to patient care.
- Currently it is mandatory to comply with the GDC CPD scheme.
- For dentists this means a minimum of 100 hours of CPD per 5-year cycle.
- By definition, verifiable CPD is an activity with clear aims and objectives as well as clear anticipated outcomes. The registrant must also be able to give feedback and receive documentary proof of the CPD activity.
- There are four development outcomes which the CPD activity must satisfy:
  - A: communication skills including consent, complaint handling, and raising concerns.
  - B: management and leadership of self and the team.
  - C: development and updating of the skills and knowledge within your area of practice.
  - D: professional behaviour skills and legal and ethical issues.
- CPD must contain a minimum of 10 hours in medical emergencies, 5 hours of disinfection and decontamination, and 5 hours in radiography and radiation protection.
- CPD should also occur in handling complaints, safeguarding, law and ethics, and early detection of oral cancer.
- CPD can be used as an opportunity to enhance your career, by learning new skills and updating existing ones, as well as demonstrating compliance with the principles of the GDC standards.
- This can be in the form of lectures, seminars, hands-on courses, or journals.
- There are many ways to increase skills and knowledge and in doing so you can build your career. Undergoing a formal postgraduate qualification can be a milestone in providing evidence of achievement in a particular area.
- Take great care when selecting your course or qualification.
- Set aims in your PDP and be clear about what it is you want to achieve.
- Evaluate the benefits of different courses and different providers.
- Unlike the undergraduate primary dental degree, which is generally a full-time commitment, there are many more options including flexible pathways and distance learning programmes.

1 GDC (2018). Enhanced CPD guidance for dental professionals. ℘ https://www.gdc-uk.org/education-cpd/cpd/enhanced-cpd-scheme-2018

- When considering postgraduate courses, it may be worth checking the documentation that is obtained and, if necessary, using the mapping document as proof.
- With regard to postgraduate qualifications, this can be more complicated. The very nature of postgraduate qualifications would mean there is a period of study, presumably with examinations to mark the end point.
- Many postgraduate courses themselves will have a generic title such as 'periodontics' or 'implant dentistry'; however, it is important to recognize that although it states a specific discipline, the extent to which the course covers that discipline can vary considerably.
- What can also vary is the amount of contact time as well as the proportion of the course dedicated to practical training both clinical and laboratory based and the amount of theoretical, lecture-based, academic, and self-directed study. This may not be abundantly clear on the course details advertised.
- Similarly, the expected degree of proficiency on completion may not be clear. Two qualifications at two different institutions may have the same degree title, with the same type of degree, and the same duration and cost, but may have different learning outcomes or focus of learning.
- If a specialist title is being sought as part of the training, it is important to identify that the training will lead to a GDC registerable specialist qualification.
- Ask questions before applying. Make clear what it is you are hoping to achieve from completing the course and if this is something that is a realistic prospect. You will be investing a lot of time and money and so it is important to make your investment worthwhile.

Personal development plan

- A PDP allows you to make the most of your CPD by planning out your learning needs and then prioritizing them [1]
- By doing this, CPD can then be sought to meet the learning needs in order of priority.
- This will allow both patient and dentist to get the maximum benefit from CPD activity.
- A PDP using SMART objectives can be set out in a table with column headers as follows:
  - Identified learning needs.
  - Relationship of the learning need to the area of practice.
  - Educational objectives.
  - How the educational activity will benefit your practice.
  - Proposed activity to meet the objectives.
  - Deadline to meet the learning need.
- The learning needs ought to be prioritized. The highest priority would usually focus on mandatory topics such as medical emergencies, infection control, and radiography and radiation protection. The next highest priority would be any identified deficiencies requiring remediation; following that, areas identified as requiring improvement and lastly, areas to enhance.

Journals

- There are numerous journals available in dentistry and within each specialty area.
- Many of these will contain peer-reviewed papers and articles on the specific subjects covered by that journal.
- Some journals only publish articles related to a specific discipline or specialty.
- Within the journals, many also have the facility to produce verifiable CPD. This would involve reading an article and answering questions, usually online.
- Upon completion, a certificate is issued based on the assumed time taken for reading and answering the questions.
- This is one of the most flexible ways of achieving CPD. There are usually only a few hours offered by each issue and they will only give a limited number of topics, which may not fulfil your PDP and so you are restricted to what that particular journal is offering.

Courses

- There are a huge number of course providers from professional societies to commercial organizations. Most NHS health education departments and deaneries will also provide a series of courses.
- The benefits of these are that you can select specific courses which best match the objectives set out in the PDP.
- All verifiable courses need to allow participants to provide feedback and should enable reflective practice.
- There will be costs associated with most courses and so it is worth taking great care in the selection of the course you choose.
- Take a look at any society or indemnity provider you subscribe to, and investigate the courses they offer, as many of these may be included in your membership, or at a discounted rate.
- There are many commercial groups that provide sponsored events which are either free or subsidized; however, it is important to bear in mind that they may be used for marketing purpose.

Online/distance learning

- There are now more courses available online, providing training in a range of disciplines.
- This will not provide direct 'hands-on' skills with feedback, but advances in online technology have allowed an exponential increase in courses being delivered remotely with great success.

Reflection

- Following the completion of a set activity, it can be mandatory to reflect on what has been gained.[2]
- It is easy to undergo various training courses without giving much thought into how a course would benefit either the professional or the patient; reflection can bring into question the reason of doing it in the first place.

2 GDC (2018). Enhanced CPD guidance for dental professionals. ℘ https://www.gdc-uk.org/education-cpd/cpd/enhanced-cpd-scheme-2018

- By reflecting on the activity, it can also give it purpose and make it more useful by evaluating how it will change practice or how it can be implemented into the workplace.
- A declaration of your CPD log, including reflection and that a PDP is in place, is necessary for GDC registration. While it is only mandatory to submit these documents if the GDC requests them, it is compulsory to declare every year that they exist.

Postgraduate qualifications

- Postgraduate qualifications are usually substantive in nature.
- Here is a list of things to consider when deciding on what qualification to choose:
  - A postgraduate qualification can be gained from a research programme or a taught programme.
  - Research programmes are more independent in nature and tend not to have research credits or modules. You are still supported by supervisors but the focus of this type of degree is your own research. Research programmes can be at master's level, such as MPhil or MRes, or to doctorate level, a PhD.
  - Taught programmes are very similar to undergraduate degrees, in that there will be a series of modules, which may make up a certain level of 'credit'. Depending on the time commitments, taught programmes will be awarded as postgraduate certificates, or diplomas, master's level, such as MSc/MClinDent, or doctorate level, such as DDS/DDSc/DClinDent.
  - Most taught programmes at master's level and above will include research and completion of a dissertation.
  - Some specialties include a research component as part of specialty training (e.g. orthodontics) and must be completed to enable satisfactory completion of specialty training and ultimately registration as a specialist on a GDC register. It is important to clarify whether the postgraduate degree you are considering will contribute to specialty training. There are strict rules about what programmes are acceptable for specialty training. For a programme to be appropriate, it must be approved by the specialist advisory committee and have the approval of the postgraduate dental dean as well as the individual dentist being eligible for a National Training Number (NTN). This should be clarified with the programme organizers prior to starting.
  - There are many programmes that offer less than full-time study. There are increasing numbers that allow for either distance learning or part-time courses, or both, to allow dentists to continue with work.
  - Some programmes allow candidates to progress from certificate to diploma to master's degree with the option of withdrawing at the end of each qualification or continuing the course to reach the next stage.
  - Where there is progression, from certificate, to diploma, to master's, the first part of the course is the certificate level which would have a series of modules to complete in the field of study. The diploma stage may consist of more advanced material with possible optional

or special study modules. To progress to the master's degree, it is generally on the completion of a module on research methodology and completion of a research dissertation.

- Qualifications can include many direct clinical aspects and may relate to a single specialty such as endodontics or disciplines such as removable prosthodontics, conservative dentistry, or aesthetic dentistry.
- While some may give recognition of new skills, others may increase proficiency in certain areas. Some qualifications may be purely academic and give no additional skills, even in a clinical discipline.

Non-clinical qualifications

- There are an increasing number of non-clinical qualifications available from institutions including those outside the conventional dental schools.
- Many of these subject areas are applicable to dentistry, though many are also useful in other healthcare fields and so there are a wide variety of institutions that offer these types of qualifications.
- Examples of subject areas include:
  - law and ethics
  - medical research
  - leadership, management, and commissioning
  - professional studies
  - medical education
  - practice appraisal
  - business.

Job applications

Applications for performers or associates in general practice

- Applying for a post in general practice is very different to applying for a training post or one in an NHS institution.
- Most practices would advertise via the classified section in a journal, by word of mouth, through other practices, or through recruitment agencies.
- When a practice does recruit an individual, they would as a minimum generally need to see the following documentation:
  - Cover letter.
  - CV.
  - Primary dental degree certificate.
  - Current certificate of registration with the GDC.
  - Proof of eligibility to work in the UK.
  - Proof of identification.
  - An enhanced certificate from the Disclosure and Barring Service (DBS).
  - A report from an occupational health service confirming status regarding blood-borne viruses.
- With the exception of the cover letter and CV, most of the documents are not used for selection purposes but are needed simply to confirm eligibility to do the job.
- Most practices would then request an interview with shortlisted candidates.

Cover letter
- Always use a cover letter and make sure it is individualized for each application.
- Address the letter to the principal rather than 'To whom it may concern' and use the principal's actual name rather than 'Sir/Madam'.
- Try to include the following where possible:
  - How you heard about the vacancy, such as word of mouth or job advert.
  - Any personal preferences that make this job right for you and how you are right for the practice, including where you are now and why you want to change job.
  - What features of the practice you like, such as the area and type of patient they attract, and how you can contribute to the practice.
  - Make sure the letter is geared to you being committed to working in that practice.
- Keep the letter as succinct as possible using a maximum of three reasons or features for anything you want to discuss. Any more than this will distract from the main points and may devalue the application. If you failed to convince them with the three most important points, then you are unlikely to convince them with any subsequent reasons.
- The letter should only be one side maximum.

Curriculum vitae
- This also has to be prepared and individualized for each job applied for.
- Try to include the following items:

- Personal details including name, address, GDC number, indemnity provider, and performer number.
- Qualification including primary dental degree and any postgraduate qualifications. Avoid using pre-university qualifications unless they are particularly relevant such as the International Computer Driving Licence. GCSEs and A levels should not generally be included unless specifically requested. State any qualifications you are working towards and the expected date of completion.
- Experience: this should be presented in chronological order starting with the most recent. Avoid any non-relevant jobs (such as a paper round in your early teens) unless you can find a good use for it. State the position and be succinct, avoiding repetition where possible in the description.
- Any prizes, awards, or distinctions and how they were earned.
- Relevant CPD activities: include any particular course that demonstrates competence in specific skills. Avoid including every CPD certificate obtained, unless it is of particular importance. If you have found that you have exceeded your required CPD amount, then prioritize CPD activity that can enhance the application.
- Particular skills or knowledge that stands out. Include any skills such as surgical wisdom tooth extraction, periodontal surgery, sedation, facial aesthetics, and particular behaviour management skills. Avoid highlighting generic skills that would be expected of a registrant.
- Publications, posters, and presentations.
- Outside interests including hobbies and social life.
- Referee details.
- It is worth making a master CV with all the details that you would want to include and keeping this updated and relevant. Editing the master CV will then become much easier for future applications.
- With regard to the skills and CPD section, focus this to each practice. Look at what the practice does—is it mainly NHS or private? If you have experience in NHS practice, it will be worth stating your current units of dental activity (UDA) target (or equivalent) and the dental health needs of the local population, to give an indication of your current performance. It is worth showcasing any special skills that make you particularly useful to the practice.
- Information on the practice and the current skill set may be found on the practice website, which may identify common areas of interest or areas in which your skills may be advantageous. Do you have any similar interests to the staff? If so, make sure this is put in.
- Sell yourself as much as possible, but most importantly *do not* lie or exaggerate your skills as your probity would be brought into question.

Interview
- Most practices will interview candidates.
- As with all interviews, first impressions count.
- Make sure you know as much about the practice as possible—try to see if you can arrange a visit with the practice prior to the interview and find out as much as you can. Simply arranging a visit can also show commitment to the job.
- Dress professionally; any portfolios or other evidence should be neatly presented and easy to access to show evidence of ability.

- While most practices will be assessing communication skills as a large part of the interview, they will also be looking to see if they can get on with the person.
- While most interviews for practices will not focus heavily on academic questions, many will investigate if your knowledge is up to date, ensuring competence.

Questions you may wish to ask

Income
- NHS/private mix.
- General/personal dental services.
- UDA target/payment per unit.
- UDA value and percentage split/sliding scales.
- Clawback per month/quarter/year.
- Private payment: fee per item/care plan (e.g. Denplan).
- Private targets.
- Laboratory costs: percentage share.
- Hygienist/therapist cost.
- Bad debts.
- NHS Pension.
- Previous associate earnings/private conversion.

Working pattern
- Flexibility on hours/days.
- On-call commitment.
- Study leave.
- Annual leave arrangements.

Patient base
- New list/established list.
- Patient demographics: age range, socioeconomic status.

Support
- Nursing: same nurse/qualified nurse.
- Hygiene/therapy support.
- Treatment coordination/administrative support.
- Advertising/website.

Surgery
- Same surgery every day.
- Age of unit/plans for upgrades.
- Left-handed unit if required.
- Equipment available.
- Shared equipment: endodontic motor/apex locator and so on and number for the practice.
- Radiography: digital/film/OPT/CBCT.
- Intraoral scanners.
- Material use:
  Shared costs or part of the percentage arrangement.
  Choice of materials.
- Computer system (e.g. EXACT, R4, Dentally, etc.).

Laboratory
- Restrictions on choice of laboratories.
- Pick-up arrangements.

Sickness/absence (extended)
- Arrangements for maternity (e.g. do you need to find your own locum cover?).

Applications for training programmes

- Applying for a training programme including DFT, DCT, or specialty training is through an online application via the Oriel website.[1]
- Individual jobs application may vary from either institution, central recruitment within the Health Education area or a national recruitment. Foundation, Core and Specialty are now national recruitment processes.
- There may also be locum appointments for training where the job is only for a specified time period and may not be the complete training programme, however the time spent may be used to contribute to training in conjunction with other programmes. These tend to be local applications, typically via NHS jobs.

Applications for NHS appointments

- Other than training programmes there are a lot of jobs within NHS organizations including the following:
  - Specialty doctor/dentist: these replaced staff grade roles. Their purpose is to provide services to the hospital including patient treatment and consultations.
  - Dental officer: these are the most junior posts in a community dental setting. They are recruited for according to service need and in accordance with the requirement of the post, which may vary from special care dentistry and sedation to oral surgery.
  - Senior dental officer: this is a community post which is more senior to the dental officer post and may need specialist status or additional qualifications or experience to achieve.
  - Clinical director: this is usually the clinical lead for the community service concerned and they are considered managerial dentists. There may be specialists that are also on this same pay band.
  - Locum appointments for service: these posts may be advertised at the training level of either a registrar or Dental Core trainee equivalent and the duties may be the same, but there is no training, and it may be for a fixed period. They can be useful for gaining experience.
  - Trust doctor/dentist: these are similar to specialty doctor appointments; however, they may have more variability in terms of pay and conditions compared to a specialty doctor/dentist.
- All of the posts listed are for service need rather than training; although there may still be an element of training provided, this is not a formal appointment for training.
- Each post would be advertised by the respective trust and they would recruit according to the needs and requirements of the service.
- Each service is different and so the exact requirements of the roles also differ; therefore, it is important to examine the job description and person specification.
- Trusts often advertise on the NHS jobs website.

1 🔗 www.oriel.nhs.uk

Training to be a specialist

Introduction to specialist training

- Any dentist registered with the GDC is entitled to practise within any specialty provided they are trained, competent, and indemnified to do so. However, you can only refer to yourself as a specialist if you are on one of the specialists lists that is held by the GDC.[1]
- For example, someone could not refer to themself as a 'specialist cosmetic dentist' as there is no such list held by the GDC and so to state specialist status in this area may make you subject to a disciplinary or fitness to practise process as this is misleading the public.
- This only applies to the use of the word specialist. Any dentist who is not on a specialist list could refer to themselves in many other ways as long it does not breach the GDC principles of ethical advertising, for example:
  - dentist with special interest in implants
  - dentist with limited practice in oral surgery
  - dentist trained with enhanced skills in periodontics.
- Current specialist titles (precise definitions can be found on the GDC website):
  - Dental and maxillofacial radiology
  - Dental public heath
  - Endodontics
  - Oral and maxillofacial pathology
  - Oral medicine
  - Oral microbiology
  - Oral surgery
  - Orthodontics
  - Paediatric dentistry
  - Periodontics
  - Prosthodontics
  - Restorative dentistry
  - Special care dentistry.
- More detailed information can be found in the Dental Gold Guide.[2]

NHS consultant

- The term 'consultant' is an NHS title, whereas a 'specialist' is one defined by the GDC.
- Post-certificate of completion of specialist training (CCST) training in a dental specialty (e.g. orthodontics, restorative dentistry) is to enable extended competencies expected of a consultant. The completion of post-CCST training does not allow the right to use the title consultant. The individual needs to be appointed to the role of consultant within an NHS organization.
- The essential criteria for appointment to a consultant post is that the candidate is a specialist. The person specification may require further training and specific competencies to be attained and to be evidenced, such as those attained during post-CCST training. Some of the dental

---

1 GDC. Specialist lists. ✎ https://www.gdc-uk.org/registration/your-registration/specialist-lists

2 Dental Gold Guide (2018). ✎ https://www.copdend.org/wp-content/uploads/2021/08/Dental-Gold-Guide-September-2021.pdf

specialties currently do not have post-CCST training, but the role of consultant is still possible based on the person specification (e.g. consultant in special care dentistry).

Specialist training programmes

- Speciality training programmes are commissioned by deaneries to deliver the specialty curriculum.[2]
- The number of specialty training posts varies according to the current workforce need in each region and the funding available.
- Candidates appointed to a specialty training post are given a NTN.
- These are all fully salaried posts and there are now no self-funded training posts.
- There are several routes to specialty training:
  - NHS ST post:
    - Appointed through National Recruitment.
    - Local appointment may occur in the UK's devolved nations.
    - Fully funded through the deanery although local trusts may fund a post if there is a local need for training.
  - National Institute of Health Research (NIHR) academic programme:
    - Academic clinical fellow or clinical lecturer.
    - Appointed locally but the candidate must benchmark through national recruitment to be eligible for appointment.
  - University appointed posts with prior agreement from the deanery:
    - Clinical lecturer posts, usually undertaking a higher research degree with a NTN.
    - Appointed locally but the candidate must benchmark through national recruitment to be eligible for appointment.

Eligibility for specialist listing

- In order to become a specialist, it is the usual requirement to have satisfactorily completed specialty training which has been approved by the deanery and will have satisfied the requirements of the ARCP.
- The individual would then be awarded a CCST and register as a specialist in addition to the usual annual retention fee (GDC).
- A separate retention fee would be paid each year to maintain registration on the specialist list.
- Historically, when the specialist lists were first introduced at the end of the last century, anyone who was able to demonstrate the appropriate, relevant experience to be considered as equivalent to a specialist was able to 'grandparent' onto the specialist list by virtue of their experience for a limited time period.
- After the grace period was over, the only route onto the specialist list would be through a ST programme.
- The specialist titles are not definitive. Since introduction, some titles have been removed, while new ones have been developed (e.g. the new specialty list in special care dentistry was created in 2008).
- When a new title has been introduced, a similar grace period has occurred to allow individuals with relevant experience to register.
- There are exceptions to this:

- There may be other courses considered equivalent to specialty training or the individual may be eligible to sit the relevant examinations.
- Other training may be applicable; however, this may be more complex to prove and additional advice should be sought from the GDC.

Availability of training programmes

- The numbers on each specialist list vary considerably.
- This is partially determined historically by the numbers that already existed in each specialty and the numbers required to meet workforce requirements.
- It is also noted that workforce requirements, both clinical and academic, do not necessarily need specialists. For example, many referrals made for oral surgery are sent to OMFS, and may be seen and treated by specialty dentists who may or may not be a specialist in oral surgery, or by an oral and maxillofacial surgeon. While there may be a great need for oral surgery services, there may be a low need for specialist oral surgeons in that region as the current workforce is sufficient to manage the need.
- Similarly, the small number of oral microbiologists means that services that require microbiological specimens to be analysed and reported on would often be performed by medical microbiologists rather than dental.
- Recruiting on the basis of workforce requirements also has an added benefit for the trainee as it means there is more likely to be available work following completion of training and the cost of training is justified.
- The availability of programmes will also vary according to the amount of funding available for training programmes.
- Specialty training posts are now generally appointed via national recruitment, where all the posts within a specialty are recruited through a single process.
- Specialties that tend to only have one or two positions available per year tend to recruit based on institution.
- The exact process in terms of application forms and interview styles varies in part due to the skills and knowledge required for each specialty and ongoing changes to recruitment processes and methods of selecting appropriate candidates. Please see the COPDEND website for information on recruitment and person specifications.[3]

Person specification

- Recruitment to specialty training now has a generic person specification with a specialty specific section.
- These are divided into three sections[3]:
  - Entry criteria: these are essential. If all of these are not met, then this will result in failure to long/shortlist. These are divided into:
    - qualifications
    - eligibility

3 🔗 https://www.copdend.org/

- ○ fitness to practise
- ○ language skills
- ○ health
- ○ career progression.
- Selection criteria: these are subdivided into essential and desirable criteria. These are used at application and interview stage and those scoring most highly on these would have their applications progressed. The areas evaluated are:
  - ○ qualifications
  - ○ career progression
  - ○ clinical skills—clinical knowledge and expertise
  - ○ academic and research skills
  - ○ personal skills
  - ○ probity—professional integrity.
- Specialty specific criteria: these are subdivided into essential and desirable criteria. These are used at application and interview stage and those scoring most highly on these would have their applications progressed. The areas that may be evaluated are:
  - ○ career progression
  - ○ commitment to specialty—learning and personal development.
- An important tip would be to start looking at the person specifications early in your career, as some aspects may take considerably longer to achieve than others, and so it is important to plan in advance.
- Please note that recruitment is an ever-changing process. For the most up-to-date information please visit the COPDEND website.[3]

Generic person specification

Entry criteria (essential)

Qualifications
- Bachelor of Dental Surgery (BDS) or equivalent recognized by the GDC.

Eligibility
- Be eligible for registration with the GDC by the time of appointment.
- Be eligible to work in the UK.
- Have the ability to travel to sites as required in order to fulfil the requirements of the whole training programme.

Fitness to practise
- Is up to date and fit to practise safely.
- Satisfactory enhanced DBS check in England and Wales/Disclosure Scotland (PVG) in Scotland/Access NI in Northern Ireland or equivalent.

Language skills
- Applicants must have demonstrable skills in written and spoken English, adequate to enable effective communication about dental topics with patients and colleagues as demonstrated by one of the following:
  - Undergraduate training in English or IELTS overall 7.0 and no less than 6.5 in all other areas.

Health
- Meet professional health requirements (in line with GDC 'Standards for the Dental Team').
- Be physically and mentally capable of conducting procedures over several hours which demand close attention.

Career progression
- Be able to provide complete details of the employment history.
- Has evidence that their career progression is consistent with their personal circumstances.
- Has evidence that their present level of achievement and performance is commensurate with the totality of their period of training.
- Has notified the TPD of the specialty training programme they are currently training in if applying to continue training in the same specialty in another region.
- Not have previously relinquished or been released/removed from a specialty training programme, except under exceptional circumstances.
- Not already hold, nor be eligible to hold, a CCST in the specialty applied for and/or must not currently be eligible for the specialist list in the specialty applied for.

Application completion
- *All* sections of the application form completed *fully* according to written guidelines.

Selection criteria

Essential qualifications
- As above for 'Entry criteria'.

Desirable qualifications
- MFDS/MJDF or equivalent at the time of application.
- Other qualifications held at time of application.

Essential career progression
- As above for 'Entry criteria'.
- Has evidence of experience in more than one dental specialty/clinical setting.
- Commitment to the specialty with clear career objectives.
- On an NHS primary care organization Performers List or able to meet requirement for listing when training/post involves primary care placement that requires listing.

Desirable career progression
- On an NHS primary care organization Performers List or able to meet requirements for listing.
- Has evidence of undertaking appropriate courses commensurate with career progression and intentions.

Essential clinical skills
- Demonstrates good patient care skills.
- Capacity to apply sound clinical knowledge and judgement to problems.
- Ability to prioritize clinical need.
- Demonstrates appropriate technical and clinical competence and evidence of the development of diagnostic skills and clinical judgement.

Essential academic and research skills
- Understanding of the principles and relevance of research in evidence-based practice.
- QI:
  - Demonstrates understanding of the principles of audit/clinical governance/QI.
  - Evidence of participation in QI/audit/service evaluation.

Desirable academic and research skills
- Evidence of relevant academic and research achievements (e.g. degrees, awards).
- Publications.
- Conference presentations/posters.
- QI:
  - Evidence of leading at least one QI/audit/service evaluation project.
- Teaching:
  - Evidence of delivering undergraduate or postgraduate teaching or teaching dental care professionals.
  - Teaching qualification (e.g. Postgraduate Certificate in Education, or other teaching training).

Essential personal skills
- Communications skills:
  - Capacity to communicate effectively and sensitively with others.
  - Able to discuss treatment/oral health options with patients/stakeholders in a way they can understand.
- Problem-solving and decision-making:
  - Capacity to think beyond the obvious, with analytical and flexible mind, bringing a range of approaches to problem-solving.
  - Demonstrates effective judgement and decision-making skills.
- Empathy and sensitivity:
  - Capacity to take in others' perspectives and treat others with understanding; sees patients as people.
  - Demonstrates respect for all.
- Managing others and team involvement:
  - Capacity to work effectively in a MDT.
  - Demonstrate leadership when appropriate.
  - Capacity to establish good working relationships with others.
- Organization and planning:
  - Capacity to manage time and prioritize various tasks and commitments, balance urgent and important demands, and follow instructions.
- Vigilance and situational awareness:
  - Capacity to monitor and anticipate situations that may change rapidly.
- Coping with pressure and managing uncertainty:
  - Demonstrates flexibility, decisiveness, and resilience.
  - Capacity to operate effectively under pressure and remain objective in highly emotive/pressured situations.
  - Awareness of own limitations and when to ask for help.

Essential probity—professional integrity

- Takes responsibility for own actions.
- Demonstrates honesty and reliability.
- Demonstrates respect for the rights of all.
- Demonstrates awareness of ethical principles, safety, confidentially, and consent.
- Awareness of importance of being the patients' advocate, clinical governance, and the responsibility of an NHS employee.
- Demonstrates altruism—evidence of the ability to attend to the needs of others with an awareness of their rights and equal opportunities.

Specialty specific criteria

Restorative dentistry

Career progression

- Has evidence of achievement of Foundation competencies from a UK DFT programme or equivalent.
- Demonstrates the competencies required at the end of UK DCT1 (i.e. outcome 1) at the time of interview and DCT2 at the time of post commencement (or equivalent).

Commitment to specialty (essential)

- Evidence of commitment to the specialty—learning and professional development. Examples may include:
  - membership of an appropriate specialist society
  - evidence of leading a QI/audit project in restorative dentistry
  - evidence of progression in skills and attributes appropriate to restorative dentistry following completion of DFT.

Commitment to specialty (desirable)

- Demonstrates experience in the specialty. Examples may include:
  - appropriate professional portfolio and employment post
  - appropriate professional logbook history
  - case/poster presentations at local or regional meetings
  - undertaken CPD appropriate to restorative dentistry.

Orthodontics

Career progression

- Has evidence of achievement of Foundation competencies from a UK DFT programme or equivalent.
- Demonstrates the competencies required at the end of UK DCT1 (i.e. outcome 1) at the time of interview and DCT2 at the time of post commencement (or equivalent).

Commitment to specialty (essential)

- Demonstrates insight, interest, and commitment to pursuing a career in the specialty of orthodontics.

Commitment to specialty (desirable)

- Should have wide training in a number of specialties commensurate to their post-qualification experience.
- Experience in maxillofacial surgery and experience in paediatric dentistry.

Paediatric dentistry

Career progression

- Has evidence of achievement of Foundation competencies from a UK DFT programme or equivalent.
- Demonstrates the competencies required at the end of UK DCT1 (i.e. outcome 1) at the time of interview and DCT2 at the time of post commencement (or equivalent).

Commitment to specialty (essential)

- Demonstrates competencies in the DCT2/3 curriculum in paediatric dentistry.
- Demonstrates good communication skills with children, young persons, and parents/carers.
- Evidence of specific paediatric dentistry skills (e.g. management of trauma, medically compromised children).
- Demonstrates commitment to paediatric dentistry.

Commitment to specialty (desirable)

- Experience in orthodontics.
- Experience in restorative dentistry.
- Experience in oral surgery.
- Experience in the public/salaried dental service.
- Experience of delivering clinical/academic training/teaching in paediatric dentistry.

Oral surgery

Career progression

- Has evidence of achievement of Foundation competencies from a UK DFT programme or equivalent.
- Demonstrates the competencies required at the end of UK DCT1 (i.e. outcome 1) at the time of interview and DCT2 at the time of post commencement (or equivalent).

Commitment to specialty (essential)

- Has experience of a substantive post working in oral surgery/OMFS.
- Has documented experience of inpatient care and management of emergencies in a hospital setting.
- Has validated logbook evidence of appropriate experience.
- Shows realistic insight into oral surgery and the demands of a career in surgery.
- Shows critical and enquiring approach to knowledge acquisition, commitment to self-directed learning and a reflective/analytical approach to practice.

Commitment to specialty (desirable)

- Attendance at, or participation in, national and international meetings relevant to oral surgery.
- Publications and/or presentations on relevant oral surgery topics.
- Demonstrates knowledge of the training programme and a commitment to own development.
- Participation and attendance on courses to develop skills on the oral surgery curriculum (e.g. IV sedation, immediate life support).
- Membership of appropriate specialist society/associations.

Oral medicine

Commitment to specialty (essential)

- Shows realistic insight into the specialty and the demands of a career in oral medicine.
- Experience in oral surgery, OMFS, or one of the additional dental specialties at DCT level or equivalent.

Commitment to specialty (desirable)

- Diagnostic experience in an oral medicine unit at DCT level or equivalent.
- Attendance at, or participation in, national and international meetings relevant to oral medicine.
- Membership of appropriate specialist society/associations.

Special care dentistry

Career progression

- Has evidence of achievement of Foundation competencies from a UK DFT programme or equivalent.
- Demonstrates the competencies required at the end of UK DCT1 (i.e. outcome 1) at the time of interview and DCT2 at the time of post commencement (or equivalent).

Commitment to specialty (essential)

- On an NHS primary care organization Performers List or able to meet requirements for listing when training/post involves primary care placement that requires listing.
- Has evidence of direct clinical experience of special care dentistry in a community or hospital setting.
- Ability to travel independently to various clinical sites during training including on domiciliary visits.

Commitment to specialty (desirable)

- Has evidence of attendance at courses or CPD activities relevant to special care dentistry.
- Postgraduate qualification in special care dentistry.
- Has evidence of experience in the provision of oral healthcare under conscious sedation techniques.
- Has evidence of experience in the provision of oral healthcare under GA.
- Member of special care dentistry specialist societies.
- Immediate life support completed in last 12 months at time of application.

Dental and maxillofacial radiology

Commitment to specialty (essential)

- Shows realistic insight into the speciality and the demands of a career in dental and maxillofacial radiology.
- Experience in oral surgery, OMFS, or one of the additional dental specialties at DCT level or equivalent.

Commitment to specialty (desirable)

- Experience in dental and maxillofacial radiology at DCT level or equivalent.

- Attendance at, or participation in, national and international meetings relevant to dental and maxillofacial radiology.
- Membership of appropriate specialist society/associations.

Oral and maxillofacial pathology

Commitment to specialty (essential)

- Shows realistic insight into the specialty and the demands of a career in oral and maxillofacial pathology.
- Experience in oral surgery, OMFS, or one of the additional dental specialities at DCT level or equivalent.

Commitment to specialty (desirable)

- Diagnostic experience in an OMFP unit at DCT level or equivalent.
- Attendance at, or participation in, national and international meetings relevant to OMFP.
- Membership of appropriate specialist society/associations.

Dental public health

Commitment to specialty (essential)

- Working knowledge of NHS health services.
- Understanding of the breadth of public health provision.
- Understanding of the role of dental public health within the wider health service and beyond.

Commitment to specialty (desirable)

- Understanding of trends in health and healthcare provision.
- Understanding of clinical governance.
- Undertakes appropriate CPD, such as courses on research methods/statistics/critical appraisals/evaluation/management.
- Demonstrates interest in QI.

Qualifications (desirable)

- Postgraduate qualification in dental public health or public health (e.g. MSc in Dental Public Health, Diploma in Dental Public Health, Master of Public Health).

Career progression (essential)

- Evidence of experience of clinical activity in more than one sector of dental service provision (e.g. hospital, salaried, and general dental service).

Career progression (desirable)

- Clinical experience beyond that provided by DFT/DCT (or equivalent).
- DCT post or equivalent in dental public health or previous experience of dental public health.
- Evidence of involvement in oral health promotion/preventive dentistry.
- Evidence of involvement in dental epidemiology.
- Experience of committee work.

Career progression

Career progression in general practice

See ℘ Career opportunities in general dental practice in the Dental Foundation Training Chapter.

Career progression—specialist pathway

See Fig. 13.1.

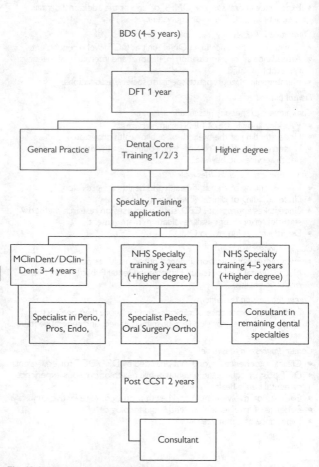

Fig. 13.1 Flow chart to show pathway for specialty route.

Index

For the benefit of digital users, indexed terms that span two pages (e.g., 52–53) may, on occasion, appear on only one of those pages.

Notes
Tables, figures, and boxes are indicated by *t*, *f*, and *b* following the page number
Abbreviations found in the index are as found in the text.
vs. indicates a comparison.